# Saving Babies?

T0385600

*Fieldwork Encounters and Discoveries*

A Series Edited by Robert Emerson and Jack Katz

# Saving Babies?

*The Consequences of Newborn Genetic Screening*

STEFAN TIMMERMANS AND
MARA BUCHBINDER

THE UNIVERSITY OF CHICAGO PRESS     CHICAGO AND LONDON

The University of Chicago Press, Chicago 60637
The University of Chicago Press, Ltd., London
© 2013 by The University of Chicago
All rights reserved. Published 2013.
Paperback edition 2015
Printed and bound by CPI Group (UK) Ltd,
Croydon, CR0 4YY

24  23  22  21  20  19  18  17  16  15      2  3  4  5  6

ISBN-13: 978-0-226-92497-7 (cloth)
ISBN-13: 978-0-226-27361-7 (paper)
ISBN-13: 978-0-226-92499-1 (e-book)
10.7208/chicago/9780226924991.001.0001

Library of Congress Cataloging-in-Publication Data

Timmermans, Stefan, 1968–
  Saving babies? : the consequences of newborn genetic screening / Stefan Timmermans and
Mara Buchbinder.
      pages ; cm. — (Fieldwork encounters and discoveries)
  Includes bibliographical references and index.
  ISBN-13: 978-0-226-92497-7 (cloth : alkaline paper)
  ISBN-10: 0-226-92497-1 (cloth : alkaline paper)
  ISBN-13: 978-0-226-92499-1 (e-book)
  ISBN-10: 0-226-92499-8 (e-book)  1. Newborn infants—Medical examinations—Social
aspects—United States. 2. Newborn infants—Diseases—Diagnosis—Social aspects.
3. Genetic screening—Social aspects—United States. 4. Medical screening—Social
aspects—United States. I. Buchbinder, Mara. II. Title. III. Series: Fieldwork encounters and
discoveries.
  RJ255.5.T555 2013
  618.92'01—dc23

                                2012019820

⊗ This paper meets the requirements of ANSI/NISO Z39.48-1992 (Permanence of Paper).

TO JESSE
AND JASPER

# Contents

Acknowledgments    ix

Introduction: The Consequences of Newborn Screening    1

CHAPTER 1.    The Expansion of Newborn Screening    34

CHAPTER 2.    Patients-in-Waiting    65

CHAPTER 3.    Shifting Disease Ontologies    97

CHAPTER 4.    Is My Baby Normal?    121

CHAPTER 5.    The Limits of Prevention    152

CHAPTER 6.    Does Expanded Newborn Screening Save Lives?    182

Conclusion:    The Future of Newborn Screening    212

Notes    241

References    265

Index    295

# Acknowledgments

Imagine a screening program performed at birth for very rare conditions. The rationale for the program is prevention: early detection promises to save babies from a sudden death. Sound appealing? Now, add that medical scientists did not know much about the conditions being screened, that it is not actually that easy to diagnose an infant based on screening results, and that the link between screening and preventive treatment is not clear. Even after a disorder is picked up with screening, some infants will still develop complications and others will die as a result of the disorder. Still, the program is state-mandated and in most locations does not require informed consent: parents are presumed to agree with screening unless they opt out. Clinicians cannot ignore the results either, because the state requires them to follow up with parents. To further complicate the issue, let's locate this screening program in a country known for persistent health inequities—a country where access to care and the quality of care remain overdetermined by market forces and a country that persistently trails behind other industrialized nations in comparative health indicators. A country, in short, in which a positive screen does not automatically mean access to care.

This country, of course, is the United States and the program is universal newborn screening. This program expanded in 2005 to screen virtually all newborns in the United States for more than 50 rare genetic conditions. This book examines how newborn screening was expanded and how families and clinicians experienced positive newborn screens in the aftermath of this expansion. Out of all of the possible health services that could have been made universally available, why did US health policymakers opt for expanding newborn screening? How do parents and clinicians act upon a positive screen when the results remain uncertain? In what follows, we examine the intended and unintended consequences of the expansion of newborn screening.

Our deepest gratitude goes to the families and clinicians who allowed us to journey with them on the winding roads of newborn screening. Due to confidentiality restrictions, we cannot thank them personally. We hope, however, that they recognize themselves in the experiences we recount and that our writing captures the high stakes of taking care of an infant with a positive newborn screen. Our research team included John Heritage, Rocio Rosales, and Arianna Taboada. John helped with grant writing, data collection, and helpful feedback on the analysis. Rocio was responsible for recording clinical consultations with Spanish-speaking families, and both Rocio and Arianna interviewed Spanish-speaking families in their homes. We received funding from the UCLA Faculty Senate, the UCLA Center for Society and Genetics, the UCLA Interdisciplinary Relationship Science Program, and the National Science Foundation. We thank Jan Stets and Pat White at NSF for their support. We are grateful that the manuscript has found a home in the Fieldwork Encounters and Discoveries series at the University of Chicago Press and we thank Doug Mitchell for his effusive encouragement and Tim McGovern for the steady navigation of our manuscript. We also thank series editors Jack Katz and Bob Emerson and two reviewers, both of whom identified themselves—Carole Heimer and Rayna Rapp—for their helpful feedback.

This book came to fruition during Mara's first year in the Department of Social Medicine at UNC–Chapel Hill. She is grateful for the support of her department colleagues, especially department chair Gail Henderson, for granting her teaching release that provided her with the freedom to write. She also benefited from conversations about newborn screening with colleagues at UNC's Center for Genomics and Society, especially Debra Skinner, Don Bailey, Myra Roche, Cindy Powell, Eric Juengst, Arlene Davis, and Rebecca Walker. Mara completed work on the manuscript with the support of a scholarly residency at the Brocher Foundation in Hernance, Switzerland.

Several individuals have commented on portions of the manuscript. We thank Rene Almeling, Renee Anspach, David Armstrong, Carole Browner, Peter Conrad, Joe Dumit, Carrie Friese, Tine Gammeltoft, Sahra Gibbon, Neil Gong, Lianna Hart, Stefan Helmreich, Klaus Hoeyer, Sharon Kaufman, Andy Lakoff, Sandra Soo-Jin Lee, Annie Lyerly, Emily Martin, Tara McKay, Sebastian Mohr, Michael Montoya, Sarah Nettleton, Emily Noonan, Hyeyoung Oh, Diane Paul, Adriana Petryna, Aviad

Raz, Barry Saunders, Merav Shohet, Bob Simpson, Debra Skinner, Mette Svensen, Karen-Sue Taussig, Iddo Tavory, Eric Villain, Kalindi Vora, Steven Wainwright, Andrew Webster, Ian Whitmarsh, Clare Williams, Norton Wise, Amy Zhou, and Jianfeng Zhu for their thoughtful suggestions and engagement with our work. We are particularly grateful to Stephen Cederbaum, Hannah Landecker, and Sara Shostak, who read the whole manuscript and offered detailed, helpful comments.

Stefan presented this research at the Wenner-Gren Symposium on the Anthropology of Potentiality organized by Karen-Sue Taussig and Klaus Hoeyer; the New England Consortium of Metabolic Programs; the annual meeting of the National Society for Genetic Counseling; and the sociology departments at Northwestern University, University of Pennsylvania, University of Southern California, University of California-Berkeley, Columbia University, King's College London, and the University of York. Mara presented this research at UNC's Center for Genomics and Society, the 2011 ELSI Congress, and meetings of the Society for Medical Anthropology and the Society for Psychological Anthropology. We both presented this research at UCLA's Center for Society and Genetics and at the annual meetings of the American Anthropological Association, the American Sociological Association, and the Society for the Social Studies of Science. We thank the participants and audience members for stimulating comments.

We are also impressed that Piero Rinaldo, Rodney Howell, and Michael Watson keep up with the social science literature. We hope our writing has enriched their understanding of what is happening in newborn screening clinics.

This study highlights the precariousness and preciousness of family. Stefan thanks Ruth Baxter for her unwavering support and contagious sense of humor. Merel suggested spicing up the reading list with books about dragons, magic, and rangers, and Jasper proposed adding some Lego sculptures. He thanks them for their diversion, entertainment, and love. Mara thanks her parents, Harriet and Marty Yogel and Stephen Buchbinder, for their care and love, and the extended sibling clan for reinforcing the importance of the kinship ties that lie at the heart of this book. Mara is grateful for a steady stream of healthy skepticism and countless helpful suggestions from Jesse Summers. She thanks Jesse, above all, for his wisdom, humor, compassion, and love.

An earlier version of chapter 2 was published as "Patients in Waiting: Living between Sickness and Health in the Genomics Era," in *Journal of*

*Health and Social Behavior* 51, no. 4 (2010): 408–423. Portions of chapter 3 were published in two earlier papers: "Newborn Screening and Maternal Diagnosis: Rethinking Family Benefit," in *Social Science and Medicine* 73, no. 7 (2011): 1014–1018; and "Expanded Newborn Screening: Articulating the Ontology of Diseases with Bridging Work in the Clinic," in *Sociology of Health and Illness* 34, no. 2 (2012): 208–220. We gratefully acknowledge permission from Sage, Elsevier, and Blackwell Publishing to reproduce portions of these articles in revised form.

# Introduction

## *The Consequences of Newborn Screening*

Holding up a $20 bill dramatically at a 2008 press conference, model and actress Renee Baio demonstrated the cost of screening a newborn baby for rare genetic conditions to the gathered journalists. With her husband, actor and director Scott Baio—best known for his role as Chachi Arcola on the TV sitcom *Happy Days*—Renee Baio had founded the Bailey Baio Angel Foundation to promote the expansion of newborn screening in the United States and to provide support for families of children diagnosed with organic acidemia oxidation disorders.[1] The organization was named after their daughter Bailey, who screened positive for glutaric acidemia type 1 (GA1) at birth. People with this condition cannot metabolize the amino acids lysine, hydroxylysine, and tryptophan and accumulate one or more toxic metabolites in their blood. The accumulation of these metabolites can lead to a metabolic crisis, an illness episode marked by vomiting, lethargy, difficulty feeding, and irritability that can result in brain damage, coma, or even death. Even without such a crisis, GA1 patients may experience developmental delays, poor growth, and muscle spasticity. Although there is variation in the symptomatic manifestation of the condition, geneticists consider it a very serious disease.

The Baios had called this press conference to urge legislators to adopt expanded newborn screening. The United States has had a newborn screening program in place since the 1960s but, as is typical for US healthcare, individual states determine which conditions to screen for. Between 1970 and 2000 great discrepancies developed, with some states screening for 3 conditions while others screened for up to 36 conditions. In 2006, the American College of Medical Genetics issued a report calling all states to screen for 54 conditions.[2] These recommendations were championed by several advocacy organizations—including the March of Dimes and the parent advocacy organization Save Babies Through Screening Foundation, Inc., with whom the Baios later joined forces.

The rationale for expanding newborn screening is powerful. The appeal resides in secondary prevention. Rather than treating children with devastating metabolic conditions, screening advocates hope to forestall the onset of symptoms. Newborn screening identifies infants who have a condition but are still asymptomatic and offers them preventive measures that may postpone symptom development.[3]

Strangely, however, the Baios' encounter with newborn screening did not fit this public health rationale. We interviewed Renee and Scott Baio about their own experience with newborn screening in 2009, 20 months after Bailey's birth.[4] When we arrived at their house, Bailey welcomed us, clutching a SpongeBob SquarePants doll. Sitting in their glass-enclosed breakfast room, Scott and Renee explained how they "went through hell" during the first 10 weeks of Bailey's life. Accustomed to talking to journalists,[5] they told us their story without much prompting. The couple had been dating for about two years when Renee found out she was pregnant, the day after Scott's father passed away. Scott was 45 and Renee was in her early thirties. They married when Renee was six months pregnant.

In the 11th week of her pregnancy, Renee started to bleed. An ultrasound showed that she was pregnant with twins. Several days later, however, she lost one of the fetuses. She recalled, "I go back to the hospital because I'm still spotting two or three days later and there just starts to be a mass of blood. It's a small mass of blood and then as one sac's getting smaller, the mass of blood is getting bigger. And then there was no second heartbeat. It just dissolved itself. I passed one and kept the other." Renee stayed on bed rest for a few weeks until she entered the second trimester. She explained that losing the twin "was very emotional. As a mother you want to know why. Why did you lose this baby; why?" Scott added: "I didn't know which end was up. She's telling me we're having twins and I'm just sort of getting over the fact that my father died and we just miscarried a baby." Renee recalled that Scott was not emotional during the pregnancy "until he laid eyes on [Bailey] and then it was instant change." This turnaround did not last long.

On day five of Bailey's life, the Baios received a phone message instructing them to visit their pediatrician's office to repeat a blood test. Bailey "tested positive for something" but the pediatrician refused to say what it was. A nurse from the state newborn screening program followed up several days later with a phone call to make sure that they had retested the baby. Playing dumb, Renee said she wasn't sure how to spell the name of the condition. The nurse spelled g-l-u-t-a-r-i-c a-c-i-d-e-m-i-a type 1. Renee had previously researched phenylketonuria (PKU) because that was, at the time, the most common metabolic condition identified through newborn screening. The name glutaric acidemia did not ring a bell. Scott and Renee confronted their pediatrician with the diagnosis and asked her whether it was worse than PKU. The pediatrician said that she wished the nurse had not told her the name of the condition because they would discover the worst-case scenario on the Internet. She admitted that "yes, it was worse than PKU," but she also added that the diagnosis was not firm yet.

The news took a toll on the recently created family. Renee recalled that Scott "was afraid to bond with [Bailey] once we got the positive [screening result]." Scott agreed that he "had a hard time." Renee recalled, "He did not want to hold Bailey." Scott explained, "Because I thought she was going to die. And then I didn't want to open my heart up and get completely crushed for the rest of my life." The positive result also caused tension in their marital relationship. Renee said, "My family lives in Tennessee. So of course, this is their grandchild. They want to know what's going on. I had her five weeks early—emergency C-section. They weren't here for that. And they're calling me. They want know what's going on and now they're concerned. So I wasn't allowed to have him hear me talk on the phone or he would bust in to the baby's room and he would say, 'She effing has it.' It was a rage, is what it was. I think I was on the verge of a nervous breakdown because here I'm trying to nurse this baby and bond with this baby." She added, "I thought for sure if she had it I would be a single parent."

For 10 excruciatingly long weeks, Renee and Scott waited for the results of a skin biopsy that would determine whether Bailey had GA1. Bailey's newborn screen value for glutarylcarnitine (C5DC), the biological marker for GA1, was 0.35 μmol/L, which was the cutoff point for GA1 at the time. With other conditions, newborn screening program officials might have wavered over whether to contact the parents about values lying at the cutoff point, but because GA1 is considered such a serious condition, the geneticists initiated follow-up testing. They specifically retested blood plasma and urine for C5DC, and again, the blood levels were slightly elevated. The next step was to do a skin biopsy and test for the genetic mutations implicated in GA1. However, only one laboratory in the country processed these biopsies and because the sample was taken right before the Thanksgiving holiday, the sample was not even sent there for two weeks. The Baios waited anxiously. Their geneticist tried to reassure them based on Bailey's apparent normal development but Scott wanted a clean bill of health based on genetic results.

Renee was prepared to put everything on hold until Bailey was out of the danger zone: "I was physically ready to hunker down in that baby's room for six years. Because the geneticist said that if you can get through the first six years without any metabolic crises, no fever, no vomiting, then you have somewhat of a chance. I was ready. I was ready to have everyone wear masks when they come in. I would just hunker and keep her in that room for six years. And me not leave. That's what I was ready to do." The couple started a crash course about GA1, requesting dietary supplements that could prevent symptom development. Renee explained: "All of it was tough. It was tough going for me to get the special formula downtown. It was tough for me to go the pharmacy to get the compound. It was so hard to go get it because every time I would go get it, it was a reaffirmation that my kid might be sick."

Renee attributed her decision to stop breastfeeding at six weeks to the stress of not knowing. At that time, the pediatrician suggested treating Bailey for "failure to thrive" because she wasn't gaining sufficient weight. The treatment involved supplementing Bailey's diet with extra protein, which could exacerbate the GA1 if Bailey did indeed have it. Renee reflected on the options she faced: "Okay my kid is going to be failure to thrive and she's either going to starve to death or we have to give her protein and I could be potentially causing my child brain damage." She felt she had failed as a mother.

Finally, in January 2008, the results came in. Renee recalled:

We had an appointment for Monday, January 13th. I told the nurse, "If the tests come in, I don't care if it's a Wednesday, Thursday, Friday; please just tell us. Just call me on the phone. Call me. Call me. Call me." I begged her and I'm calling her sometimes twice a day. Then on that Friday, January 11th, there was a celebrity baby gifting suite over in Beverly Hills. We decided to go because we went through her first Thanksgiving, her first Christmas, our wedding and everything was just kind of—we were numb. And so Scott said, "Let's go," because we knew that that Monday was our D-Day. So he said, "Let's just go and let's just try to enjoy it." We went through all the motions and got the free baby gifting things. While we were there, I got the phone call, but I didn't hear my cell phone ring. We're in the valet and I'm like, "Oh my God." So I tried to call my voice mail and that's the one day that T-Mobile was upgrading their voice mail. We get home and they had left a message on the home phone. I tried to call the voice mail box here at the house and just as she's getting ready to tell me, she goes, "Hi, this is Carla from newborn screening." The phone went dead because it had been off the charger. So I've gotta run to the other end of the house and Scott and my older daughter are like, "What'd they say? What'd they say?" So I had to run to the other end of the house to get the other phone, run back to the baby's room and they said, "Hi, this is Carla from newborn screening. I just want to let you know that it was a false positive and your baby is fine." And then I hit the floor.

At the time of our interview, the Baios' relationship was still recovering from this near brush with disease. Renee reflected: "We went from a relationship of two years of never arguing, never having any type of friction between us, nothing negative really ever. Maybe about the dog being in the kitchen or just small stuff. But it went from that to totally living together, him losing his father, me pregnant and losing a baby. And then we've got this baby that's potentially sick. It was just boom, boom. We're still trying to climb out of it. It almost ruined our marriage."

The experience with newborn screening galvanized the Baios to start a charitable foundation. Scott had pledged that if his daughter did not have glutaric acidemia, he would devote his energy to setting up a foundation for children with the disorder: "It's like an underground disorder. A lot of people don't know about it, they've never heard about it. A lot of people don't know when they bring their baby home what the heel stick is for."

*   *   *

The Baios' experience goes to the heart of this book. From a public health or medical perspective their ordeal does not count for much: Bailey's case was included in a state database of false positives and this measure represents the only official record of her screening experience.

What is medically invisible ends up being deeply meaningful socially, however. The encounter with newborn screening shaped Scott and Renee's young marriage, their charitable work, and their relationship with their daughter. The Baios are unique in their ability to leverage their celebrity status to create a charity complete with publicists and easy access to the press. Their experience is more typical, however, in how their daughter's newborn screening results came as a deep shock, how their baby did not show any symptoms but might have harbored a life-threatening condition, how they lived in suspense for months before finding out whether their child had a disease, how they were willing to go to great lengths to do the best for their child, how they treated something that ended up being a nondisease as a disease for a short period of time, and how even though Bailey had been cleared of disease, some lingering questions about her elevated levels remained.

If the Baios' harrowing experience does not register in the official program statistics, what narratives drive newborn screening policy? The common approach in medical and advocacy circles is to tell the story of the scientists who made newborn screening possible and to focus on dramatic patient stories as indicators of medical salvation. In fact, that is how the Baios talk publicly about newborn screening. Every month, their foundation website highlights an "angel," a child diagnosed with an organic acidemia disorder. Scott and Renee report heart-wrenching stories about infants with devastating conditions who had the misfortune of being born in states that did not screen for these conditions. If only they had been born in a neighboring state, the message goes, these children might have been saved. This is an emotionally powerful narrative that forms a benchmark for evaluating the efficacy of newborn screening. But it is not the only narrative. The Baios' own experience does not, in fact, fit in. Renee and Scott are careful not to present themselves as the face of organic acidemia disorders because, in the end, their daughter was not diagnosed with one.

In this book, we will highlight a fuller spectrum of effects that newborn screening has created for families and clinicians. We do not make the case for or against newborn screening. If anything, we found strong support for screening. The Baios' channeling of a difficult experience into pro-screening activism is telling of the appeal of newborn screening. All parents in our study, regardless of the final outcome, remained steadfast in their support of the screening program, although some would have preferred a different communication process or more supportive services.

We happened to be in the right place at the right time to observe newborn screening unfolding. In California, the setting of our research, expanded newborn screening had only been in place for about two years when we began our study in November 2007. This is how the process works. The state Department of Public Health ensures that every baby born in California receives a heel prick to collect a small amount of blood between 24 hours and six days after a baby's birth. Babies born at home without medical supervision are tracked through the county registrar to make sure that they receive the screen. The birth registrar provides the parents with an informational brochure that explains how to get their infant screened, and also informs the newborn screening program of any births that occur outside hospital facilities. The program is able to screen 99 percent of the 1,500 babies born in California each day with only 1 percent inadequate samples.[6] The California experience is typical for the United States: currently, more than 99 percent of the more than four million newborns born annually are screened for more than 50 rare genetic conditions.[7]

Newborn screening is de facto mandatory because parental consent is not required except for in the District of Columbia and two US states: Maryland and Wyoming.[8] Parents in 30 states, including California, can opt out of screening for religious reasons, and in 13 states parents can opt out for any reason.[9] The default position, however, is to screen every newborn. In fact, one state without religious exemption has removed a child from parental custody to conduct newborn screening.[10] Hospital personnel present the heel prick as a routine matter during the hospital checkout procedures, along with other bureaucratic forms and handouts about feeding and well-baby visits.

Typically, a nurse will stab the child's heel with a sharp triangular-shaped piece of metal. The nurse squeezes the heel until a drop of blood forms. The first drop is wiped away and the second drop is blotted upon a special card. These cards are sent to state laboratories to be processed. Most parents never hear from the newborn screening program because the blood sample screens negative. In those cases, the newborn screening program sends the screening results to the hospital and the physician listed on the screening form, usually a primary care physician or pediatrician.

If a blood sample screens positive for a target condition, the results are followed up through a network of clinical care coordinators that work for the state newborn screening program. (Note that "positive" refers to a result that lies outside of a predetermined normal range: the value is either higher or lower than that of the average infant.) First, the clinical care coordinator will contact the child's primary care provider to ask for a follow-up test. If no physician is listed on the birth certificate, coordinators rely on a network of state public health nurses to track the family down. The physician's office calls the parents and schedules the follow-up test: a confirmatory blood test, and often a urinalysis, depending on the condition. In the majority of the retested cases, the follow-up test is negative and the physician is informed that there is nothing to worry about. If the values still remain positive, the clinical care coordinator refers the patient to a regional specialty follow-up center under contract with the state, where a member of the clinical staff schedules a clinic visit to conduct additional tests and, if necessary, initiate treatment.

This is where we came in. This book draws on our ethnographic research in one specialty follow-up center in California. The clinic we studied specializes in the treatment of children's metabolic disorders.[11] For nearly three years, we followed 75 families whose children's newborn screening results lay outside of a preset normal range. We attended the weekly outpatient clinic, observed and recorded consultations between geneticists and families, sat in on staff meetings, and examined patients' medical charts. We also interviewed clinicians, parents, and policy actors about their experiences with newborn screening. This book tracks the intended and unintended consequences of expanded newborn screening for clinicians and families, both in and out of the clinic.

## How to Study Newborn Screening?

Proponents of expanded newborn screening have imbued newborn screening with tremendous potential for benefits. Take this quote from the influential American College of Medical Genetics report that helped to catalyze the expansion:

> States and territories mandate newborn screening of all infants born within
> their jurisdiction for creating treatable conditions that may not otherwise be
> detected before developmental disability or death occurs. Newborns with these
> disorders typically appear normal at birth. The testing and follow-up services of
> newborn screening programs are designed to provide early diagnosis and treat-
> ment before significant, irreversible damage occurs. Appropriate compliance
> with the medical management prescribed can allow most affected newborns to
> develop normally.... As the model for public health-based population genetic
> screening, newborn screening is nationally recognized as an essential program
> that aims to ensure the best outcome for the nation's newborn population.[12]

With every phrase in this passage, newborn screening is enriched with benefit potential. The goal is the prevention of "developmental disability or death" and "significant, irreversible damage." The mechanism of "early diagnosis and treatment" followed by "appropriate compliance with the medical management" leads to the promise that "most" infants "develop normally." Four additional elements are key. First, *hidden danger*, meaning that without newborn screening no one would suspect that the infants were at risk: "newborns with these disorders typically appear normal at birth." Secondly, *urgency*: "early" intervention is necessary. Thirdly, *universality*: as a "public health-based population genetic screening" program, all infants should be screened. And finally, "testing and follow-up" suggests that screening by itself is insufficient but a *lifelong, integrative, systemic approach* is required to achieve health benefits.

When we compare this account with the Baios' experience, we find that the policy logic of secondary prevention does not adequately capture the multiple meanings that newborn screening held for the family after hearing that Bailey was flagged with a possible disorder. The danger of losing Bailey when she looked and behaved fine affected every aspect of the Baios' relationship as a recently married couple and a newly constituted family. Scott indicated, "I didn't want to open my heart up and get completely crushed for the rest of my life."[13] Although both parents were willing to put their lives on hold to save Bailey, they were not sure that their relationship would survive the bout with a serious metabolic disorder. A positive newborn screen thus triggered a broad array of actions, only some of which fall under the intended goal of prevention.

Prevention did not fully explain the work of clinicians, either. While the policy logic of secondary prevention is oriented toward population outcomes, the job of clinicians is both more mundane and more complex because they respond to individual patients in the here and now. This means that sometimes they aim to prevent the onset of disease, other times they try to talk parents out of going overboard with preventive measures, and on still other occasions they face the difficult task of communicating that prevention is not going to save a baby.

After witnessing our first encounters between parents and clinicians, we realized that policy visions do a poor job of capturing the effects of newborn screening in the clinic. Prevention is too limited and too vague a framework to explain the clinical outcomes of newborn screening: it is only one possible outcome at the end of a lengthy trajectory. Our approach in this book is to examine the broad range of intended and unintended consequences and the daily effects of screening as they unfolded in the clinic. We follow how people act and react, and if these actions prevent the onset of diseases, we are interested in the specific kind of prevention that newborn screening achieves in the lives of infants and its effects on the larger healthcare field.

Here, we are on the lookout for the *consequences* of newborn screening, an approach drawn from pragmatist theory. These consequences include the ability of newborn screening results to produce emotions, prompt courses of action, suggest justifications, revise previous understandings of disease, and make dietary decisions reasonable. This means that we do not presume to know what newborn screening is and then track its impact on people's lives. Rather, it is through its practical consequences that newborn screening exists and is imbued with specific meanings. *Newborn screening is what it does.* We are interested in the practical difference newborn screening makes: what is the added value you obtain from a positive screen? Actions and experiences are the concrete imprints of the impact of newborn screening that constitute what newborn screening is about.

One implication of this approach is that we take a broad perspective on relevant consequences. Newborn screening technologies connect the biological body at the molecular and symptomatic level with macro factors such as the third-party payer health insurance system in the United States. Screening and test results, possible symptoms of developmental delay, and metabolic crises are not inevitable, predictable, or well-understood entities: they become opportunities for further interpretive actions. In turn, regulatory actions to reimburse dietary supplements directly affect both bodily processes and opportunities for medically sanctioned action. In fact, the micro and macro, the social and physiological converge. We do not decide a priori which consequences are salient, but instead follow the impact of newborn screening wherever it may lead.

Situations of friction, in which habitual ways of thinking and doing no longer seem to work, are of particular interest because they call for improvisation and innovation. Such anomalous situations invoke what the pragmatist philosopher Charles S. Peirce called *abduction*, an inferential creative process that produces new hypotheses and modes of action. For Peirce, people constantly perform abduction in their everyday life, continuously recalibrating their expectations of the future when they face surprising phenomena. We put a child to bed, hear a loud "boink" noise, followed by crying, and presume that the child fell out of bed. In everyday life as in science, such conjectural hunches require corroboration with further evidence. Peirce distinguished two kinds of surprise: novelty, or a new experience, and anomaly, or an unexpected experience. Peirce conceptualized the process of abduction as both a logical inference and a flash of insight occurring when one's mind wanders.[14] We do not need to follow Peirce's speculation about the cognitive foundation of insight. Indeed, a more sociological approach would attend to the cultural schema and available resources that make such flashes of insight more likely.[15] Healthcare providers and parents facing puzzling clinical situations have developed transposable problem-solving repertoires.[16] Abductive insights prompt a process of trial and error to verify one's hunches that may result in new knowledge about disease, new patient categories, and new modes of managing patients. The unexpected, creative consequences of expanding newborn screening drive our analysis.

A focus on the creative potential of consequences does not imply a naïve inductivism in which the meanings of newborn screening emerge continuously de novo out of an experiential flow. Clinics, healthcare systems, and families all have their routines, habits, and cultures. With unexpected events, however, these old ways of dealing may fall short and new actions and knowledge may develop, at times somewhat reluctantly, due to resistance. As pragmatist philosopher William James wrote, "To a certain degree, therefore, everything here is plastic,"[17] meaning that even historically established ideas and practices need to prove their utility and relevance for the situation at hand. Then, even with unexpected events, a narrowing of experiences and actions may occur. What was an emergency becomes a recurring situation, and solutions and resources carry over from one instance to another. Some actions and experiences may develop into habits that suggest more appropriate responses. And at some point, there may become a standard way of managing the unexpected—perhaps a point where people have trouble imagining that there were ever other ways of reacting. Such routinization may occur even if people do not desire the reproduction of particular modes of dealing with problems. From a pragmatist perspective, then, at the most elementary level, a positive newborn screen is a prompt for collective action that runs against or along with established ways of dealing with issues. Newborn screening results become meaningful through the consequences they have for people, and it is through studying the consequences that we have access to the meanings, beliefs, and truths of newborn screening.

## Acting under Uncertainty

The organizing mechanism of newborn screening is knowledge: knowing that a child has a metabolic disorder prior to symptom development should translate into preventive action. If diagnosis takes too long, it may be too late. Thus, newborn screening is expected to provide accurate knowledge and control over a process that without technological intervention would lead to serious health consequences.

In the everyday world of parents and clinicians managing a positive newborn screen, however, presumably definitive knowledge gives rise to uncertainty. The Baios' interview contains many statements about the experience of knowing, not knowing, and the inability to undo knowledge that they might rather have not known. They faced the vexing issue of figuring out what the condition was. Scott recalled that Renee "really needed to know [the implied diagnosis]. They don't tell you anything. They said that there's an abnormal read." Renee concurred: "We weren't told anything; nothing at all, nothing, nothing, nothing." When she managed to extract the disease name from the nurse, the concern became knowing too much from unreliable sources. Their pediatrician warned that if they "get onto Google, it tells you the worst-case scenario." Instead, Internet searches helped Renee level the playing field: she brought the knowledge she learned online to the geneticist who was surprised that she requested specific treatments. Mostly, however, Scott and Renee talked about "not knowing what to do" but opting to treat Bailey as if she had the condition because, Renee added, "as a mother, that's what I am comfortable with." Interposed were critical questions whether Bailey's failure to thrive was due to the GA1 treatment.

Renee and Scott were not alone in their struggle with knowledge generating more uncertainties. Their geneticist was "most confident" that Bailey did not have the condition, but Renee recalled him saying, "'You need to go by the science. You have to go by the testing. You have to go.' But I had everything in me saying this child doesn't have it." The geneticist thus intuitively knew that Bailey did not have the condition but still needed authoritative scientific knowledge. When the geneticist told her that Bailey did not have GA1, Renee wanted to know whether her daughter was a carrier. The geneticist told her that it did not matter, but Renee said: "It does matter, right. That's why I want to know." Finally, when Scott and Renee questioned why this was happening to them, Scott recalled that a physician told him, "We're all just guessing. Sometimes we get it right, sometimes we get it wrong. That's why it is called practicing medicine. We're learning as we go."

Newborn screening is a technology expected to provide actionable knowledge, yet it generates uncertainty in the clinic: clinicians and parents face questions about what is known, what knowledge is sufficient for the situation at hand, what is knowable yet unfathomable, and how uncertainty relates to science and intuition. Uncertainty, referring here to doubt about how to act, is a well-known challenge in healthcare.[18] Pioneering medical sociologist Renee Fox highlighted medical uncertainty as an endemic characteristic of contemporary medicine. Drawing from her studies on medical school socialization, medical experimentation, and organ transplantation, Fox focused on the social and moral meanings of medical uncertainty for physicians and patients, and on their collective responses.[19] What makes uncertainty special in the medical field, according to Fox, is the fact that medicine is associated with basic and intimate aspects of the human body and psyche. Medical uncertainty has a deep moral and existential dimension: it provokes fundamental questions about whether lives are worth living, about balancing potential with risk, and about weighing danger against benefit.

Fox emphasized that uncertainty could not be dispelled with scientific or technological advances. She drew attention to the recursive nature of uncertainty: while technologies may address some forms of uncertainty, they seem bound, inevitably, to uncover previously unrecognized forms of uncertainty or to produce new ones. Indeed, the recursive nature of uncertainty has been well documented in studies of medicine, health services, and wellness more broadly. Evidence-based medicine (EBM), for example, consists of the critical evaluation and ranking of all available scientific evidence to address specific clinical questions. While EBM is directly oriented to obliterating uncertainty within medicine's quickly changing knowledge base, the implementation of EBM in clinical settings requires new statistical skills that are in short supply in medical settings.[20] Research has shown that when presented with novel antidepressive drugs, clinicians engage in personalized clinical trials to double-check recommendations[21] and rely on senior academic colleagues for the most updated information.[22] Clinicians also struggle with weighing individual patient parameters against population-level profiles and integrating new protocols with other forms of knowledge.[23] While EBM may have reduced the uncertainty resulting from an outdated biomedical knowledge base, it has also generated new form of uncertainties related to the implementation of standardized guidelines.[24]

Considering the recursive nature of uncertainty, we may expect that while newborn screening is a technology-driven response to diagnostic uncertainty, it will create new uncertainties in unanticipated arenas. Biomedical uncertainty highlights gaps in knowledge due to a rapidly changing knowledge base and a continuous stream of medical innovations with far-reaching, but little understood, intended and unintended consequences. Such uncertainty is inevitable whenever new technologies produce previously unavailable knowledge about patients. This knowledge provokes questions about the technology's reliability, about its relationship to other forms of knowledge, and about its usefulness for taking clinical action.

Biomedical uncertainty contains a number of critical dimensions that will guide our examination of the consequences of newborn screening. One such critical dimension relates to the *forms* of uncertainty following newborn screening. The specificity of uncertainty matters greatly: uncertainty differs by source, issue, and locus.[25] The source of biomedical uncertainty may come from expressing information as probabilities with questionable reliability or adequacy of risk estimates; ambiguity due to conflicting opinions, imprecision, or lack of information; the novelty of information; or its complexity (e.g., genetic test results contingent on environmental factors or interactions between various treatments). Genetic information raises different uncertainties depending on the purpose of testing. The early adopters of direct-to-consumer genomic services, for example, tended to assess the predictive power of their personal genetic risk profiles skeptically in light of their family history and undertook few life changes based on their genomic information.[26] In contrast, the majority of women who carried the fragile X gene interviewed in one study decided not to have a biological child to avoid passing on the gene.[27] Their choice, however, was complicated by ambivalence about the consequences for the size of their own families and about other people's choice to opt for children despite the risks of fragile X. The issue at stake in biomedical uncertainty may also range from diagnosis, prognosis, and causal explanations to treatments and side effects. Since biomedical uncertainty depends on exposure to information and an ability to act on it, its locus may include clinicians, patients, or both in interaction. Some parties may lack knowledge about what they should know; in other situations ignorance may be shared across multiple parties, or may shift within and among groups over time.

Another critical dimension is *what to do* about biomedical uncertainty. How do clinical staff and families manage uncertainty in the interactional space of the clinic? Because uncertainty reflects a lack of knowledge, which impedes action, one prevailing theme in the biomedical literature is a "will to know": the idea that the proliferation of information reduces uncertainty. From this perspective, the stress, maladaptive behaviors, and general malaise of uncertainty need to be countered by a search for and full disclosure of all available information. Uncertainty becomes an affront against a modernist promise of control in medicine. Indeed, studies of uncertainty due to screening or undiagnosed symptoms demonstrate a strong desire to know among patients and health authorities.[28] However, this widespread "ideology of uncertainty reduction"[29] ignores that knowledge is a moving target, situated in the contingencies of the situation at hand.

Uncertainties require management, but the reduction of uncertainty through information gathering is only one of many appropriate responses. Even with a family history of highly heritable conditions, relatives of people with Huntington's disease opt not to undergo predictive testing with remarkable frequency.[30] Also, in the process of deciding to test within the context of family history, people weigh knowing against being known:[31] disease-related knowledge may lead to stigma, insurance discrimination, and a future curtailed in other ways. Social scientists have observed cases in which patients, especially those with poor prognoses, actively sought out and clung to uncertainty because not knowing drew out hope and lingering possibilities for recovery.[32] Other situations involve a preoccupation with determining what is not known rather than choosing biomedical interventions: the traditional nondirective model of genetic counseling emphasizes educating about uncertainties rather than imposing decisions. Then, there is the issue of knowing too much. Information overload reveals the enormity, complexity, contradictions, and endless qualifications in the medical literature.[33] Doing something may require sorting through and simplifying competing explanations and suggestions. There may be some knowledge that you regret having, knowledge that leads to a loss of innocence and enjoyment. Finally, resources to act also matter. The relevance of preventive information is greatly diminished if you cannot afford the recommended measures.

A third critical dimension is how uncertainty challenges the *interactions between patients and clinicians.* The hallmark of medical professionalism is the use of expert knowledge on behalf of patients. Biomedical uncertainty may backfire onto the messengers, clouding the patient-clinician interaction with blame and distrust.[34] At a time of increased patient consumerism and persistent biomedical uncertainty, patients may "doctor shop" until they find a physician who tells them what they would like to hear, look for information outside the clinical interaction, engage in online or interpersonal support groups, and even organize to resist medical authority and produce alternative ways of knowing.[35] However, while a trusting patient-clinician relationship can no longer be taken for granted, resistance and conflict is not the only possible response to biomedical uncertainty. Clinicians may counter uncertainty with compassionate support, extensive availability, reassuring communication, and other attempts to provide care congruent with the patient's best interests while acknowledging the limits of medical knowledge.[36] In fact, they may bridge uncertainty and vulnerability with trust and care.[37]

Much of the social science literature views uncertainty as a deeply entrenched and problematic characteristic of a modernist Zeitgeist demanding more knowledge, competence, and coping strategies.[38] An emphasis on uncertainty may give the mistaken impression of a suffocating malaise among patients, families, and clinicians. The opposite is true. Precisely because it irritates the phenomenology of business as usual, uncertainty energizes intense and imaginative action: it generates revisions of knowledge about disease and entire patient populations, creative work-arounds to provide treatment under stifling insurance restrictions, questioning of organizational procedures, new alliances and divisions of labor, and so forth. While deeply unsettling, uncertainty is also an inventive force.[39] Uncertainty leads to creativity especially because the stakes are high for those involved. At the same time, these innovations are not necessarily beneficial or satisfactory for all but may create new stratifications of disease or reinforce existing social inequities in who gets access to healthcare.

## Medical Technologies in the Clinic

The tension between the proliferation of knowledge and uncertainty about what action to take frames the consequences of expanded newborn screening in the clinic. What, then, triggers biomedical uncertainty? In Bailey Baio's case, the element that set this cycle in motion was a single number. The key difference between Bailey and more than 99 percent of newborns was that a biological parameter, C5DC, registered a screening value of 35 μmol/L, which was the cutoff value for GA1 at the time. This particular value represents the intersection of various innovations in newborn screening. It reflects an established relationship between a biomarker and a disease, and an understanding of a particular range of normal values. It also reflects the use of a new technology in newborn screening: tandem mass spectrometry. This technology drove the expansion of newborn screening because it allowed the measurement of multiple bio-markers using a single blood sample.[40] Prior to tandem mass spectrometry, adding a condition to the screen required the creation of a separate disease-specific assay. The adoption of tandem mass spectrometers in newborn screening has profoundly increased the number of biomarkers that can be screened. Although tandem mass spectrometers remained off-site, their presence in the clinic was palpable through lists of numbers reflecting biochemical values.

The introduction of innovative technologies into clinical settings is a particularly vulnerable time in a technology's life cycle.[41] The implementation phase entails a handover from the people designing, packaging, and marketing a technology to the users of the technology, although the distinction between user and designer remains blurry.[42] Designers—in this context everyone involved in bringing a technology to the clinic—charge the technology with potentiality. They imagine an ideal scenario in which people will use the technology to achieve preset goals.[43] In the case of newborn screening, assumptions about shared interests across diverse populations, parental aspirations for the health of their child, clinical competencies, and ideal users were inscribed to varying degrees in operating protocols and the materiality of the tools.

Of course, the designers' assumptions are necessarily incomplete, idealistic, and simplistic. Underspecification of users and infrastructures is necessary for the technology to reach a broad constituency and adapt to diverse settings.[44] Technologies specifically require buy-in or the active submission to some shared goals, but they vary in the extent to which they allow flexibility or demand adherence to formal rules.[45] Too much flexibility or formality in the wrong places can doom technologies.[46] Take, for example, a French photoelectric lighting kit, specifically created for use in Africa.[47] Although beautifully designed, this technology proved useless because it required a nonstandard plug unavailable in Africa and because the technology was only repairable by experts with specialized tools. Therefore, in spite of great need, this technology found neither users nor use. Contrast this with the Zimbabwe Bush Pump, another tool designed in and for Africa.[48] This brightly colored device used to pump clean water from wells in rural Zimbabwe was designed for a simple production process and easy repair. The device proved even more flexible than anticipated: users tinkered with its construction so that it kept functioning when critical bolts fell out or the user community changed. The success of the Bush Pump rested with its adaptability to settings with widely diverging tools and skill sets and community arrangements for water procurement. For other technologies, however, too much flexibility can lead to their undoing.[49]

The effects of technological scripts can thus only be understood in their relationship to real-world situations. Working out technological prescriptions necessarily implies a form of "situated action."[50] That is, working with technologies is contingent on specific, moment-to-moment unfolding circumstances that, in turn, are constituted through actions. In clinics, technological knowledge may be resisted, subverted, or ignored, and its social and cultural significance must be adapted to the situation at hand.

Technology adoption is not simply a dialogue between users and designers: competitors and regulators contribute as well.[51] For medical technologies, governmental regulators play an important role in approving or suspending the use of technologies. The regulatory process inevitably sets standards for knowledge acquisition by specifying the kinds of evidence needed, for example, to establish the efficacy and safety of new pharmaceuticals.[52] Local regulations at the level of the state or even an individual insurance company may affect the financial viability of a technological innovation by specifying reimbursement policies. Every time a competing technology is introduced, a new budget cycle rolls around, a contract is up for negotiation, or a lawsuit is filed, the technology's likelihood of adoption may be greatly affected.

Technologies work by the grace of textured networks of interlinked parties and the smallest detail may undermine a technology's functionality. The circle of people implementing technologies expands beyond designers, users, regulators, and competitors to countless other actors that are necessary to make technologies realize their objectives but are too mundane, esoteric, or remote to warrant official specification and attention. These actors remain invisible until a breakdown somewhere in the technological logic indicates their critical collaboration. They may include the nameless courier bringing blood samples to the laboratory, technicians calibrating machines, a journalist writing a piece on health technologies, or legislators taking a stand against financial waste in healthcare.[53] Anyone may become a barrier and complicate the implementation of technologies or even make the entire technology moot.

In the clinic, screening techniques work as technological portals: when biochemical values fall outside a preset normal range, they summon people with a message to do something about the threat of pathology. Whether they want to or not, families and clinicians then enter a world in which screening results feature as pressing issues that must be dealt with.

This new world, however, will be a world partly of their own making. Realizing the added value achieved by screening technologies depends on the alignment, submission, negotiation, and transformation of an expanding array of actors. Our approach examines technologies-in-action: newborn screening as one element that contingently brings other elements together in new configurations of biosocial life.[54]

The critical role that changing technological scripts played in expanded newborn screening can be illustrated with Bailey Baio's case. In 2008, the year that Bailey was born, a C5DC value equal or higher than 0.35 µmol/L triggered a follow-up test for GA1. By 2010, the cutoff value had been changed to 0.60 µmol/L. If Bailey had been born in 2010, she would never have been picked up by newborn screening. Her life and her parents' lives—including the period that Scott characterized as "three months of living hell"—would have been completely different.

## Screening and Prevention

The Baio family is now a leading advocate for newborn screening in the United States. We wonder, though, what Renee and Scott would have done if they had been asked to provide consent for newborn screening. Would they even have agreed to have Bailey screened? This is a moot question because newborn screening is de facto compulsory. The uniqueness of this situation cannot be exaggerated. In the United States, few health services or public health programs enjoy the same government resources and commitment as expanded newborn screening. In fact, recent legislative mandates to vaccinate young women for human papillomavirus generated tremendous controversy.[55] We might have expected a market model in which companies make an expanded newborn screen available to parents willing to pay a fee. In an era infused with bioethical concern about patient autonomy and genetic discrimination, it seems almost inconceivable that the overwhelming majority of infants are screened for *genetic* conditions without informed consent, especially since these conditions are very rare, poorly understood, and not infectious diseases. The compulsory setup of newborn screening signals an extraordinary belief in the power of screening.

The word "screening" spans the contradictory meanings of concealing and revealing something with a screen. The term refers to hiding someone or something from prying eyes and to sifting an element of interest out of a larger group. As is common in public health, newborn screening follows the second meaning in its efforts to reveal hidden disorder. Medical screening involves an inevitable balance between sensitivity—the ability to correctly identify true cases—and specificity—the ability to weed out negative cases. Ideally, a screen is 100 percent sensitive and specific, which means that it identifies all the positives and only the positives. In reality, a strict focus on sensitivity will generate false positives, while an emphasis on specificity will allow true positives to go undetected. False negatives provide a misleading sense of security and void the preventive potential of screening. False positives create unnecessary alarm and are associated with adverse psychological outcomes.[56] Diagnostic testing subsequent to screening helps to clarify whether a positive is a true or a false positive. The institutional momentum in the policy world is to reveal hidden disease and thus to focus on identifying the true positives, even if the inevitable result is to increase the rate of false positives.

Historians have noted a shift in public health policy in the post–World War II period from improving population health with environmental interventions to preventing chronic disease. Increased attention to prevention followed from changes in the understanding of the natural history of diseases, in which earlier detectable pathological states coinciding with lowered thresholds for clinical diagnosis generated a gradual expansion of disease categories and new pharmaceutical markets.[57] The notion that one could offset disease by identifying asymptomatic individuals has gained currency with the advent of a risk paradigm, which aims to translate epidemiological risks into the enumeration of individual risk factors and the calculation of risk probabilities. Large clinical and epidemiological studies have since isolated biological, lifestyle, and community risk factors that might lead to higher rates of disease, prompting preventive efforts.

Identifying people at risk requires a massive infrastructure of surveillance medicine, a new form of medicine based on monitoring healthy populations rather than caring for the sick that emerged in the early twentieth century.[58] Surveillance medicine has relied on large-scale screening campaigns, of which mammography and pap smears are paradigmatic examples. As physician historian Robert Aronowitz has observed, "Defined by pathologists but sustained by screening campaigns, different cervical and breast precancers have been discovered."[59] Such precancers, along with conditions such as hypercholesterolemia and hypertension, have moved from disease symptoms to risk factors to self-contained diseases. The result is not only an expansion of disease categories but also a cascading of diseases in which surviving one condition becomes a risk factor and a preventive target for other conditions.[60]

In recent years, screening has garnered increasing public attention with controversies surrounding mammography and prostate-specific antigen (PSA) screening guidelines making major newspaper headlines.[61] Screening has also moved into the genetic domain, with advances in prenatal testing technologies and growing awareness of the links between genetic mutations and certain types of cancer generating demand for presymptomatic genetic testing.[62] Nevertheless, newborn screening continues to be the current face of public health genetics in the United States, reaching far more potential patients than the late-onset or prenatal screening with which much of the American population is most familiar.

Prevention through screening is attractive to health policymakers hoping to expand healthcare access while controlling costs. The reality is, however, that screening programs drive up medical consumption, particularly in the United States, where screening programs are more expensive and subsequent care is more difficult to access than in other industrialized countries.[63] Fishing expeditions for rare diseases may not be the most efficacious way to promote population health. Whether a screening program is able to deliver on the promise of prevention depends in part on the availability and accessibility of health services and efficacious therapies further downstream from screening. While advocates justify screening for its presumed efficacy, observers have also noted direct adverse effects. Among these risks are overuse and underuse of screening among various populations,[64] the inefficient use of healthcare resources for follow-up testing, a loss of privacy and confidentiality, side effects associated with undergoing the screening procedure, and contamination of screening results.

The feasibility of secondary prevention rests upon the public's participation in screening programs. Screening advocates causally tie the avoidance of worst-possible outcomes to screening programs, but research shows broader motivations among people opting in. For voluntary screening, compliance with screening recommendations depends partly on a persuasive interaction between a patient and clinician informed by policy guidelines and insurance reimbursement policies and partly on a realization that screening is either in one's own best interest or the right step to take to fulfill one's responsibility to others (e.g., when mothers undergo cervical screening at the urging of their daughters).[65] In some communities and for some individuals, screening has negative connotations. For example, early screening for sickle cell disease in the 1970s was associated with eugenic intentions since it targeted African Americans and was perceived by some as an indication of racial inferiority.[66] Because expanded newborn screening is quasi-mandatory, compliance with screening guidelines in this context may seem a moot point. Still, while mandatory screening neutralizes motivation to screen, different perceived rationales may influence how the public responds to screening and acts upon its results. In compulsory screening programs administered by government authorities, the most salient aspect of the screening program for the general public is the actual screening procedure.

The policy ambition of screening to prevent disease becomes somebody's job in clinics and laboratories all around the world. A tandem mass spectrometer produces a computer printout of numbers marked with an asterisk to indicate a result lying outside a preset normal range. To enable screening to reveal disease requires someone to pick up these figures, convey their significance to the relevant parties, and create a collaborative set of relationships aimed at preventing disease. In essence, screening is conveyed through interactions to render emotions, cognition, relationships, resources, and abstract results relevant to the situation at hand. Disease identified by screening exemplifies the observation that "disease occurs, of course not in the body but in life ... in time, place and history and in the context of lived experience and the social world. Its effect is on the body in the world."[67]

The interactional experience in the clinic encompasses screening's contradictory meanings of concealing and revealing across time. Newborn screening promises to divulge a forecast of who a child really is, but it also allows for the possibility that the result is not clinically significant. Screening alters the binary between health and sickness. Detecting and diagnosing asymptomatic individuals with a disease they might be unaware of and *could* develop in the future separate diagnosis from the experience of pain and suffering.[68] While risk factors and predictions are inevitably probabilistic, actions based on these predictions become determinate.[69] Many families cling to the hope that the screen hides a healthy child. As we saw in the Baios' situation, families aspire for their children to be deemed false positives although they remain haunted by the possibility that the results were correct after all. For children who already have developed symptoms, the preoccupying issue is to understand *how* abnormal the child will be. Here, the question of what exactly the screen picked up gives way to questions about what kind of future the parents may expect, knowing that this future will be somewhat compromised.

## Genetic Stratification

The Baios' repeated visits to genetics clinics might give the impression that tandem mass spectrometry is a genetic technology. This would be incorrect. The screen is performed by measuring the biochemical composition of analytes in the blood, rather than gene sequencing. The location of care in a genetics clinic might also suggest that the conditions targeted by the newborn screening program are genetic disorders. Strictly speaking, the conditions we studied are genetic, but their genetic nature was not always their most salient feature. More immediately relevant, the conditions are metabolic disorders—or "inborn errors of metabolism," as they are referred to in the medical community, which affect the processing of food into energy. Metabolic disorders have become linked to genetic mutations, but this association has only been made relatively recently. Although scientists realized that PKU could be inherited in the 1930s, it only became a paradigmatic genetic disorder when advocates for the Human Genome Project sought exemplars of successful therapeutic interventions for genetic conditions.[70] Although genetic factors cause metabolic disease, the relevance of the genetic nature of metabolic disease varies over time and place. Few genetic mutations are pathognomonic—that is, characteristic to the extent that their presence settles a diagnosis definitively—of metabolic conditions.

We observed geneticists using biochemical screens followed somewhere down the line with genetic tests to diagnose rare metabolic conditions associated with various genetic mutations. Is this still a study of genetics? We argue that this *is* the current face of clinical genetics. It has been close to six decades since Francis Crick and James D. Watson discovered the structure of DNA and more than a decade since the human genome was decoded. During this period, advocates of genomics spun promises that genetics would revolutionize medicine, offering cures for countless diseases. A good example is a recent book by Francis Collins, architect of the Human Genome Project and current director of the National Institutes of Health, who still anticipates the dawn of personalized medicine fueled by genomic innovations.[71] The counterpoint to this genetic hyping came from social scientists and some geneticists who decried the biological reductionism, determinism, and essentialism that would follow the "geneticization"[72] of health at the expense of social structural causes of difference.[73]

In hindsight, it seems that both the "genohype" and handwringing about genetic determinism have been exaggerated. We are now living in the era of the *routinization* of genetic medicine, in which genetic mutations tend to play an important but not necessarily leading role in clinical care. Indeed, Collins's Human Genome competitor in the commercial sector, Craig Venter, noted soberly that "decoding the genome has so far yielded nothing more than a 1–3% increased understanding of an individual's probabilities of contracting a disease" and dismissed personalized medicine as a commercially unfeasible pipedream.[74] Sociologists Carlos Novas and Nikolas Rose deflated the social science counterhype when they argued that the capacity for genetic technologies to identify people as at risk for diseases is but "one dimension of a wider mutation in personhood."[75] Similarly, philosopher Ian Hacking wrote:

> The genes of an individual determine the extreme limits of possibilities, but it is choices that create one's character, one's veritable essence, one's soul. Here is a credo for an existentialism without dogma for our time: our genetic essence is not our essence. The possibilities that are open to one, one's character and potentialities, are formed during one's life, even if for many they become petrified at an early age.[76]

If a phenomenon such as "geneticization" exists, it is foremost in a purely quantitative increase of genetic information rather than in qualitative genetic essentialism. In fact, quantitative social scientists have increasingly adopted the position that "genetic expression can only reveal itself through social structural change,"[77] and have included genetic polymorphisms in research that examines a variety of outcomes and heritability.

In genetics clinics in France, the United Kingdom, Canada, the Netherlands, New Zealand, Israel, and the United States, social scientists have found that molecular information is rarely conclusive in biomedicine but requires interpretation along with other signs and symptoms.[78] The informative value of genetic analyses is filtered through relevant disease, patient, clinician, and genetic characteristics. More important than the genetic nature is the actual content and the context in which the information was sought, given, and received. Thus, if the genetic information confirms a diagnosis after a patient has had debilitating symptoms, the results are often accepted with a sense of quiet resignation. Patients with neurological symptoms expressed relief after finally obtaining a conclusive diagnosis of a progressive, degenerative neurological disease, which would also likely be the patient's cause of death.[79] This sense of relief is unsurprising in light of the literature on contested illnesses, where the presence of unexplained symptoms might raise the suspicion of mental instability and where not knowing is often experienced as worse than having a disease.[80] If the genetic information confirms a condition associated with mental retardation—such as fragile X syndrome—but the symptoms at the time of diagnosis are not clear, patients and their caregivers may find value in the prognostic uncertainty of the results.[81] The diagnosis may well be definitive but the actual manifestation of the syndrome in the specific patient remains indeterminate. If the genetic information offers a likelihood of risk for a familial disease such as cancer, its informative value will be weighed against the observed experience of other relatives with the disease and their experiences.[82] If these relatives have a disease that is not considered debilitating on a daily basis, such as thrombophilia,[83] prospective patients may ignore the information. More important than genetic information sui generis is what social scientists called the "subjective badness" of the information or the extent to which an unwanted outcome matters to a patient.[84]

Such contextual issues are at stake not only for patients and their relatives but also for medical geneticists. Geneticists routinely qualify molecular test results in light of symptoms and morphological signs.[85] Genetic testing leads to the expansion of disease categories and requires reconciling molecular with other bases of disease.[86] Geneticists draw on various communication strategies to contextualize the probability that a patient may manifest symptoms of a genetic disorder. Thus, "mutations, far from reifying and simplifying pathological situations, expand and recompose them in different ways."[87]

Consequently, rather than a future in which genetic knowledge will save or corrupt healthcare, we have entered into an era of the routinization of genomics, a time when genetic information is one piece of information to be contextualized, interpreted, and related to other knowledge forms. What, then, is distinctive about genetic information?

Increasingly, the evidence shows that genetic information offers new wine in both old and new wineskins. Some scholars have argued that genetic data creates grounds for new group formation. Early on in the investment in genetics, anthropologist Paul Rabinow imagined "biosociality" as the creation of advocacy groups, vocabularies, narratives, practices, experts, and institutions around genetic information.[88] These biological stimuli for identity formation only partially coincide with traditional mod-

ernist categories of race, ethnicity, gender, and age: "Older cultural classifications will be joined by a vast array of new ones, which will cross-cut,
partially supersede, and eventually redefine the older categories."[89] Various patient advocacy groups have indeed sprung up around genetic conditions, such as a French organization dedicated to creating a research institute for neuromuscular disease.[90] Still, while the socially binding factor
is a presumed biological tie centered on shared genetic risk, the form of
advocacy organizing is similar to breast cancer, HIV/AIDS, and other advocacy communities.[91]

Of particular concern for social scientists is that much of recent genetic medicine is not organized around individuals with different genetic
risks but instead around well-entrenched social groups presumed to have
differential health risks. The flashpoint of contention has been the genetics of race. Sociologist Troy Duster argued early on that modern genetics
reintroduces "eugenics through the back door."[92] An extensive literature
on race and genetics shows both how genetic knowledge *could* render the
notion of distinct racial populations obsolete due to new social groupings
around genetic markers *and* how genetic knowledge *could* indicate significant biological variation between different racial and ethnic groups useful
for medical diagnosis and treatment.[93] Race and other identity features
may receive a second lease on life in the genomic era. The category of
race already has significant traction in public health, biomedical research,
and the social imagination.[94] Genetic information may lead to naturaliza-
tion as well as the denaturalization and renaturalization of social life.[95]

Kinship represents a critical area for social differentiation on genetic
grounds because genetic information tends to spill over from an individual to other family members.[96] When people related by blood ties, rather
than a singular patient, become the object of medical scrutiny,[97] social
scientists have noted the possibility of entrenchment of social ties along
biological criteria.[98] Yet, even in the kinship realm, the effects of genetic
information are diluted, subordinated to other ties, and reinterpreted,
creating a "gap between genetic information—which is often highly technical but incomplete—and meaningful knowledge, which, by definition, is
socially, not medically defined, evaluated, and acted upon."[99] Rather than
a geneticization of the family, a "familarization of genetics" exists among
people tested for the genes for late onset Alzheimer's disease, "in which
risk estimates are absorbed into and embedded within pre-existing beliefs
about who in the family will succumb to AD."[100] The selective uptake of
genetic information is further mediated by the nature of disease and the

meaningfulness of the genetic information. The persuasiveness of the information is stronger for rare single gene disorders[101] than for genetic susceptibility testing, such as the genes implicated in breast cancer. Genetic information may create a genetic kinship proximity which can tighten the bonds between relatives because it provides a shared risk, drive them apart when they disagree about the need for testing, leave already distant family ties distant, or be subverted altogether for other ties that bind.[102]

How to capture genetic stratification? We view the collection of genetic information via newborn screening as an opportunity to classify people along new criteria.[103] Human conditions are interactive and dynamic, Ian Hacking argued, because classifying people into categories, such as diagnostic ones, affects the people classified, and changed self-understandings in turn loop back onto the properties of the classification, leading to modifications, which then again affect the people classified. This cycle is perpetuated because the category becomes a way of relating to the self and others—an attributed novel identity that requires appropriation. The classification changes when it becomes part of a population of people, an infrastructure of institutions, knowledge production, and experts. The category receives traction; it becomes an account to justify actions and becomes a way to express accountability to self and others for actions taken and omitted. It becomes a choice consideration with moral overtones. When a new categorization receives traction in people's lives, it has a high likelihood of changing the original category. Geneticists learn things about conditions that they did not know before. The changed knowledge base affects not only the knowledge of the disease but also how geneticists approach newly diagnosed patients.

The work of anthropologist Lynn Morgan offers a wonderful example of a feedback loop radically changing the understanding of a categorization to the point that past properties are unrecognizable in the present.[104] Morgan was shown a decaying collection of about a hundred preserved fetuses in the storage room of her university's biology department. To contemporary eyes saturated with popular cultural images of fetuses as either icons of life or specters of death, the careless collection in mason and mayonnaise jars might evoke strong emotions. Yet Morgan discovered that for a period of time in the first half of the twentieth century, these embryos were exclusively viewed as scientific specimens rather than protohumans. Embryologists searching for the earliest and best-preserved specimen treated fetuses as autonomous, free-floating scientific materials, disregarding the reproductive policies that created the supply of fetal tissue and ignoring the women and their incomplete pregnancies who made these samples possible. Today, the remainders of these collections have become culturally toxic: no institution would want to house a fetal collection, and these collections tend to quietly disappear when they are rediscovered.[105] Morgan shows that, ironically, our current views of fetal images originate from the work of the embryologists who decontextualized the fetuses as autonomous entities. Cultural entrepreneurs making popular movies about fetal development have imbued the fetus with human agency, will, and determination.[106] This exemplifies Hacking's looping effect, in which people appropriate categories that end up changing the category itself. In this case, natural kinds turned into deeply social kinds. Categories offer a new worldview, but making this worldview stick in popular culture dynamically modifies the categories.

In the context of newborn screening, we see the growing availability of molecular information as an opportunity for human classification and differentiation that needs to be made to "stick" in order to become clinically and socially meaningful. Making the genetic information bond may lead to the creation of new forms of social belonging or reinforce existing sociopolitical regimens of differentiation.

* * *

Newborn screening offers an emblematic site for a close examination of the interplay between technological innovation, screening, and clinical genetics, and the uncertainties they provoke in US healthcare. Newborn screening forms a unique instance of a universal health service within a medical system with deep access and quality inequities and concerns about rising costs. The program's aim of saving babies from rare disorders will depend on the participation of an entire population. Most screened infants will receive no direct benefit but will leave a blood sample with a state agency. The extent to which screening is beneficial for the infants picked up at birth will depend on how the information provided by screening links to preventive actions. Newborn screening is also a test case for the long anticipated translation of genetic knowledge from the laboratory into the clinic. In the genetics clinic, we witnessed clinicians working out the relevance of genetic information for diagnosis and treatment and the possible emergence of biosocialities. Above all, as the Baios testified, newborn screening constitutes a previously unavailable opportunity for parents to do everything possible to give their child the best future at a frontier of medical knowledge.

The key take-home message at this point is that no consequence of newborn screening is preordained. Policymakers and screening advocates have promised that expanded newborn screening produces distinct individual, familial, and societal benefits: expanding the screening program will prevent disease, save lives, influence reproductive decision-making, and reduce healthcare costs. Whether any of the policy aspirations materialize remains an open question. The process of implementing expanded newborn screening offers a privileged entrance point to examine a spectrum of moral choices before they settle.[107] Once diagnosis and treatment are routinized, it is difficult to imagine alternative courses of action. Yet, as sociologist Everett Hughes reminds us: there was a time that different routes could have been taken. It could have been otherwise.[108]

## The Setting and the Study

This book is based on an ethnographic study of a genetics clinic conducted between November 2007 and July 2010. We observed 193 clinic visits with 75 families and recorded the consultations on a digital audio-recorder.[109] We aimed to observe all clinic consultations with newborn screening patients whose families spoke either English or Spanish. The newborn screening patients were interspersed in a general genetics clinic that met one afternoon per week in an academic hospital, but the newborn screening patients formed a distinct group. When discussing these patients in staff meetings, the geneticists introduced them by their age and announced that they "had been picked up by newborn screening." The clinic enrolled about two new newborn screening patients a month and conducted follow-up appointments with an additional two to four patients per week. The clinical coordinator notified us in advance if patients were scheduled that met our inclusion criteria. Consequently, we missed very few patient visits.[110]

Often, we began the recording when the family entered the examination room, which could be an hour or more before they saw the geneticist. For first-time visits, we used that time to interview families about how the results were delivered and what they knew about the child's potential disorder, and for returning families, we asked them for updates on how the child was doing. At the end of each clinic day, the staff met to discuss patients and get feedback on treatment plans, particularly for challenging cases. We observed these weekly team meetings as well. Almost all of the parents provided permission for us to view their children's medical records.

We also formally interviewed 27 families in their homes. Our study population was racially, ethnically, geographically, and socioeconomically diverse, including parents who were movers and shakers in the entertainment world and highly educated professionals, as well as computer technicians, factory employees, and other blue-collar workers. Consequently, our interviews—and our trusty GPS devices—took us to many different neighborhoods scattered across Southern California's sprawling landscape. We visited towering houses with swimming pools out back and modest apartments where children's toys cluttered the crowded living space. Two research assistants, Rocio Rosales and Arianna Taboada, traveled up to several hours to interview Spanish-speaking families in our study, some of whom worked as migrant farm laborers in California's fertile central coast.

For practical reasons, we allowed families to choose who would be present for the interview. As is common in the literature on children with special medical needs, most of our interviews were conducted with the child's mother, or in one case, a grandmother who provided most of the child's day-to-day care. However, we did manage to interview three fathers and three couples jointly. When combined with the fact that fathers were present at clinic visits more often than they were not, we have been able to include a broader range of fathers' perspectives than is typical for studies in this area. Interviews included questions about the family's background, their experience with newborn screening, their knowledge and understanding of the genetic condition, the consequences of the newborn screening results for family life, and the child's medical treatment. Between clinic visits, we conducted informal phone interviews with other families in the study, and we repeatedly interviewed the medical team members both formally and informally. We analyzed this data following the principles of abductive analysis in which methodological steps of coding of data and memo writing occur in dialogue with a social science literature.[111]

* * *

A very influential member of the genetics team was the clinical coordinator, Monica Wu, who was the clinic's point person for the families of children receiving a positive newborn screen. She typically discussed a course of action with the geneticists but then ordered tests, dealt with insurance issues and pharmacies, contacted families and pediatricians, and scheduled clinic visits. She not only kept track of everything but also kept everyone and everything on track. For diet-related issues, she turned to a dietitian. Over the course of our study, the team rotated through various dietitians when the clinic's long-term and much beloved dietitian retired and funding limitations made it difficult to replace her. The last dietitian was Lucy Chin. Monica also collaborated with a social worker, Denise Moskowitz, when families needed help accessing services, including public insurance programs or social services available to families of children with special medical needs. Other staff members included three genetic counselors, one of whom was a rotating intern. The genetic counselors were involved in the initial triaging of newborn screening families and overall management of the clinic.

The geneticists included a core team of four physicians: Dr. Jean-Pierre Dati, Dr. Gabriel Flores, Dr. Mark Silverman, and Dr. Sarah Malvern. Following the customs of the clinic, we will refer to the physicians by their last names and to the other staff members by their first names throughout the book. Dr. Silverman followed most of the clinic's newborn screening patients. He was the gray eminence of this group of physicians. Over the course of his career, he had witnessed the growth of medical genetics. Some of his extensive research career had been intertwined with newborn screening. He was involved in a newborn screening pilot program in the early 2000s and had testified to California legislators to advocate for the expansion of newborn screening. During our research, he participated in the state's regulation of newborn screening. He was also an active participant on a Listserv on which medical geneticists discussed issues related to newborn screening.

Dr. Silverman was a renaissance intellectual and something of a character. He read widely in diverse genres, including classical literature, detective stories, history, and biographies, and was an avid listener of classical music and opera. His clinical uniform included a bow tie, suspenders, and a belt, and he could not resist a pun or a joke. After observing him for three years, we concluded that his sense of humor worked via association. Anything could trigger a joke—a name, a word, a color, a gesture, or an observation—and if it was triggered, it had to come out. When we mentioned buying beets at the farmer's market, he punned that "we didn't want to miss a beat." Most of the time, these associations were made in good jest but occasionally, patients and staff found them inappropriate. The list of puns and jokes could distract from the matter at hand. As happens to many physicians at some point, some patients asked to be seen by another doctor, but Dr. Silverman also had a loyal following among many families.

The other physicians each had a limited number of newborn screening patients assigned to them, but they could still be responsible for any of these patients when they were on call and the patient experienced a metabolic crisis. Dr. Dati was in charge of the genetics service. He ran the staff meeting and had research interests in the genetics of sex development. Dr. Flores was a native Spanish speaker and the most junior member of the group. Dr. Malvern was in charge of the craniofacial clinic and spent the least time in the genetics clinic. She assigned medical students and residents to follow a specific geneticist. Each of these physicians ran an independent research laboratory. They also collaborated with clinicians from a local Health Maintenance Organization (HMO) and were assisted by a rotating cast of fellows and visiting physicians. Among the genetics fellows, we observed Dr. Anippe Nazif and Dr. Ella De Vries at several points in their interactions with newborn screening patients.

Ethnography presumes "us" studying "them." Ethnographers study others, most often "down" when studying people with less power, or occasionally "up" when research subjects are powerful.[112] Except for the obvious clinical expertise of the genetics team, the boundary between us and them was not always clear-cut. Unlike Charles Bosk's pioneering study of genetic counseling,[113] we were not invited to study the clinicians but once we invited ourselves, we felt welcomed by the team. Dr. Silverman in particular repeatedly stated that our presence increased the staff's awareness of how families experienced newborn screening. Several members of the genetics team were well versed in social science research methodology and, somewhat surprisingly, knowledgeable in social science literature. Several of the physicians actively participated in a colloquium series organized by a consortium of social scientists and biological scientists, either as invited speakers or as audience members. Dr. Dati had co-taught courses with a sociologist and read extensively in the sociology of sex and gender. When we started our study, Dr. Silverman bought Stefan's book *Postmortem*. He discussed his reading not only with us but also with several families and during a staff meeting. Dr. Silverman described for one set of parents the increased awareness that having us as social observers brought to his clinical practice: "But he's [referring to Stefan] made me very conscious of the fact that we sometimes don't succeed in communicating what we think we're doing. We're just not that good. And so it's humbling to be observed. And not observed so much as—because he didn't criticize our efforts. He didn't say, 'You're really screw-ups,' or anything like that. He just said that the patients, as we talked to them, see the world somewhat differently from you, which is good. It's pretty good. You know, it's been very valuable for us."

The warrant of this book goes further than the immediate reflexive value of our presence to the clinicians we studied. We examine the consequences of newborn screening on people's lives beyond the official discourse of cost-effectiveness, prevention, and lifesaving. In the next chapter, we provide a historical review of how the expansion of newborn screening broke precedent with earlier attempts at population screening. From there, we will follow families and geneticists making newborn screening work in the clinic.

## CHAPTER ONE

# The Expansion of Newborn Screening

The United States is one of only two industrialized countries without a national newborn screening policy.[1] Instead, individual states determine screening targets. When newborn screening began in the early 1960s, state newborn screening programs grew slowly and unevenly. Consequently, by the turn of the twenty-first century, significant discrepancies had appeared between states in the number and kind of screening targets, with individual states screening newborns for between 3 and 36 conditions. Whether or not a baby was tested for medium-chain acyl-coenzyme A dehydrogenase deficiency (MCADD)—a condition in which a child could become seriously ill when fasting for prolonged periods—depended on where the family lived, generating geographical health disparities.

After the turn of the twenty-first century, newborn screening became more uniform. In 2005, a task force of the American College of Medical Genetics recommended screening for 29 primary conditions as well as 25 secondary disorders that would be detected incidentally while screening for the core set.[2] The centerpiece of this expansion and standardization of newborn screening was the implementation of new technologies that enabled screening for multiple conditions with one blood sample. Although the recommendations became controversial for reasons that we will explore shortly, various advocacy and professional organizations lobbied to turn the recommendations into state policy. In only a few years, all states began screening for the core set, and some states began screening for additional disorders beyond the recommended panel. Observers refer to this event as *the expansion of newborn screening*.

In the remainder of this book, we will focus on the broad and varied consequences of expanded newborn screening, but in this chapter we introduce some of the stakeholders and the decisions that made this expansion possible. Our reason for attending to this implementation process is that it offers a powerful benchmark for examining the work in the clinic. We will argue that the recurring problems that families and geneticists encountered in the clinic were largely hardwired into the way the expansion of newborn screening was implemented. The setup of newborn screening affected which conditions could be screened, how quickly parents could be informed of the results, who would help them interpret and understand the results, who would pay for screening, and what the ensuing medical care would be like. Newborn screening advocates considered evidence selectively while acknowledging that they did not have the answers for some scientific issues that would be crucial for implementation. They ignored pertinent characteristics of the US healthcare system and left many aspects of executing expanded newborn screening up to local actors, regardless of whether these actors were up to the task. They presumed a standard script in which a patient would be identified with and treated for a life-threatening condition, but many patients with metabolic disorders now face ambiguous conditions or disorders for which treatment remains insufficient. The expansion of newborn screening with its priorities and silences thus set the stage for interactional uncertainties when geneticists discussed screening results with parents.

## The Origins of Newborn Screening

Medical review articles invariably locate the origins of newborn screening in the work of Robert Guthrie, a microbiologist and screening advocate.[3] While experts agree that Guthrie initiated newborn screening, opinions are mixed as to whether his approach struck the appropriate balance between science and advocacy. Over time, Guthrie's work has come to signify a historical lesson of either a successful public health initiative or the dangers of unbridled screening. The story goes like this.

After the birth of a child with mental retardation and a niece diagnosed with phenylketonuria (PKU), Guthrie became active in the local chapter of the National Association for Retarded Children (NARC, now the Arc of the United States[4]). Parent activists founded this grassroots organization in the 1950s to fight discrimination against children with mental retardation in public schools and to provide alternatives to institutional care. The organization counted physicians among its members and its advisory boards, but they were primarily involved because of per-

sonal and family experiences with mental retardation. While serving as
vice president of a local NARC chapter, Guthrie was approached by a director of a local children's rehabilitation center who was looking for an
easier way to check phenylalanine levels in children with PKU who had
been put on a restricted diet. People with PKU, a rare autosomal recessive
genetic condition, are deficient in the enzyme needed to break down the
amino acid phenylalanine. Consequently, phenylalanine builds up in the
body and may cause mental retardation and other symptoms. A phenylalanine restrictive diet was an experimental form of PKU treatment developed in Britain and published in the early 1950s.[5]

Guthrie's original research was on cancer, but he shifted his research
to PKU screening as a way to prevent some types of mental retardation.
He and his assistant, Ada Susi, developed a bacterial inhibition assay that
enabled presymptomatic diagnosis of PKU using neonatal blood. Guthrie
realized that if plasma phenylalanine levels could identify affected children, the technique could also be used as a screening method for undiagnosed children. The attraction of developing a screening method was that
the condition could be discovered prior to the onset of irreversible symptoms and mental retardation might be prevented. In the method Guthrie
developed, blood was collected via a heel stick prior to hospital discharge
and then blotted on a piece of filter paper and mailed to a laboratory.
There, a technician punched out a small disk of filter paper and placed it
on an agar gel plate containing bacteria and a bacterial growth inhibitor.
If the sample contained extra phenylalanine, the inhibition was overcome
and the bacteria grew. The amount of growth, visible to the eye within a
day, was proportional to the phenylalanine level. The screen was interpreted by comparing the diameter of the growth colony on each sample
disk to the colonies of a series of reference disks with standard phenylalanine content. In healthy people, phenylalanine levels are usually under
120 μmol/L, but the assay was sensitive enough to detect serum phenylalanine levels of 180–240 μmol/L. When an elevated level was detected,
the laboratory notified the infant's physician, who explained the result to
the family. Before Guthrie's assay, the only alternative screening method
was the urine ferric chloride test developed by Willard Centerwall in 1957,
which measured phenylpyruvic acid based on fresh urine in a diaper. This
"wet diaper" or "nappy" test was relatively unreliable, although the US
Children's Bureau, housed in the Department of Health, Education, and
Welfare, had recommended it as the preferred testing method for infants
at risk for PKU (e.g., infants with affected siblings) prior to the Guthrie

inhibition assay because no better option was available.[6] The wet diaper test was only reliable six to eight weeks after birth, when brain damage might already have occurred, and thus was not suitable for population screening.[7]

In 1961, President John F. Kennedy made federal funding available for research about mental retardation, and Guthrie's PKU research drew the attention of the Children's Bureau. The idea of trying to prevent mental retardation rather than rehabilitating afflicted patients was appealing to the Children's Bureau, which funded a pilot study in 1962 that screened 400,000 infants in 29 states for PKU. The study used Guthrie's bacterial inhibition assay to test blood and urine for phenylalanine, and established the superiority of the blood test over the urine test. Guthrie's major technological contribution to PKU screening was thus to create a test that would screen for phenylalanine levels in the blood rather than in the urine and to develop bloodspot technology which facilitated an easy screening infrastructure. Once the hospital-laboratory connections had been established, most states involved in the Guthrie field trials continued to screen for PKU after the end of the study. By 1964, four states had laws requiring PKU screening.

PKU screening was met with resistance by some public health researchers and metabolic researchers who doubted that population screening for a rare disease such as PKU was efficient. Metabolic experts advising the California Department of Public Health, for example, argued against the state coordinating a field trial because the mechanism of PKU, the reliability of the Guthrie test, and the effectiveness of dietary treatment were unknown.[8] Since treating PKU with a low-phenylalanine diet had only been introduced in the United States in the mid-1950s, relatively few infants had aged sufficiently to predict their cognitive and developmental functioning while on the diet. Although the diet suggested biochemical success insofar as it lowered phenylalanine levels, its long-term impact on mental retardation was unknown. Only in 1967 did the Children's Bureau fund a study that established the long-term physical and cognitive benefits of a low-phenylalanine diet when initiated early on. In addition, controversy remained for more than a decade about when to start the diet and how long the patient should stay on it.

The California state advisers also argued that the vast majority of mentally retarded people did not suffer from PKU and that this community needed social support rather than scientific intervention.[9] Indeed, research using the Guthrie assay and other predictive technologies showed that less than 1 percent of institutionalized mentally retarded people had PKU. Screening for PKU was thus unlikely to make a dent in this population. This low yield posed a problem for population screening. In Massachusetts, newborn screening proponents were fortunate because the program identified the first case of PKU after only 1,000 infants were screened and found nine cases in the first 53,000 samples. It then took another 50,000 samples to find the 10th case. If it had taken this long to find the first case, enthusiasm for screening might have been dampened. Massachusetts became the first state to pass legislation mandating newborn screening for PKU and the only state without organized medical opposition to this legislation.[10] In Washington, DC, no infants were diagnosed within the first three years of mandatory screening, and health officials concluded that they had better use for the resources.

Generally, the American Medical Association (AMA) and its state organizations opposed mandatory screening as an infringement of physicians' rights to regulate their professional practice. The AMA was concerned about regulatory intrusions into the patient-physician relationship. By the early 1960s, the AMA had been fighting government intrusion for several decades on various fronts—including public health clinics, private insurance, Medicare and Medicaid legislation—to preserve physician autonomy and a lucrative fee-for-service system.[11] In 1967, the American Academy of Pediatrics cautioned against adopting underdeveloped screening programs too quickly.[12]

In the face of such resistance, Guthrie, the son of a salesman, became an "evangelist" for universal PKU screening.[13] He circumvented professional objections by working directly with parents, legislators, and the press, and encouraged the National Association for Retarded Children to develop model legislation and lobby for state laws mandating newborn screening. A nameless sociologist hired by the National Academy of Sciences in the early 1970s documented the tug of war between the medical profession and the local ARC chapters to influence legislators in 12 states.[14] In Florida, a woman whose child's PKU was not detected early pushed for a bill mandating screening. She teamed up with Maxine Baker, who had been elected to the Florida House of Representatives, to introduce a bill. Although the state medical association opposed the bill, the Florida Chapter of the Association for Retarded Children and some pediatricians supported it. In 1965, a bill was passed that made PKU screening in Florida voluntary. In 1971, an amended law made PKU screening mandatory since the voluntary screening was an insufficient incentive to screen infants.[15]

Grassroots mobilization generated legislative successes in spite of resistance from organized medicine. By 1965, 27 states mandated newborn screening and by 1973, an additional 16 states followed suit. An important aspect of this early legislation was that in most states informed consent was bypassed. Parents could object to the screening, but already in 1975 one source stated that "parents are frequently not informed of the test or their right to object."[16] Furthermore, only 25 of the 43 states provided for medical treatment in their legislation, and only 7 states provided treatment free of charge.

In the decades after PKU screening began, various tests were gradually added to newborn screening to justify the low yield of PKU screening and the extensive infrastructure required. Using the same technology, Guthrie and other researchers developed screening tests for congenital adrenal hyperplasia, hypothyroidism, and toxoplasmosis. The intervening decades also saw the advent of two-tiered screening to lower the likelihood of false positives.[17] With a successful demonstration of two-tiered screening for congenital hypothyroidism, screening for other conditions such as hemoglobinopathy followed.

From the 1970s through the 1990s, there were various attempts to strengthen universal newborn screening in a more systematic fashion. The federal government initiated legislation in 1976 to support screening for genetic diseases and provided limited funding to pay for screening costs and research. The federal government also developed standards for laboratories and screening tests. The Council of Regional Networks for Genetic Services distinguished five system components of newborn screening that included the screening itself, follow-up for positive results, diagnosis, long-term therapy, and an evaluation of the entire system to make sure that benefits were realized for the newborn, family, and society.[18] This approach spelled out algorithms, technical requirements, regulatory structures, and quality assurance monitoring for each component of the entire system. Still, newborn screening remained largely a state responsibility with individual states choosing the panel of screening targets and organizing payment, education programs, opt-out policies, and follow-up procedures.

## PKU Screening as a Cautionary Tale

Universal screening for PKU was the first large-scale population screening program in the United States. It became a cornerstone public health initiative that required close collaboration with healthcare professionals and a well-developed infrastructure integrating laboratories, state health agencies, hospitals, clinical centers, and families. In the following decades, various stakeholders retold the story of the implementation of PKU screening to make broader points about genetic screening, expanded newborn screening, and even the eternal nature-nurture debate.[19] PKU and later sickle cell disease became good case studies through which to think about genetics and screening. Rather quickly, some medical professionals drew a cautionary lesson from the introduction of PKU screening. Evaluated against the standards of contemporary biomedical innovations, these professionals argued, the advocates for PKU screening had been lucky. Considering the scientific unknowns, the program might easily have failed in its main goal of preventing mental retardation. Proponents had been advocating screening for a condition that was not well understood.

Population screening required a reassessment of PKU. One key issue was the relationship between elevated phenylalanine levels and mental retardation. Once screening began, researchers found that elevated phenylalanine levels did not automatically result in mental retardation. Some infants whose newborn screens displayed slightly elevated phenylalanine levels had older siblings with similarly elevated phenylalanine levels but without mental retardation.[20] Later, researchers distinguished between classic PKU and benign hyperphenylalanine, the latter of which did not require dietary modification. In addition, some children who did not have PKU still developed mental retardation because their mothers, who had PKU, did not follow the recommended diet during gestation: the children were affected because of the teratogenic effect of phenylalanine.[21] Maternal PKU was considered an unintended consequence of the success of screening and resulting deinstitutionalization of people with PKU. Few women with PKU gave birth when spending their lives in institutions, yet after screening and early intervention, many of these women went on to have children. According to medical professionals, such women risked undermining the benefits of screening if their phenylalanine levels were high during pregnancy: "Given average reproductive rates, the frequency of new cases of PKU-related mental retardation could return to its former level after only one generation if no treatment is available to protect their offspring."[22]

The promotion of PKU screening also depended on the success of the low-phenylalanine diet as an effective treatment. Yet understandings of dietary regulation were somewhat rudimentary when mandatory screening was implemented. Some children with false positive results or with what later was recognized as hyperphenylalanine were put on low-phenylalanine diets unnecessarily, depriving them of a crucial amino acid for proper development, which, paradoxically, could also lead to mental retardation.[23] Furthermore, the benefits of detection might have been squandered if the test was performed too early (in the first hours of life) or too late (month three or four). In addition, the accuracy of the Guthrie test was not established until 1974. To avoid false negatives, the cutoff point for a positive screen was initially set low. Consequently, the test resulted in an initial false positive rate of 90 percent.[24] These issues had not been worked out by the time screening was implemented, and the push for testing might have backfired if detection, diagnosis, or treatment had failed to fulfill the promise of preventing mental retardation. The origin of PKU screening also offered a lesson about the power of advocacy: "The public, including patient advocacy organizations, has more political power than the medical community, and may impose testing without an evidence base."[25] Critics concluded that in the future, scientific uncertainties should be worked out first and public health officials should develop a healthcare infrastructure for treatment before investing in newborn screening.[26] PKU screening had worked because the pieces had fallen into place eventually, but the initial programs, according to observers in the next generations, had been built on hope, luck, and activism rather than a solid scientific base.

The professional caution narrative dominated a series of authoritative reports issuing guidelines for implementing genetic screening after the highly anticipated decoding of the human genome. Each report drew cautious lessons from the implementation of PKU screening. For example, a 1975 report from the National Academy of Sciences, *Genetic Screening: Principles, Practice, and Research*, dissected in three chapters what was neglected in the implementation of PKU screening and drew lessons for the introduction of additional genetic screens.[27] The committee characterized the adoption of mandatory PKU screening as "fragmented, uneducated, and hurried decision-making"[28] and observed with hindsight: "It is clear that those involved in [PKU] screening in the early days did not anticipate many problems and failed to see the necessity of documenting their successes."[29] The message was that a more measured, scientifically supported approach with adequate quality control, and buy-in from health professionals was preferable.

In 1994, the Institute of Medicine (IOM) report, *Assessing Genetic Risks: Implications for Health and Social Policy*, added the accumulated wisdom from newborn screening for sickle cell disease in African Americans, which revealed similar issues as PKU screening. Screening for sickle cell disease failed to distinguish between carriers and full-blown cases of the disease. Knowing one's carrier status had few medical benefits but led to stigmatization and discrimination. Some in the African-American community perceived the screening as a targeted form of genocide since carriers were warned against reproducing. This impression was further perpetuated by the fact that some states targeted "high-risk" ethnic groups rather than screening the entire population. Screening also started in the early 1970s but only in 1986 did a randomized clinical trial establish that penicillin prophylaxis reduces infant and childhood mortality for sickle cell disease. The IOM committee found that since 1975 "various diseases had been added to newborn screening programs without careful assessment of benefits and risks."[30]

In 1998, the Task Force on Genetic Testing, an advisory group reporting to the NIH's National Human Genome Research Institute, issued a report titled *Promoting Safe and Effective Genetic Testing in the United States*. In a lengthy appendix about the history of PKU, the report stated: "The history of PKU shows that it is easy to exaggerate the ease and efficacy of treatment and to understate the costs. . . . Once the idea of newborn screening became established, the program could be rapidly routinized and, once routinized, easily expanded for other purposes."[31]

What did these reports advise to avoid a repeat of the PKU screening experience? In a word: caution. According to these reports, population screening should only be implemented under stringent conditions. For our purposes, three points of an established historical consensus are critical. First, in 1968, JMG (Max) Wilson and Gunnar Jungner articulated the World Health Organization (WHO) "gold standard"[32] that population screening is only permissible when it addresses an "important health problem" for which an "accepted treatment was available." Wilson and Jungner noted that "phenylketonuria is extremely uncommon but warrants screening on account of the very serious consequences if not discovered and treated very early in life."[33] Of course, PKU screening was well under way by the time these criteria were formulated. The primary thrust of the Wilson and Jungner WHO principles was that, above all, the patient should benefit from screening. Geneticists, bioethicists, pediatricians, and others echoed the basic assumption in all subsequent reports. The 1994 IOM report, for example, adopted the principle that "a person should not be used as a means for the benefit of others,"[34] drawing a line at screening infants for the benefit of parents' reproductive decision-making and the development of scientific knowledge.

Second, the scientific advisory bodies that authored the different reports demonstrated great sensitivity to the issue of parental informed consent. In its 1983 report, *Screening and Counseling for Genetic Conditions*, the President's Commission for the Study of Ethical Problems in Medicine and Biomedical and Behavioral Research argued in favor of confidentiality, autonomy, knowledge, well-being, and equity. The commission posited that "mandatory genetic screening programs are only justified when voluntary testing proves inadequate to prevent serious harm to the defenseless, such as children, that should be avoided were screening performed."[35] More precisely, the commission "finds no basis in the maximization of social utility that justifies compulsory participation in genetics programs."[36] The 1994 IOM committee struggled over whether screening for established conditions such as PKU and hypothyroidism should be mandatory or voluntary. While the committee had embraced the principles of voluntary consent to screening, some committee members thought that mandatory newborn screening was preferable in light of potential public health benefits. The committee compromised: "It is appropriate to mandate the *offering* of established tests."[37] The Task Force on Genetic Testing made a strong case in its 1998 report that informed consent should be required for all genetic tests. Regarding newborn screening, the task force noted: "If informed consent is waived for a newborn screening test, the analytical and clinical validity and clinical utility of the test must be established, and parents must be provided with sufficient information to understand the reasons for screening."[38] This discussion took place in a period of budding awareness of bioethical issues, including increased attention to past research abuse and the growing importance of informed consent and institutional review boards.[39]

Third, the consensus among these different reports was that the expansion of newborn screening should not be driven by technological innovations but rather that the focus should be on building a medical infrastructure for follow-up testing, affordable treatment, and health services. Wilson and Jungner had emphasized that screening should be cost-effective and should be part of a long-term commitment to follow-up care.[40] The 1994 IOM report was the first to raise the issue of "multiplex" technologies for newborn screening. Such technologies enable the simultaneous screening of multiple conditions with one blood sample. The committee cautioned against adopting these technologies without the necessary infrastructure in place. The report from the American Academy of Pediatrics made the strongest argument for viewing screening as part of a comprehensive system of follow-up and quality assurance centered around the "medical home," a term the academy has refined over time to highlight the importance of evidence-based primary care as a critical partnership between healthcare providers, patients, and their families.[41]

If the consensus was strong, why, then, was there such a proliferation of reports? One reason was the shared opinion among the authors that the implementation of PKU, sickle cell disease, and other screening programs could be improved. In addition, PKU was increasingly viewed as a harbinger of the future due to rapid developments in the field of genetics following from the Human Genome Project. Another reason was the growing influence of the discipline of bioethics on regulatory oversight in medicine. The Human Genome Project set about 3–5 percent of funding aside for bioethicists, legal scholars, and social scientists to study the ethical, legal, and social implications (ELSI) of the increasing availability of genetic information. This funding stream generated attention to the potential harms of genetic screening, especially the danger for insurance discrimination, stigmatization, and violations of privacy. Since relatively few examples of actual genetic applications existed, genetic screening became a prime subject of bioethical contemplation. The take-home lesson distilled from the PKU experience was that patients should benefit from screening and that a comprehensive approach to disease prevention was required. Expanding screening should proceed cautiously.

## PKU Screening as Success Story

Sociologist of science Leigh Star[42] and scholars interested in social movements have drawn attention to the important question of spokespersonship, noting that science gives authority to some and silences others, and that disease advocates may appropriate, counter, and dilute the language of science. For 40 years, the dispassionate reports written by bioethicists, public health researchers, and geneticists toed a cautionary line regarding genetic screening, but missing were the voices of patients, advocates, and other stakeholders. The history of PKU had clearly shown that professionals were not the only interested party in newborn screening. Advocacy organizations such as the Arc of the United States, the March of Dimes Foundation, and various disease-specific foundations established by par-

ents of affected children also claimed a strong stake in newborn screening.[43] Yet although the 1975 National Academy of Sciences report called
for advisory boards containing professionals and laypersons, lay organizations did not have a formal voice in subsequent reports. In the aftermath of
the 2000 American Academy of Pediatrics report calling for a system-wide
approach to develop screening, the March of Dimes Foundation made
newborn screening a policy priority and began to work directly with legislators to standardize screening.[44] When the US Health Resources and Services Administration commissioned the Secretary's Advisory Committee
on Heritable Disorders in Newborns and Children in 2003 to advise the
US Secretary of Health and Human Services on the most appropriate application of universal newborn screening, Jennifer Howse, the president
of the March of Dimes Foundation, was a "liaison member" of the committee, and parent advocates were invited to speak during the public comment period.

As an example of the contrast between advocacy narratives and the
scientific reports, here is the June 8, 2004, testimony of Jana Monaco, rep-
resenting the Organic Acidemia Association and the National Coalition
for PKU and Allied Disorders, to this committee.[45]

Most importantly, I am here for my six-year-old son, Stephen, the third of four
children, and to tell you about the harsh reality of undetected inborn errors of
metabolism. Three years ago today, I was sitting in Stephen's ICU room trying
to determine when to discontinue life support. Ten days earlier, Stephen had
contracted a typical stomach virus. However, I found him the next morning
in an unresponsive state that no mother should ever have to endure. He was
transported from one hospital to another. His tests indicated severe acidosis,
leading them to suspect a metabolic disorder. The initial tests eliminated certain ones, but others had to be sent out. Twenty-four hours later, Stephen was
diagnosed with isovaleric acidemia, a very treatable disorder found through
reliable testing.

Unfortunately, Stephen's diagnosis came too late. He had slipped into a
coma. While preparing for an MRI, Stephen went into seizures. Within minutes
of returning to his room, he had crashed before our eyes. After a great deal of
intervention, Stephen was clinging to life on a respirator. The MRIs revealed
swelling around the brain stem and extensive damage throughout his brain.
As you can imagine, we were devastated at the thought of losing our son. How
could such a happy, healthy, energetic, normal child come so close to death in
such a short time?

While we were trying to come to terms with his prognosis, we discovered that Stephen was a walking time bomb waiting to ignite and that this whole situation was preventable had he benefitted from comprehensive newborn screening at birth. We had also linked a similar episode at 18 months with the disorder, but the doctors failed to recognize the signs and symptoms. They had acted within the standards of care for a small community hospital, standards which we now know had a direct impact on his future. Hindsight is brutal.

Stephen started to show signs of progress, and after three and a half weeks he received a gastrostomy tube and was removed from the respirator. He was then transferred to Kluge Children's Rehab Center in Charlottesville, Virginia for six long weeks. Since then, Stephen has made progress. However, he is far from the little boy that we once knew. He requires total care, continuing to be fed via G-tube. He cannot walk, talk, sit up, nor hold his head up without support. He is also legally blind. Stephen takes four anticonvulsant medications, yet still has three to four seizures per day. Due to his neurological state, hiccups last four to five hours and usually result in a hospital stay because of GI bleeding. He recently had surgery called an orchiopexy to bring his testicles down that retracted due to spasticity.

Our days are filled with therapies and numerous doctors' appointments. I spend many phone hours settling insurance disputes. His medical costs have exceeded the million dollar mark and continue to climb. Stephen is now under the school system with an IEP and has been assessed at the functional level of a two-month-old. We are waiting for his second wheelchair, at a cost of about $5,000. I ask you, is this cost effective?

Gone are Stephen's opportunities for a normal life because our government and health system continue to debate the cost-effectiveness of universal newborn screening. Stephen's fate was already determined because he was born in Virginia, where only eight disorders are screened for. Had he been born in North Carolina, where the list includes 36, Stephen would be in a normal kindergarten class this year instead of occupying a special education slot.

It is a travesty that Stephen is a statistic at the hands of bureaucracy and lack of knowledge within the medical community. While the debate continues, more babies and children are going to die or share Stephen's fate. Yet the equipment and knowledge to avoid this already exists. The life of my Stephen and the thousands like him born each year should not be so devalued. These disorders can be debilitating and deadly if not caught.

A testimony to the significance of early detection is our 20-month-old daughter, Caroline. With the knowledge we gained with Stephen, Caroline was diagnosed with the same disorder through prenatal testing. Early diagnosis enabled the doctors, one being Dr. Carol Greene, to establish a protocol of care prior to her birth. With a restricted protein diet and medications, Caroline is doing very well and developing normally. She is a typical happy, healthy toddler, thanks to early detection. Unlike Stephen, she will have a normal childhood, and she will have dreams.

Although Stephen has suffered severe brain damage and dreams have been lost, we know that his life has a purpose, and we will see to it that it is fulfilled. Thank you to the advisory committee for your attention and dedication towards expanded newborn screening.

These powerful testimonies formed an important strategy for advocates dedicated to expanding newborn screening. They marshaled the emotive power of threats to infants and premature, preventable deaths to provoke political action. Feminist theorist Sara Ahmed introduced the term "affective economies" to reference the dense networks of sentiment that circulate throughout social formations and help to regulate sociopolitical activity at a supraindividual level.[46] "In such affective economies," Ahmed notes, "emotions *do things*, and they align individuals with communities— or bodily space with social space—through the very intensity of their attachments."[47] Preventing the deaths of babies may well be the ultimate trump card in such an affective economy. The political currency flowing from these emotionally dramatic arguments should not be underestimated; it may help to reframe a decades-long history of cautious expansion. These testimonies build on a stark contrast between disaster and salvation to imply a straightforward causal logic: screening prevents morbidity and mortality if politicians can muster the political will to implement a screening program.[48] They also rendered screening actionable by pointing to a fundamental geographical inequity in screening. Rather than putting a face on statistics, the dramatic testimony can trump statistics altogether. Rather than caution, they implied urgency. And instead of concern about resources and infrastructures, the testimonies profiled the social and financial cost of taking care of a disabled and terminally ill child.

We do not want to imply that these testimonies by themselves are sufficient to change the course of screening history, but when filtered into the political arena through professionalized advocacy organizations such as the March of Dimes, they form an important discursive counterweight to the cautionary lessons drawn from PKU screening. For health advocates, the main takeaway message from the implementation of PKU screening was that newborn screening saves lives. In fact, among the advocacy organizations that worked to expand newborn screening was the Save Babies Through Screening Foundation, Inc. This organization advocated for a federal law titled "Newborn Screening Saves Lives" (signed into law in 2007), which establishes grant programs to provide education in a broad array of congenital disorders, training in newborn screening technologies, and coordination of follow-up care.

Less dramatic, but equally insistent, were the testimonies from industry representatives from small start-up and well-established companies and universities that developed or offered screening technologies. They generally made their services available for any expansion of newborn screening. They, too, were invested in turning PKU into a success. Some of these companies teamed up with advocacy groups to amplify their messages.

The counterview thus regarded newborn screening as an unmitigated triumph and imposed a moral imperative to screen: "Few things we do in preventive medicine have been as remarkably successful as has been newborn screening."[49] The cautionary version of PKU's history acknowledged its successes but highlighted a whole set of unresolved and persisting problems. In the counternarrative, the emphasis was reversed. Advocates noted that not all of the issues with PKU screening had been worked out prior to its implementation, but once it was instituted, it succeeded in preventing mental retardation for a small but highly vulnerable population. Once the technology was put into place by a passionate grassroots organization with a charismatic spokesperson and sympathetic professionals, the science and the infrastructure followed. Indeed, the proponents of expansion celebrated the marriage of patient advocacy with visionary health professionals to promote screening in light of opposition from clinicians.[50] From this perspective, PKU screening was largely a success story that mandated replication for unnecessary deaths and morbidity to be averted.

## The American College of Medical Genetics Report

Due to the lack of a comprehensive federal policy on newborn screening, by the beginning of the twentieth-first century, states varied widely on the kinds of screening tests they offered. Some tests were added due to pressures or lawsuits from well-connected parents or advocacy organizations,[51] other programs relied on advice from expert advisory committees, while in other states expansion was the prerogative of the state's

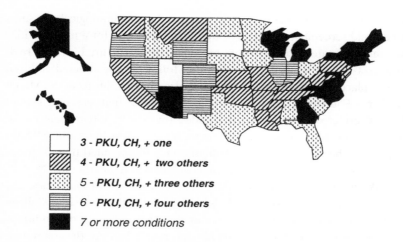

3 - PKU, CH, + one
4 - PKU, CH, + two others
5 - PKU, CH, + three others
6 - PKU, CH, + four others
7 or more conditions

FIGURE I. US Newborn screening in 2000. *Source:* AAP Newborn Screening Task Force 2000, p. 392.

public health director. Consequently, by the turn of the millennium, the number of screened conditions varied from 3 to 36, as seen on the map (see figure I).

Every state screened for PKU and congenital hypothyroidism. More than 40 programs screened for sickle cell disease and 48 for galactosemia. Some states included tests for congenital adrenal hyperplasia, homocystinuria, maple syrup urine disease, and biotinidase deficiency. A few states also included screening tests for cystic fibrosis, tyrosinemia, additional metabolic disorders, and other conditions such as congenital infections. Forty-one states screened for sickle cell disease universally, but three states only screened high-risk ethnic groups. By this time, approximately 4,000 newborns per year were identified with a genetic disorder, but some observers feared that more than 1,000 newborns with detectable conditions went undiagnosed.[52]

In 2000, the Health Resources and Services Administration (HRSA) funded the previously mentioned American Association of Pediatrics to review the state of newborn screening. This task force called for greater federal involvement in newborn screening. The report offered a nuanced appraisal of the need to expand newborn screening, noting that "not all conditions are good candidates for newborn screening."[53] It also called for developing model state regulations to guide the implementation of newborn screening programs. While acknowledging the accomplishments of newborn screening over the past decades and the technological pressures to expand screening, the report emphasized the need for a measured investment in state-based newborn screening infrastructure based on realistic cost-benefit analyses to ensure that follow-up for affected children was in place. The report was sharply criticized by officials from the March of Dimes Foundation, who objected to the premise that screening should be cost-effective and instead demanded that the report evaluate each available test to recommend uniform screening across the country.[54] Subsequently, the March of Dimes Foundation recommended that all states screen for a core set of nine conditions in addition to hearing loss.[55]

Taking up the call from the American Association of Pediatrics task force and other professionals, HRSA next funded the American College of Medical Genetics (ACMG) to recommend a uniform set of conditions to standardize state newborn screening programs. In 2005, the committee recommended a core panel of 29 conditions that should be included in every state's newborn screening program as well as a secondary group of 25 targets that were part of the differential diagnosis of the core panel and would be identified by screening for the core set. The ACMG task force also determined that newborn screening was not advisable for an additional 30 conditions for which there was either no screening test available or for which the evidence for screening was limited.

The ACMG report constituted a major departure from earlier reports on newborn screening and genetic testing. The American Academy of Pediatrics had reviewed the field only a few years earlier and concluded that there was insufficient evidence for a uniform screening panel. The Massachusetts Newborn Screening Advisory Committee had similarly concluded that there was sufficient evidence in favor of newborn screening for only 10 conditions and had opted to conduct two pilot studies to gather data about an additional 20 conditions that appeared promising.[56] Advisory groups in Australasia, Belgium, and the United Kingdom, among others, also came up with a much more limited list of recommendations.[57]

How, then, could the ACMG come up with strong recommendations for 29 core and 25 secondary conditions? The primary aim of the ACMG task force was to justify the expansion of newborn screening, and the scientific evidence was deployed creatively to reach that goal. Depending on one's perspective, the ACMG constituted a bold and creative innovation in a field paralyzed by a lack of data and urgent needs, or it constituted a travesty of science for advocacy and policy purposes. The report constituted a break with recent history in at least three areas: (1) expanding the beneficiaries of newborn screening, (2) promoting multiplex technologies, and (3) creating evidence for decision-making. We will review these developments in turn, focusing on the elements that had the greatest impact in the clinic.

## Expanding Beneficiaries

Since the Wilson and Jungner report, public health policymakers have agreed that the patient being screened should be the main beneficiary of population screening. The ACMG committee expanded the potential beneficiaries to include family members and the broader society, an example of "benefit creep."[58] In contrast to earlier reports warning about genetic discrimination in health insurance and the difficulties of interpreting carrier information, the ACMG committee argued that families might like to know about conditions for which no treatment existed because it could shorten the "diagnostic odyssey" of consulting multiple physicians following the development of symptoms, as well as provide information useful for future reproductive decisions.[59] In addition, a child's diagnosis could indicate a genetic risk for others in the family.

The presumptive societal benefits were mostly scientific. Diagnosing conditions with unclear clinical evidence or few treatment opportunities in infants who would otherwise remain undiagnosed for long periods of time could be useful for understanding the "natural history" of rare genetic conditions. It might provide information about the earliest patterns of development and create opportunities for testing treatments earlier.[60] In addition, population screening could have cost benefits for the overall healthcare system. The important conceptual innovation was not only that the number of beneficiaries expanded but also that a screen could be justified if it provided scientific or family benefits *even if screening did not benefit the individual patient.*

Using the example of screening for developmental disabilities, behavioral scientist Donald Bailey and colleagues pointed to added benefits of newborn screening: earlier therapeutic interventions, access to services helpful for children and families, sensitivity to consumer preferences for information, and increased knowledge about disorders. "Benefit historically has been construed too narrowly," they argued, "considering only those circumstances in which the infant's health is much improved as a result of earlier treatment."[61]

In the ACMG report, the benefits of screening were evaluated independently from each other, although individual benefits were weighted more heavily. The committee's scoring instrument allocated a maximum of 2,100 points for each condition under consideration. A maximum of 100 points were awarded when early identification provided clear benefits to family and society. The indicators of societal and familial benefit included education, understanding prevalence and natural history, and cost-effectiveness. The familial and societal benefits were distinct from the "overriding criterion" of the individual benefit of early intervention, which was worth 200 points.[62] The core indicator of whether a screen would benefit a patient was the efficacy of treatment. The ACMG report acknowledged that only 4 core conditions had treatments with the potential to prevent all negative consequences, while another 10 conditions had treatments that would prevent most negative consequences. For the majority of conditions (15), only some negative consequences could be prevented, meaning that treatment might only influence a subset of outcomes, provide incremental improvement, or prove effective in some individuals. Yet despite the limits of individual benefit, the committee found that early identification provided clear family and societal benefits for most of the conditions (26) in the core panel. Thus, familial and societal benefits influenced the inclusion of some core conditions in the recommended panel.[63]

Surprisingly, the ACMG committee did not address the hot-button topic of earlier reports: should newborn screening require parental informed consent? Even the argument for forgoing informed consent for PKU screening because the treatment is straightforward and the consequences of untreated disease are too dire had been deeply controversial in the past.[64] The committee's expansion of mandatory newborn screening beyond the criteria associated with PKU constituted a radical departure from earlier reports, yet the committee had little to say about how these changes should affect informed consent. The authors simply noted that states have different consent/dissent procedures. In a written commentary that defended the ACMG conclusions, one of the report's authors stated that "obtaining consent is not an easy issue."[65]

Critics of the expanding conceptualization of newborn screening benefits and beneficiaries came from the fields of public health, genetics, and bioethics.[66] They pointed out that the "ACMG working group adopted the new criteria [of benefit] with little discussion or justification and immediately began using them to select the new uniform panel, which was then released as a *fait accompli*. . . . For some of the new conditions, it is less obvious that newborn screening for the condition is truly part of an adequate level of care, or if it is, that it should take priority over other ethically urgent healthcare not readily available to all children at the time."[67] These concerns were tied to the mandatory natures of newborn screening and privacy and confidentiality issues: "If the rationale is a family benefit . . . then the ethical requirement is clear: parents should be informed and allowed to make their own decisions."[68] Critics also took issue with the notion that avoiding the diagnostic odyssey is best done through population screening, noting that testing when symptoms appear may be more effective than screening an entire population.[69] Generally, the critics argued that "detecting disorders that have no proven treatment or for which treatment is helpful is just not as urgent as detecting PKU."[70] In fact, expanded newborn screening may be more akin to diabetes susceptibility testing than PKU screening, presenting a completely different set of potential harms "centered around the probabilistic nature of the information, potentially maladaptive parental reactions to this level of uncertainty, and perceived breaches of the autonomy of the child being tested."[71]

### Accommodating Tandem Mass Spectrometry

The ACMG committee explicitly acknowledged that its recommendations were driven by the increased reliance on multiplex technologies in genetic screening: "New technology has been one of the driving forces in the evolution of newborn screening programs in the United States and is a critical factor in the evaluation of a condition to determine how appropriate for screening it is."[72] What was the new technology on the block? "Multiplex testing technologies are emerging that can simultaneously identify multiple analytes from a single analytical process."[73] This technology is "appealing for several reasons, including sensitivity for detecting ion species in low concentration, ability to quantify results relative to internal standards, high-throughput and precision, and the opportunity to simultaneously measure multiple ion species."[74] In fact, the expansion of newborn screening could be described as an example of a technology seeking a set of applications in much the same way that pharmaceutical developments stimulate new patient markets.[75]

Multiplex technologies allow laboratory technicians to screen for multiple disorders simultaneously using a single specimen. With previous testing methods, such as chromatography[76] and bacterial inhibition assays, screening for new disorders required a separate assay, instituting the principle of "one test–one disorder." This fostered a conservative approach to expanding screening targets because every new condition required an investment of resources. By 1990, however, researchers showed that tandem mass spectrometry could be used to identify metabolic disorders and lauded its ability to screen quickly for multiple disorders at once.[77]

A mass spectrometer measures the weight of numerous metabolites in a single drop of blood. In tandem mass spectrometry, two mass spectrometers are connected together by a collision cell. The tandem mass spectrometer works as a coin sorter, first sorting and then counting the coins. The collision cell disaggregates molecules after one of the mass spectrometers has weighed and sorted them. The other mass spectrometer sorts and weighs the pieces of the molecules that are of interest to screeners. Levels of specific metabolites lying outside a preset normal range indicate the possibility of metabolic disorders because the enzymes responsible for the breakdown of amino acids are lacking and the compounds accumulate in the blood in toxic levels. The technology can detect more than 50 disorders in a three millimeter bloodspot in less than two minutes.[78]

By 2006, 21 states had already begun to use tandem mass spectrometry in their newborn screening programs, and an additional 12 states were considering implementing it.[79] At the same time, private companies such as PerkinElmer Genetics had been marketing more comprehensive newborn screening based on tandem mass spectrometry to hospitals, states, and directly to patients since 1994. Some observers feared that the privatization of newborn screening could undermine the public health objectives of newborn screening.[80] By 2001, some states—including Mississippi and Illinois—made it mandatory to inform parents before and after a child's birth that screening for disorders not included in the state newborn screening program was commercially available.[81]

The ACMG task force constructed its selection criteria to favor the inclusion of disease categories that could be screened with multiplex technologies. Screening criteria compatible with multiplex platforms quickly added up. Out of a maximum of 2,100 points, 200 points were allotted to conditions for which multiple conditions were detectable by a single test, while multiple analytes relevant to one condition in the same run, other conditions identified by the same analytes, overall analytical cost, and high throughput[82] were each worth 50 points. In addition, technical criteria not specific to tandem mass spectrometry included feasibility of detection via neonatal bloodspots or by another simple, in-nursery method, which was worth an additional 100 points, and the availability of a sensitive and specific screening test algorithm, which was good for an additional 200 points. A third of the total score thus depended on the technical feasibility of screening methods with the highest score allotted to conditions compatible with tandem mass spectrometry.

Both the authors of the ACMG report and their critics acknowledged that the technology was only one element in a broader screening infrastructure. Critics and proponents also recognized that making tandem mass spectrometry work on a national scale would require substantial troubleshooting, standardization of laboratory protocols and clinical guidelines, and, especially, fine-tuning the sensitivity and specificity of the technology. Yet where the critics thought that these additional elements should be in place before expansion, the proponents simply noted the need for developing the infrastructure.

### Do-It-Yourself Evidence

The ACMG task force also faced the problem of a weak evidentiary base from which to make recommendations. While the ACMG report broadened the familial and societal beneficiaries of newborn screening, it evaluated scientific evidence more narrowly than earlier reports, which had examined scientific criteria as well as cost-effectiveness, notification systems, follow-up, insurance reimbursement, and quality assurance. Since the Wilson and Jungner report, every committee had advocated a systems approach to newborn screening, integrating the technology into a broader spectrum of healthcare resources and priorities. The ACMG group, in contrast, avoided entangling technology with money, resources, and healthcare priorities by dividing the committee into two expert groups. This division of labor put clinicians and scientists in charge of creating scientific rankings of the screening targets, leaving a more heterogeneous second group consisting of clinicians, government officials, laboratory directors, and family representatives to focus on the infrastructure. In the past, of course, infrastructural problems and healthcare costs had tempered enthusiasm for expanding newborn screening, but the separation of the scientific issues from those affecting healthcare delivery had the effect of decontextualizing the viability of screening.

Even with an exclusive focus on scientific evidence, the task facing the scientific expert group was daunting. Ideally, conditions should be included in newborn screening based on a solid understanding of their incidence, their "natural history"—that is, a description of the uninterrupted progression of the disease from onset until recovery or death—treatment interventions, and the performance characteristics of tests (e.g., selectivity and sensitivity). For genetic conditions, this evidence was lacking due to the rarity of the conditions, multiple genotypic etiologies, the rapid implementation of treatment after diagnosis, and the variation in cutoff values for some disease markers.

The committee overcame the lack of scientific evidence by imposing expert opinion. They used a two-step process to accomplish this. First, based on literature review, a survey of individuals active in newborn screening (including "consumers," a catchall term for nonexperts), and feedback from broader groups of stakeholders, the expert group developed the aforementioned 2,100 points scoring system. The scoring system gave great weight to a potential screening target's compatibility with multiplex technologies, disease incidence, treatment, and the potential benefits of screening. The treatment category included cost (for 50 points) with two possibilities: expensive (> $50,000/patient/year) or inexpensive. Generally, however, the scoring system considered few systems characteristics, although the group identified "multiple barriers to implementing an optimal screening and follow-up program."[83]

Second, the expert group created a database for 84 potential newborn screening targets, again relying on a combination of literature and expert review. The group created fact sheets based on the literature. Two experts in the field then evaluated the fact sheets for the strength of the evidence in favor of screening. This information was then combined with a broad, purposive survey of international disease experts who scored a number of conditions based on the predetermined scoring criteria to obtain a final score for each condition. The committee suggested a cutoff point of 1,200 out of 2,100 points for a condition to be included in the core panel or the secondary target category. Conditions with a score under 1,000 were not considered appropriate for newborn screening at this point. The difference between the core and the secondary target categories was the availability of an efficacious treatment and a well-understood natural history, but conditions could also become part of the secondary target group if they were initially considered inappropriate for newborn screening but were identifiable via the multiplex technologies.

This methodology came under withering criticism from public health researchers, bioethicists, and physicians.[84] The expert group's evaluation took place in the era of evidence-based medicine, during which a set of procedures for how to make clinical recommendations based on scientific evidence had long since been institutionalized.[85] At the most elementary level, evidence should be evaluated based on its scientific strength, encapsulated in the "hierarchy of evidence."[86] The highest level of evidence in this hierarchy is obtained in randomized controlled clinical trials. Most evaluation systems consider prospective studies as offering the next highest standard of evidence, followed by retrospective data. Expert opinion constitutes the lowest standard of evidence. A review committee analyzes the available data and answers specific questions based on an evaluation of the evidence. If the evidence is lacking or weak, no recommendation is made.[87] Authorities of one of the federal offices charged with making evidence-based recommendations—the US Preventive Services Task Force—determined that the ACMG's evaluation process and criteria lacked transparency and rigor and the expert group lacked sufficient methodological expertise. These critics insinuated that the expert group "has given up on good scientific evidence and relied on extrapolation and supposition," basing its recommendations largely on "colloquial evidence."[88] In a blistering critique, the critics concluded that most conditions now recommended by the ACMG would not pass the standardized criteria required in health policy decision-making:

> Based on the ACMG fact sheets and the validation reports characterizing the evidence, we believe that if the ACMG list of core conditions were evaluated using the USPSTF approach, a few would be recommended with an A or B grade, meaning that there is at least fair evidence that the benefits outweigh the harms. Perhaps a few more would receive C grades; the evidence is at least fair, but what the evidence shows is that benefits and harms are too closely balanced to support an across-the-board recommendation about introducing the service. The majority, however, would be given an I: there is insufficient evidence to recommend for or against. . . . The ACMG recommendation that these conditions be adopted by all state newborn screening programs is premature.[89]

Critics further charged that the committee consisted of strong advocates for expansion rather than a variety of unbiased parties, the survey lacked an analytical framework, the sampling of respondents was biased toward lay advocacy groups, the literature review was not performed systematically, and the scope of the project was unduly restricted.[90] With regard to the last issue, the lack of cost analysis was particularly questionable. Scientists affiliated with the British National Health Service had published a report in 2004 showing that, with the exception of PKU and

MCADD, there was insufficient evidence and cost-effectiveness to support tandem mass spectrometry technologies for newborn screening in the UK healthcare system.[91] In the United States, however, cost-effectiveness is often neglected within health policy discussions, due to cultural anxieties about healthcare rationing.[92] The ACMG report simply noted that results of a cost-benefit analysis would be published separately but that "most newborn screening programs reduce overall costs."[93]

* * *

In a classic example of what sociologist Diane Vaughan has called the "normalization of deviance," the ACMG committee expanded the ethical and policy principles for including conditions in newborn screening.[94] Normalization of deviance refers to the process whereby well-entrenched criteria are gradually eroded to the point that conditions previously considered deviant become acceptable. Vaughan found evidence for this phenomenon in her analysis of the conditions that enabled the Space Shuttle *Challenger* be launched with O-rings that should have been deemed ineffective according to engineering standards. She documented the paper trail leading to the reclassification and normalization of the O-rings.[95]

In the healthcare field, organ and tissue transplantation offers another example of the normalization of deviance.[96] Organ and tissue transplantation was originally instituted under stringent guidelines that were considered inviolable, including restrictions on the age and health of the donor, deference to the forensic death investigation system, and a prohibition on payment for donation. Over the past decades, the weaknesses in solid organ procurement and subsequent shortage of organs for transplantation have led to a gradual erosion of each of these restrictions to the point that practices that were once considered unethical are now considered acceptable: age limits and health standards of donors have been relaxed, and organ and tissue organizations have fought the forensic community about access to potential donors.[97]

A similar shifting of restrictions on the traditional beneficiaries, the systems approach to screening programs, and scientific evidence occurred in the expansion of newborn screening. Thus, the ACMG report catalyzed expanded newborn screening by privileging multiplex technologies, ignoring most systems aspects of newborn screening, expanding the beneficiaries of genetic screening, and generating evidence through expert opinion.

## Implementing Expanded Newborn Screening

Out of all of the reports written by various advisory bodies, the ACMG report was both the most controversial and the most influential. The report was available for a 60-day public comment period in February–March 2005, but the March of Dimes Foundation had already endorsed its preliminary recommendations by September 2004, before the report was even published online and publicly accessible. The American Academy of Pediatrics and the Association of Women's Health, Obstetric and Neonatal Nurses endorsed the report in May 2005, as did the Secretary's Advisory Committee on Heritable Disorders in Newborns and Children. The ACMG report helped to usher in a wave of expanded newborn screening, fostering an attitude that screening more conditions was better. In 2005, 23 states tested for more than 20 core conditions recommended in the ACMG report. In 2006, the figure had risen to 31 states, covering more than 64 percent of all babies born in the United States. By 2007, 40 states screened for at least 20 of the recommended core conditions. By August 2008, only Massachusetts, Oklahoma, and West Virginia mandated screening for less than 20 of the recommended conditions. (Massachusetts made the screen universally available but did not require it.) By 2010, all states screened for 27 of the 29 core conditions.[98]

Behind these expansions was a planned state-by-state political advocacy movement coordinated by the local March of Dimes chapters, which included "lobbying days" of the state legislators, publicity campaigns in local newspapers, and fielding of expert and lay testimonies at hearings. In many states, March of Dimes representatives were members of state newborn screening advisory committees.[99] Advocates for expanded newborn screening also marshaled legal arguments to compel adoption of the universal panel. In *Molloy v. Meier, et al.*, a pediatric practice was found liable for its failure to order genetic tests that would have alerted parents to the existence of a heritable disorder that might have affected reproductive decision-making.[100] Although this case was about prenatal testing, legal scholars argued that the adoption of the ACMG recommendations by professional and federal agencies instituted a new standard of care in newborn screening, requiring at a minimum that screening should be made universally available.[101]

The lobbying for universal screening relied on the dramatic testimonies of parents. In fact, one of the parents in our study, Nathan Schubert, testified several times in Sacramento on behalf of expanded newborn screening. California had implemented a pilot program for expanded newborn screening in 2000 and the Schuberts' daughter Lucia participated. Five days after her birth, they received a phone call from their pediatrician. Lucia had screened positive for 3-methylcrotonyl-coenzyme A carboxylase deficiency (3-MCC), a rare metabolic disorder. "If Lucia hadn't been born at that *particular* hospital during that *particular* timeframe of that pilot program window," Nathan told us in an interview more than seven years later, "she would very likely be dead. And if not dead, perhaps severely mentally or physically retarded." Soon after, Nathan joined forces with the March of Dimes, and traveled to Sacramento several times to testify to the California state senate about the benefits of screening. With the aid of his lobbying efforts, legislation was passed that transformed the pilot study that Lucia had participated in into a permanent public health program. Nathan explained his role in this process: "And I would get up and tell our story and then end it by saying, 'I don't know where we'd be without newborn screening,' and sort of finish on that note, very emotional. And then the mic would get passed to a mom I'd never met before, and she would say, 'Actually, I would know. I know what that's like.' She would tell [what happened] when you didn't get the newborn screening, sort of the flipside, the negative, so that was just horrible. I can't tell on this tape—too many tears."

As Nathan acknowledged, this approach was persuasive with both Democrats and Republicans alike: "It's hard to go up there and say, 'By the way, this doesn't have to happen.' And then get someone saying, 'Well, I think we shouldn't do that.' So I think it was an easy argument to make." "Saving babies" through screening imbued lifesaving with political urgency and facilitated a universal humanitarian response. Due to the efforts of Nathan and others, California was one of the first states to adopt the standardized panel, which it did in 2005, even before the ACMG report was published.

*    *    *

Critics charged that "the ACMG report does not provide convincing arguments or data to conclude that the recommended panel is optimal for child welfare or the most effective use of scarce resources."[102] Yet rather than defending the ACMG process, its authors maintained that expansion was inevitable. When responding in 2008, they observed confidently:

"There is little advantage at this time to discuss whether there should be expansion of newborn screening; it is occurring briskly at this very moment."[103] Critics and advocates alike realized that the door to expansion of newborn screening was opened and the expansion was being institutionalized. Since the ACMG report was published, additional screening targets have been added, and some states have expanded even beyond the recommended panel.

## Living Expanded Newborn Screening

Expanded newborn screening has arrived. Currently, nearly 99 percent of the more than four million babies born annually in the United States are screened for a broad array of rare conditions.[104] This is one of the largest screening programs of its kind in the world. As with the implementation of the original PKU screening programs, the expansion focused on screening technologies with the expectation that the healthcare infrastructure would follow, but much of this remained an uncharted territory. Crucial residual issues of the actual screening, follow-up, and treatment had to be worked out, and uncertainty arose when families met health professionals to discuss screening results. These uncertainties did not emerge randomly but were foreshadowed in the setup of expanded newborn screening: they followed from the roads taken and not taken.

*Consequences for families.* For most parents, positive newborn screening results will still come as the proverbial lightning flash on a clear day. Public opinion research suggests that few new parents know about newborn screening.[105] This lack of awareness results, in part, from the historical precedent of mandating screening without informed consent.[106] While religious or other objections are possible in some states, few people are explicitly told that opting out is an option and the default action is to screen.

When newborn screening results are positive, uncertainty remains about the implications of the findings. One major assumption underlying the broadening of screening beneficiaries from infants to families and society is that families will welcome health information even if its meaning is ambiguous, the infant is only a carrier, or there is no treatment for the condition screened. At the same time, throughout the history of newborn screening, research has confirmed that early diagnosis may interfere with parent-infant bonding at critical moments.[107]

Once a positive screen is available, it sometimes remains unclear what can be done about it. PKU screening set a high standard for treatment because the program was justified by the promise that early intervention could offset mental retardation.[108] In expanded newborn screening, the link between early detection and treatment was considerably loosened. For example, children diagnosed with galactosemia may suffer liver failure and an early death if fed breast milk or formula containing lactose. Newborn screening and a lactose-free diet may save lives, but the children often suffer from neurological impairment, speech abnormalities, and visual problems anyway.[109] Children diagnosed with MCADD and other diseases may die unexpectedly, even after newborn screening diagnosis.[110]

*Ontological properties of screening targets.* The nature of screened conditions also remains a work in progress. The expanded newborn screening panel broadened what counts as a screenable condition with the inclusion of 25 secondary targets. How do these conditions translate into diagnoses? Even more elementary, what is a condition? This is not a theoretical question but a practical question that baffled the ACMG committee.[111] Based on how the conditions were classified, the core panel contained anywhere from 9 to 142 conditions. The low figure was based on the test platform used while the higher figure referred to the number of genetic loci. The official number of 29 reflected the opinion of the expert group. If the clinical phenotype was used, the core panel contained only 27 conditions.[112] How do genetic mutations relate to screened conditions? There are more than 500 mutations in the PAH gene that can cause highly elevated phenylalanine levels. Rare forms of PKU can also be caused by defects in at least four other genes.[113] Then, the primary marker for MCADD is also a primary marker for other conditions such as medium-chain ketoacyl-coenzyme A thiolase deficiency (MCKAT) and glutaric acidemia type 2 (GA2).[114] Screening thus reveals information that requires further interpretation.

In addition, some of the conditions added to the newborn screening panel were exceedingly rare and little information about their etiology, natural history, or clinical relevance was known. At the same time, conditions previously considered rare might not be so rare after screening has been initiated, as health officials in Australia discovered when they began screening for MCADD, short-chain acyl-coenzyme A dehydrogenase (SCADD), very long-chain acyl-coenzyme A dehydrogenase (VLCADD) and citrullinemia.[115] The genotype-phenotype link, too, was often highly variable. Not every child with the same genetic mutation manifested the same symptoms as other children, including siblings. In each of these situations, the information churned up by newborn screening results requires extensive interpretive work by families and healthcare providers to determine the properties of the screened condition and to create treatment plans.

*Sociopolitical screening infrastructure.* Expanding the number of conditions to be screened is only tipping the first domino in a line of dominoes. Screening requires a notification system for parents and healthcare providers, measures for follow-up testing, specially trained healthcare personnel to help interpret results, financial reimbursement for special diets, and long-term follow-up for diagnosed infants. All of these steps down the line from the initial screening process have financial, ethical, professional, and legal ramifications, and require the creation of new functions and the collaboration of diverse parties. The ACMG report remained mum on the broader infrastructure needed to implement the expansion of newborn screening, leaving it up to states to work out the details. Therefore, the expansion of screening inevitably bumped into the patchy character of US healthcare provision. The case of sickle cell disease had already shown how broader inequities in the healthcare system could plague screening programs: children diagnosed with sickle cell disease have not always had access to the recommended treatment. Several studies have documented that fewer than half of children affected with sickle cell disease receive the recommended prophylactic treatments.[116]

*       *       *

Following the expansion of newborn screening, states screened for more than 50 core and secondary conditions, but what these conditions were, whether they suggested any long-term health consequences for the child, and how the screening results would be integrated into the broader healthcare system remained uncertain. The ACMG report offered a clear vision for expansion but ignored crucial aspects of how this expansion would work out. Genetics staff and families needed to address these uncertainties in the clinic. We have termed this collective project of implementing the technology *bridging work*.[117] This work aims to reconcile the promise of technologies with the realities of their implementation. Bridging work fills the gap between the technology as it was envisioned by designers and the technology as it is experienced by actual users. Technologies are constantly tinkered with, but at some point there is a handover from designers to users. This transition is a vulnerable point in the lifecycle of technologies because a host of unintended consequences may stop the technology in its tracks. In many cases, medical technologies have been abandoned rather than put into practice.[118] Because newborn screening was state-mandated, however, clinicians had no choice but to implement newborn screening technologies into their work in the clinic. One of the first things they noticed was that newborn screening identified many more patients than they had anticipated. And even more puzzling, these patients were very different from the metabolic patients they had previously encountered in their clinics. We turn to how clinicians and parents dealt with these puzzling screening results in the next chapter.

CHAPTER TWO

# Patients-in-Waiting

The architects of expanded newborn screening presented the avoidance of "diagnostic odysseys" as one of its main societal benefits: "Society could benefit by a reduction in medical diagnostic odysseys that are costly to the healthcare system."[1] Diagnostic odysseys are lengthy, exhaustive, and costly ordeals during which patients with unexplained symptoms travel from one physician to the next, subjecting themselves to an endless battery of tests, often without finding a satisfactory diagnosis. Prior to newborn screening, many families of children with genetic conditions had undergone such journeys. One of the sayings impressed upon medical students is "if you hear hoof beats, think horses, not zebras," meaning that a clinician should first consider common medical diagnoses before contemplating more esoteric conditions. For patients with rare metabolic conditions, a diagnosis often came too late, all too often after a crisis with irreversible damage had already taken its toll. The promise of a quick diagnosis at birth thus provided a powerful rationale for the expansion of newborn screening. Of course, this societal benefit presumed that the diagnosis itself was unproblematic. We will show in this chapter that, paradoxically, the expansion of newborn screening has launched some families onto diagnostic odysseys of an entirely different sort.

Rather than diagnosing asymptomatic patients with clear-cut diseases, expanded newborn screening identified a distinct group of newborns with screening values lying outside a preset normal range that did not always clearly correlate with defined disease categories. We refer to these patients as *patients-in-waiting* because they hovered for extended periods of time under medical attention between sickness and health, or more precisely, between pathology and an undistinguished state of "normality." A patient-in-waiting was treated as a patient in the medical encounter but it was not always clear whether anything was wrong. The major issue facing a newborn patient-in-waiting in our study was not only whether the baby would develop a metabolic disorder but also whether the screened condition was actually a disease. At stake in clinical interactions were the social and biological characteristics of the screened condition and the status of the newborn: was this baby healthy or sick? A major consequence of expanded newborn screening was thus the management of new patient populations marred by fundamental uncertainty about the nature of screening targets. Such management went beyond identifying a patient, and included settling upon a diagnosis, monitoring developmental milestones, recognizing potential symptoms, and developing a plan for intervention. The stakes were high in such encounters. Unlike prenatal genetic technologies where interactions are dominated by the quest for the perfect child,[2] newborn screening implied imperfection after the child had been born. For genetic conditions, imperfection might mean developmental delays, neurological deficits, or sudden death.

As we saw in the previous chapter, diagnostic uncertainty was foreshadowed by the screening technologies. Tandem mass spectrometry screens for biomarkers rather than specific diseases. Consequently, the one-to-one link between disease and test present in earlier screening technologies was lost. The knowledge that a biochemical level fell outside a preestablished normal range could indicate several different disorders, or could be of ambiguous clinical value. Thus, the novelty of tandem mass spectrometry technology was that it revealed an abundance of information requiring further interpretation.

Anomalous screening results interrupted established workflows and required negotiations to grasp their clinical relevance.[3] The routine operating procedures of the genetics clinic no longer moved patients along, and geneticists and families entered an unfamiliar landscape. These anomalies exposed what Everett Hughes called "the rough edge of professional practice," where professional habits fail to satisfactorily address personal tragedy.[4] Anomalies, as pragmatists have explained, are like unexpected forks in the road. "As long as our activity glides smoothly along from one thing to another," pragmatist philosopher John Dewey wrote,

> or as long as we permit our imagination to entertain fancies at pleasure, there is no call for reflection. Difficulty or obstruction in the way of reaching a belief brings us, however, to a pause. In the suspense of uncertainty, we metaphorically climb a tree; we try to find some standpoint from which we may survey

additional facts and, getting a more commanding view of the situation, may decide how the facts stand related to one another.[5]

Without routines to fall back on, clinicians and parents deliberated over what to do next. And it is in the doing that we find the situated meanings and clinical relevance of newborn screening results. The work in the genetics clinic had a deeply practical dimension: a baby might be at risk for a metabolic disorder, but a decision would need to be made about what the baby could and should eat. An action, even a passive one such as waiting things out, was needed. Such actions reflected back on what the team thought, at that moment, of the anomalous result. In this chapter, we examine how the meaning and relevance of expanded newborn screening results emerged from the actions geneticists and parents took on behalf of patients-in-waiting.

## Patients-in-Waiting

The making of patients-in-waiting rested upon a prolonged mixture of contradictory messages about the nature of the screened disorder. For patients-in-waiting, the newborn screening results oscillated between indicating a false positive and a true disease. The pathways that linked biochemical measures, genetic markers, test results, symptoms, and treatment were unsettled. The screened conditions were irrevocably ambiguous, both biologically and socially: biologically because the clinical significance of elevated levels was not established and socially because it remained unclear how screening results would affect the child's and the family's life. As we will show, once this ambiguity was aroused, it did not easily dissipate. The sociologically fascinating observation is that this betwixt-and-between state still required action. And it was through the actions of parents and clinicians that the screening results became endowed with particular meanings. The possibility of developmental delays, neurological deficits, and sudden death was so threatening that these conditions became functional even as uncertainty about the urgency and efficacy of these measures lingered.

With newborns unable to respond to the screening results, the management of uncertainty fell to their parents. This raises the question: who is the *patient* signaled by the concept of patients-in-waiting? One of the unique characteristics of newborn screening is that parents and infant shared the patient role.[6] While the infant provided blood and urine samples and was

at risk for developing symptoms, the parents were responsible for acting upon the test results. As in many pediatric settings, the geneticists examined the infant's muscle tone, reflexes, and developmental milestones
but questioned, admonished, and reassured parents. In the genetics context, however, parents were often asked to submit their own genetic material for confirmatory analysis, which rendered them patients in quite another sense. In interviews, parents used the "we" pronoun when referring
to their children's medical experiences. This sharing of the patient role
rendered the social implications of newborn screening even more visible:
parents, under medical scrutiny, were often quite explicit about the kind of
measures they were willing to take on behalf of their child, how screening
results altered their expectations for their infant, and how these results affected their newly grown family.

In the next sections, we examine how parents and geneticists made
sense of, and responded to, diagnostic uncertainty in the context of newborn screening. We describe the patient-in-waiting odyssey as a trajectory[7]
characterized by a shocking onset, a protracted middle period with clinic
visits focused on follow-up tests that remained ambiguous, and finally, a
gradual fading away of the patient-in-waiting status for the genetics team
if not for the parents.

## Onset

Eight days after her son's birth, Wendy Levinson received an alarming phone
call. It was the day of Jacob's bris, the Jewish ritual circumcision that occurs
on the eighth day of life, and the table was laden with pastries and drinks for
the family and friends set to arrive in just an hour. Her father-in-law had flown
in from Philadelphia, and other family had driven from Las Vegas. But when
Wendy answered the phone, she was told that she needed to bring Jacob to the
hospital immediately.

A few days earlier, she had been notified that Jacob's phenylalanine levels
were elevated. It could be a false positive, she was told, but she was asked to
bring him in for retesting. Wendy and her husband went back to the lab and
had Jacob's blood drawn. They were not very worried. Jacob seemed fine, and
they did not think there would be a problem. "I just had a fine feeling," she
recalled.

Yet on the morning of the bris, the nurse from the genetics clinic called
and told Wendy that Jacob's levels were still elevated. They wanted to see him
immediately in case he had phenylketonuria (PKU). Wendy described her re-

action: "I, at that point, was devastated. I mean, we were like—we didn't know what to think. We were horrified. We were, you know, we—we—I was a mess . . . I broke down." So they canceled the bris, and went to the hospital.

"The rabbi was actually very understanding," Wendy noted. "He said the baby's health is most important, and everybody was understanding. But it was just difficult."

When they went to the hospital, Dr. Silverman and Monica Wu, the nurse coordinator affiliated with the newborn screening program, explained the results. They were reassured by the fact that Jacob's levels were still relatively low for someone with PKU, which could be a sign that he had hyperphenylalaninemia, a milder form of the disorder. Nevertheless, Wendy remembered, "They said, 'Your baby has PKU.'"

Wendy continued, "I saved all the material from the hospital, and it's like what is this? And actually the first time that they had suggested that he might have PKU, you go back to read the material and it's like, a blurb. And basically it says, we test for this. PKU is this, and basically in a nutshell, if, you know, because of a deficiency in an enzyme, your—your child can become mentally retarded. And then you go on the Internet and it's like, if the levels are like this, you know, he'll become retarded. So, I'm like, what?! He's losing IQ points by the second. And I'm like, oh, my gosh! I'm looking at him, and he seems fine. Is his brain, you know, getting destroyed by the protein that's in my breast milk? And, you know, I was . . . it was really very, very nerve-wracking. So, I can only describe it all . . . the best way to describe the whole situation is an emotional rollercoaster."

Just as most people remember where they were during major disasters, parents remembered where they were and what they were doing when they received the phone call about their child's results. Typically, a nurse from the regional newborn screening office notified the pediatrician or primary care physician, who in turn called the parents to inform them about positive screens and to ask for a follow-up test. Unfortunately, some physicians' offices made these calls at the end of the day. If they could not reach the parents and needed to leave the information in a message, parents had to wait until the next day to have their questions answered. Even then, most of the parents in our study indicated that their physicians knew little to nothing about these rare conditions. Dr. Flores acknowledged to one family: "I guarantee you, no doctor in the greater metropolitan area, except here, is going to know what you are talking about because it is a very rare disease." If the pediatrician was unknown or unavailable, some families learned about their child's results from a representative from the state newborn screening program. These phone calls were not ideal either because parents received bad news from someone they had never met. Occasionally, the family could not be located and the newborn screening program called upon public health nurses to track them down.

The initial positive results of newborn screening came as a *shock* to almost all parents. They had been focused on pregnancy and delivery and understandably gave little thought to rare genetic conditions.[8] Although parents were offered informational brochures about newborn screening, many parents did not remember receiving this information. Wendy Levinson's description of the experience as an "emotional rollercoaster" can be explained in part by the way that she, and other parents, learned about positive results. The contradictory messages often began with the very first communication. Representatives from the state's newborn screening program instructed pediatricians not to scare parents unduly. They offered qualifiers, saying, as they did to the Levinsons, that the initial levels probably indicated a false positive result. In the same conversation, however, parents were urgently advised to retest the same day. "STAT," as one father vividly recalled. Depending on the suspected condition, the request to retest could be accompanied with preventive measures such as not letting the newborn sleep for more than three hours without feeding, avoiding breastfeeding, or using a soy-based formula. Parents also received instructions about possible symptoms and warning signs.

Parents told us that they felt "devastated," "surprised and shocked," "freaked out," or "scared" by the newborn screening results. They referred to the initial phone call as: "horrible," "giving the new mom a heart attack," "my nerves were shot," or "didn't know what to think." Similar to Wendy Levinson's fear that her son was losing IQ points by the second, another mother recalled how even during the initial phone call her thoughts immediately went to the worst possible outcome: "The gal on the phone tells me, 'Oh, your daughter tested positive for a carnitine transporter deficiency.' Okay, I'm not a scientist. That just sounds really scary, and immediately the tears go. She's just talking, talking. And she asks, 'Are you crying?' I'm like yeah I'm crying because I don't know what kind of a life my daughter is gonna have. You know? I don't know what this is." Another mother reported feeling that her son was "brand new and what if he dies?"

Wendy Levinson took the initial news quite well because she believed her son was doing fine. Still, even she panicked when she heard the let-

ters *P K U* and searched the Internet for additional information. The aim
for a careful balance between encouraging parents not to panic and ensuring that they take the condition very seriously was destabilized when
parents conducted an *online search* or *consulted any kind of information*
provided by healthcare providers because these sources identified the
worst-case outcomes.[9] One mother recalled: "I was devastated at first because I didn't know what the heck it was.... First they said that he was
positive, and I didn't know for what, so that of course was horrible. Then
they told me, and I still didn't know. She just told me they got it tested
again. So I just wanted to research it myself on the Internet."

Once they had a diagnostic label, parents learned that in the worst-case
scenario hyperprolinemia could be associated with schizophrenia, MCADD
patients could die a sudden death, untreated PKU could lead to mental
retardation, carnitine deficiency could cause muscle weakness—including
weakness of the heart muscle, and glutaric acidemia type 2 could be life-
threatening. Parents of a child with a possible biotin deficiency recalled
learning online that the condition "can cause mental retardation, blindness, loss of hearing, seizures, and even death." Geneticists warned parents not to trust the information they found because Internet message
boards offered limited and outdated information about rare genetic conditions. Dr. Silverman explained the bias to a family: "It's like the news:
when someone has illicit sex it makes it to the paper. When someone is a
good husband, they don't want to write an article about it."

Parents' experiences of diagnostic uncertainty thus originated in wildly
disparate mixed messages from a variety of sources following a positive
newborn screen. Working with pediatricians, state newborn screening personnel tried to reassure families that the results likely indicated nothing
serious, but a quick search for information produced a long list of hor-
ror stories. Before families even saw a geneticist, the momentum across
a wide diversity of families was to take the condition seriously. Newborn
screening infrastructure was set up to persuade parents that the results demanded immediate retesting and required preventive measures. Shocked
by the unexpected news, most parents complied with retesting and visited
the genetics clinic with the hope that a resolution could be found.

Parents' reactions to a positive newborn screen were not uniform across
families but depended instead on the context in which the news was received. Some infants had older siblings with serious disabilities; other families had crippling financial and social challenges. For each of those groups,
having a child with screening results that could in the distant future lead

to a disease was not always the most pressing concern in light of the immediate stressors facing them. In a few families, the child with a positive newborn screen followed an older sibling diagnosed with the same condition. These families had a good idea of what was awaiting them. At the other end of the continuum were families who had suffered for years with infertility problems and miscarriages, for whom this was to be the last chance at having a child. A mother sobbed, "Eric and I have worked really hard to have our kids and having children has not been easy for me. I worked really hard for both of them."

*Clinic Visits*

The initial anxiety-provoking communications described in the last section were typical for all parents contacted for a positive newborn screen. A screen only flags the possibility of a diagnosis and requires more specific follow-up tests to rule out a false positive. At this point there were three possible trajectories (see figure 2).

First, in the overwhelming majority of cases, the retesting revealed that the initial screen was a false positive. In these cases, the parents did not typically meet with the genetics team because the pediatrician conducted the repeat test (dashed line). These families might have been kept in suspense for a week or so but they were reassured about the likelihood of a false positive. When the families were extremely anxious, they had an opportunity to meet with the genetics team. Our study contained nine families with such single clinic visits.

Second, in 24 cases, the retesting or sequencing demonstrated the unambiguous presence of a well-established disease (solid line). These are the true positives. Patients in the category of true positives sometimes developed symptoms even before they received newborn screening results or suffered a metabolic crisis in the first years of life. Sometimes, they remained asymptomatic, but there was no ambiguity that they had a well-established disease. This group of true positive patients contained seven children with classic PKU. When parents asked questions, geneticists were able to give authoritative answers and provide standard treatment protocols.[10]

The third scenario entailed patients-in-waiting because the confirmatory follow-up tests did not provide resolution and the ambivalent messages continued (dotted line). Forty-two infants in our study fell into this category. The trajectory of patients-in-waiting resembled a "rollercoaster,"

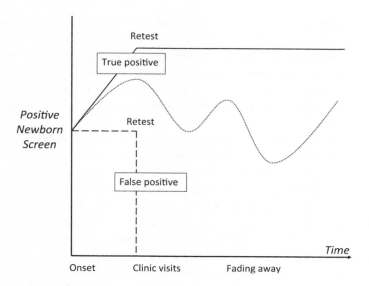

FIGURE 2. Newborn screening trajectories.

with ups and downs that called into question whether the infant had a condition and what the condition really meant. The weeks or months of suspense could be an intensely anxious period for these parents and during that period the newborn remained, in the eyes of the parents and the genetics team, a patient-in-waiting. By the time these families were referred to the genetics clinic, they had been turned into a captive audience, hoping for a clear explanation of what was going on. Those families still counting on a false positive saw their hope vanish when the referral came with the request to submit to more tests: "They told us that it was maybe a false positive, and so we sort of relaxed and thought, 'Well, okay, well, maybe this happens all the time.' And then, again, we get this, 'Oh, no, you have to get another test.'"

It is critical to point out that while patients-in-waiting correlated with certain diagnostic conditions, *the patient-in-waiting category is not a distinct biological or genetic classification.* It is not the case that all patients diagnosed with a particular disorder were automatically kept in limbo. Patients-in-waiting were made in interactions marred by uncertainties about the nature of disease and depended on geneticists' communication styles and work routines and families' healthcare experiences, receptivity, and anxiety levels. Because the patient-in-waiting trajectory was characterized by mixed messages, communication problems could influence the experience, such as when a geneticist was unable to convey details about the disease when communicating through an interpreter with a Spanish-speaking family. In addition, outstanding experiences with healthcare providers (either good or bad), expectations about the child's life, and other challenges facing the family could mediate how families interpreted the staff's mixed messages.

The encounter with the genetics team remained the family's primary source of knowledge about the genetic condition. To back up their recommendations, the geneticists often referred to studies that were recently published or still in press, or to personal conversations with leading researchers. Parents often quickly learned more than their pediatrician about the genetic conditions, but they did not surpass the knowledge of the geneticists. Typically, however, even the geneticists did not have all of the answers, shaping the liminal state of a patient-in-waiting.

Becoming a patient-in-waiting was not a subtle process. The uncertainty of how to interpret newborn screening results colored the clinic interactions. Consider this example from our fieldnotes of a first consultation between a foster mother and a geneticist regarding a child with elevated proline levels:[11]

Most babies enter the medical system soon after a positive newborn screen, but Ana Lancerio was lost to follow-up for six months. Her parents received a referral to a metabolic specialist but since they struggled with drug problems, they did not keep the appointment. At seven months, social services placed the baby with an aunt, Isabella Bonilla. Isabella learned about the newborn screening results when she brought Ana to the hospital for a routine appointment, and made contact with the genetics clinic.

Normal proline levels for newborns fall between 100 and 350 μmol/L but Ana had a level of 1261 μmol/L. Like most parents, Isabella googled "hyperprolinemia" but did not learn much about the condition. When the geneticist, Dr. Dati, found out that he had a baby with hyperprolinemia on his schedule, he turned to us and said that he had not seen a hyperprolinemia case before.

When Dr. Dati talked to Isabella, he stated, "From my perspective, it is quite reassuring. First of all, her proline levels are high but they are not super high." He indicated that if it were not for newborn screening, he would never have detected it.

Dr. Dati next explained that hyperprolinemia came in two variations: "The first one is simply a biochemical finding. It is a random finding. No symptoms, nothing." He added that the difference between type 1 and 2 does not depend on proline levels alone but also on mutations in different genes. He continued, "The ultimate way of figuring this out would be to test the genes. Those tests are not available clinically. They are available on a research basis."

Isabella asked when symptoms could be expected to appear, and Dr. Dati answered that they should manifest in the first year of life. When Isabella pressed the question of whether the symptoms could appear later, Dr. Dati admitted, "They could. We don't know. I can't guarantee anything but the fact that she is developmentally perfectly on target is a good sign." Isabella asked about warning signs besides seizures. Dr. Dati explained that they should be attuned to regular developmental landmarks such as sitting, walking, and babbling in time.

At the staff meeting later that day, the geneticists also disagreed about a fundamental question: whether hyperprolinemia was a true disease that required any kind of clinical action. Dr. Flores shook his head and said, "It sounds *loco* to me."

This first clinic visit introduces many of the typical issues facing patients-in-waiting. *Diagnostic uncertainty due to lack of scientific knowledge:* As Dr. Dati explained to Isabella, little was known about hyperprolinemia because few children with this condition came to medical attention prior to newborn screening. *Fundamental question of false or true positive:* Ana had elevated levels but they were not as elevated as is typical for patients who express symptoms of hyperprolinemia. She resided somewhere in limbo between pathology and normality. *Mixed messages:* Dr. Dati necessarily communicated mixed messages about the condition, emphasizing the potential seriousness with qualifiers suggesting that in her case it was not likely very serious. *Unanswered questions:* Isabella was concerned and looked for clarity, but her questions were met with evasive answers because Dr. Dati did not know the answers. Most of the symptoms that could indicate the beginning of a problem remained rather vague and nonspecific. *Questions about the status of the disease:* The team questioned the utility of testing because there was no treatment anyway. The question facing the clinicians and the family was not only whether Ana had hyperprolinemia but also whether it was a true disease.

## Repeat Testing Remains Inconclusive

In newborn screening, the expected sequence of events to resolve diagnostic uncertainty is to conduct confirmatory blood or urine tests, followed by DNA sequencing for the genes associated with the condition if genetic information can affect the diagnosis or treatment. Note, however, that for hyperprolinemia DNA sequencing was not commercially available at the time that Ana's elevated proline levels were identified. Increasingly focused testing should bring genetics staff closer to a diagnosis. Geneticists have practiced this modus operandi over several decades with other patients they see in the clinic.[12] As specialist consultants, the geneticists' bread and butter was to provide a diagnosis. They received referrals to examine patients with physical anomalies, cognitive delays, or other unusual features that could indicate a genetic disorder. In those cases, the geneticists checked the configuration of symptoms or abnormalities and then determined which genetic test to order. If the test confirmed a diagnosis, the patient would be followed in the clinic. Although a genetic test was rarely sufficient on its own,[13] phenotypic signs without molecular confirmation were deeply baffling, if not entirely unusual. The staff organized appointments based on test schedules or discussion of test results. Confirmatory tests thus structured most genetics encounters. Consequently, the genetics staff's approach to ambiguous newborn screening results followed established routines, without, however, the hoped-for resolution. For patients-in-waiting, the resolve of confirmatory testing was wanting, and a sequence of inconclusive retesting defined the length of the trajectory.

The duration of the patient-in-waiting trajectory was greatly influenced by the waiting period for test results to be returned. Confirmatory testing took time. Families might hesitate about some tests. For some tests, Monica had to obtain prior insurance authorization. The family had to go to the lab for a blood sample. The sample had to be sent to the right facility. The results had to come back and the family scheduled for a new clinic visit. Still, the defining feature of the patient-in-waiting trajectory was that the test results failed to provide diagnostic closure within the clinical encounter. "I don't know if it's black or white, or we're still in gray," a father explained, "Her tests have failed. Her two tests have failed." Dr. Silverman agreed: "Well, there's an unusual result." An unusual result implied that the follow-up tests did not exclude the possibility that something was wrong, but the results were not serious enough to indicate a clear-cut disease.

The dynamics of inconclusive retesting were at play for James and Sheila Honan. Their son Mike's newborn screening results showed slightly elevated levels of C5-DC acylcarnitine, the biomarker indicative of glutaric acidemia type 1 (GA1)—the same condition under consideration for Bailey Baio. On repeat acylcarnitine profile testing in blood plasma, the levels were normal in the blood serum but still about six times as high as expected in the urine. When sharing this news with the Honans, Dr. Flores provided a mixture of good and bad news and then offered molecular testing as a solution for the conundrum of diagnostic uncertainty. He said, "So what tends to happen is that the babies do okay. And particularly in the first five years of life is when the highest risk occurs for having problems. And when they mostly get in trouble is when they get sick. So the baby gets sick and doesn't eat. Then what happens is the body starts breaking down its own protein and releases all those amino acids, all those units that he cannot use for energy. So then the acid accumulates and keeps going up, up, up. That goes to the brain and causes damage. Well, unfortunately, the damage is irreversible. So the idea is to catch it early so that we can give him nutrients to prevent him from breaking down his own protein. And as long as we do that, then we'll prevent the brain damage. Now the elevation that we saw here is very slight. We usually see a much higher elevation in patients who have the very serious form of the acidemia. So what we would like to do today is to confirm that the elevation really means that he has a genetic change in his DNA, which encodes the instructions for everything that our body does."

Dr. Flores laid out two different logics while acknowledging, as was typical for patients-in-waiting, that these logics were not 100 percent reliable. The first was the principle of increased pathology, in which lower elevations likely correspond to a reduced disease risk. A lower level *should* indicate a lower risk but whether it really does remains unclear. The strict cutoff point used in newborn screening is likely an instance of misplaced concretism—a precise number that insinuates quantitative authority but actually results from social convention, and in the case of newborn screening, reflects a balance between caution and risk. The challenge for such numbers is to "preserve the integrity of information without a priori standardization."[14] What is certain is that one crisis could cause irreversible brain damage. But even if the disease was serious, preventive measures were possible. Bad news followed good news, but lingering uncertainties undermined the quality of either news because Dr. Flores did not know whether Mike was truly affected.

The second logic referred to the sequence of repeat testing to reduce diagnostic uncertainty. After confirmation of the biochemical tests, genetic mutation analysis should provide clarity about the severity of disease. The acylcarnitine levels served as markers for GA1 and by conducting molecular tests, the geneticists should be able to determine whether the mutations associated with the condition were present. Yet this logic could also fail. Dr. Flores admitted: "Now I have to warn you that even if the result comes back, there's two possibilities. One is we'll do the test and we don't find any changes in the DNA. Great, he's off scot-free. We don't worry. We don't need to see you anymore. But it could be that—remember our instructions come from Mom and Dad. Right? So you get one copy of the gene from Mom and one from Dad. So as long as you have one copy working, you're fine. It's when both of them don't work, then you have a problem. Right? So it is possible that we may find, in him, one of the two mutations or changes, but not find the second one. In that case, we may have to do further testing to confirm really if he has it or not."

The mutation analysis worked, in a diagnostic sense, only if it did not detect anything or if it identified two known mutations associated with GA1. If DNA testing uncovered no mutations, Dr. Flores would feel reassured that Mike was unlikely to have the disease, although theoretically, it would be possible that he had two completely unknown GA1 genetic mutations. In this instance, Mike would likely be classified as a false positive. Two known mutations would confirm that Mike definitely had GA1, and he would move from a patient-in-waiting to a true positive. Ambiguity would be perpetuated, however, if the test showed only one mutation, because then two scenarios would be possible: Mike might only have one mutation, in which case he would be a carrier, or Mike might have a second mutation that had not yet been identified. In this case, Mike could be at a higher risk for disease. Finding only one mutation could thus perpetuate the diagnostic odyssey.

In Mike's case, this is exactly what happened: molecular analysis identified only one pathological mutation. At the next meeting, Sheila Honan responded to the test results with, "So, we're still in this ambiguous stage." A genetics fellow, Dr. De Vries, pulled out the test results and explained, pointing to the paper: "It says here that they found one undocumented variant which makes this change. And they're saying that this change has been reported to be causative for GA1. The second plausible mutation was not identified. This could mean that he's just a carrier or it could mean that he has a second mutation that they weren't able to find." The possibility of an unknown and undiscovered mutation left open the possibility that Mike was still at risk for a metabolic crisis.

The geneticists decided to check Mike's acylcarnitines again to see whether he still had elevated levels. If the C5 level was no longer elevated, he was likely a carrier. James Honan wondered why they would go back to a test that had already been carried out: "I get so mixed up—but is that the same as the initial blood test we did when they were checking for the elevated carnitine level?" Dr. De Vries answered: "Yes, just to see if he's still excreting these things that are high. If it's better, maybe it could point us more that he's just a carrier." Dr. De Vries suggested that if the levels had gone down, Mike was likely at a reduced risk, although her tentative phrasing implied that this would not be conclusive evidence. In fact, rather than test results adjudicating between pathology and normality, results primarily became meaningful over time. The new acylcarnitine levels would be compared to the previous ones, and if the levels had gone up, there was likely something going on; if they remained the same or went down, the geneticists would be more reassured that Mike was likely a carrier.

The Honans recognized the inconclusiveness of this repeat testing regimen. At the next conversational turn, James returned the discussion to the therapeutic implications of the condition in spite of inconclusive follow-up testing: "Now, I'm assuming that any symptoms would be basically nonexistent until he got older. I mean, actual symptoms. The only real danger at this point is if he gets sick." As Mike's father articulated, for patients-in-waiting the core message was continued vigilance for the onset of symptoms, in spite of extensive retesting.

## Establishing Clinical Relevance

For some patients-in-waiting, diagnostic ambiguity centered on the question of whether they truly had a condition. For other families, repeat testing indicated that the child had the condition but its clinical relevance remained unclear. Now that the infant was diagnosed with a metabolic condition, how would the condition affect his or her life?

Geneticists distinguished a metabolic diagnosis from a true disease to emphasize that even with the condition, the child would not necessarily become ill. Thus, Dr. Silverman explained to a couple for whom extensive retesting showed it more likely than not that their son had 3-MCC, "But I believe, the reality is that he has a condition not a disease. Do you understand the difference? A condition is less serious, less important. But it's a real condition, we're completely sure. He has a deficiency with an enzyme." Dr. Dati made a similar distinction to a couple whose child was positive for MCADD: "It's not really a disease in the sense of you have a little kid at home who is sick. He's not sick. He's just fine. He's healthy, and he's gonna be healthy most of the time except when he gets sick, like the flu or the cold, which other kids get sick the same way. It's just when this happens, you just have to pay a little more attention. But he's a healthy child."

For some conditions, including hyperprolinemia, SCADD, and 3-MCC, the geneticists wondered whether the diagnosis had any clinical relevance. Dr. Malvern explained to a couple whose daughter had been diagnosed with SCADD that the ontological status of the condition was up for grabs: "SCADD is one of the genetic disorders that is kind of an enigma to us. We understand the disease that's associated with the mutation and how its impact is. But SCADD, even the person who has described the disorder has come to a point where he said he is not sure that these mutations really caused the disease process." The geneticists had similar conversations with the parents of children with 3-MCC and hyperprolinemia. In such cases, even if a diagnosis had been confirmed, it did not always have clear clinical ramifications.

When faced with questions about clinical relevance, the geneticists consulted their colleagues at other institutions to help guide their actions. This strategy did not always lead to a resolution. Duarte galactosemia is one variant in a family of galactosemia disorders in which the child's ability to process lactose is compromised, which can lead to mental retardation and even death. However, children with Duarte galactosemia seemed to escape metabolic crises, and the geneticists wondered whether this particular variant was pathological. In terms of treatment, the geneticists were uncertain as to whether infants with Duarte galactosemia required a diet of soy-based formula, as was typical of other galactosemia variants, or whether they could be breastfed. In a meeting with one couple, Dr. Silverman admitted that the field was divided: "It's interesting, we have a List[serv] here of metabolic specialists worldwide, and frankly if you were to ask these specialists, 50 percent don't treat Duarte galactosemia compounds at all, and 50 percent put them on soy formula." To another family, he stated, "This is one of those situations where it's the most frustrating for parents because as physicians and scientists we don't have a clear answer." Parents picked up on the lingering uncertainty in the field. A father complained to us, "Well, the concern is, to be honest, lack of research. No one can tell me what it is. I want advice to know exactly and nobody knows. There seems to be a correlation that seems to help but no one tells how exactly and how much. . . . I don't truly understand it all, and as I mentioned, I try to educate myself, and ask questions, and no one seems to really have the answers." Thus even if they had a diagnostic label, the lack of consensus about what to do or even whether to do anything at all rendered some conditions ambiguous medical objects.

## Social Traction

In spite of diagnostic and treatment ambiguity, over the months of retesting the positive screening results *received traction as the focal point of a set of practices* in the lives of the families and in their interactions with the genetics team. Even if confirmatory testing was inconclusive, it did not dispel the possibility that something could be wrong with the child. Physicians erred on the side of caution, leaving emergency measures in place and admonishing parents to watch the child vigilantly for listlessness, periods of fasting, or vomiting. These measures generated traces of paperwork that turned ambiguity into a bureaucratic disease entity[15] and created a set of routines and repeat consultations for the parents and geneticists.

Because little is known about rare genetic conditions even among healthcare providers, the geneticists invariably prepared an emergency letter for all parents to present to emergency department providers in case the child should become ill. Parents received instructions on how and when to use the letter, such as the following: "The more important thing is what we're going to give you today, which is called the emergency letter. And what it is, is a letter that describes exactly what I talked about to you right now, but also instructions to doctors in case he [the child], God forbid, were to ever get sick. There's a chance that he could get in trouble. How? Well, usually in this condition if you don't eat for a long period of time, you cannot use energy properly. Then your sugar level can go down very fast. And in babies in particular it can go very fast. If you're older you have more of a chance to help yourself. But in a baby who has to feed very frequently, it's dangerous to stop eating because you're vomiting all the time or you're just feeling icky and you don't want to eat. So anytime he gets sick and you feel like he's sleepy, lethargic, like you can barely wake him up, he's not breathing right, anything like that, you need to take him to the emergency room." Geneticists reviewed these emergency procedures and warning signs at almost every clinic visit. Depending on the condition, the parents could also be asked to provide more frequent feedings or to give dietary supplements. Such precautions further settled the condition as a real disease in the lives of many parents of patients-in-waiting.

Geneticists were often quite aware that they could cause the family to take an as-yet ambiguous condition too seriously. Consequently, they couched their admonitions with a strong message that the baby was healthy, except for the additional risks posed during periods of fasting. Dr. Flores concluded his educational message with one family: "Just be very alert but just keep treating him like he is. The other thing I don't want you to do is start to put him in plastic wrap and isolating him from the whole world. Everybody wash their hands. No, just treat him like he is. Do take him for walks and stuff. It's just being more alert about any changes in what he looks like." Dr. Silverman similarly told another couple, "As far as what we can tell, you have a healthy child with a slight biochemical abnormality." Note, however, that even these putative reassuring messages are mixed with careful qualifiers.

In spite of these encouragements about health, the precautionary measures rendered the disorders functional in family life. In the case of Ana, the possible hyperprolinemia patient described previously, the disorder gained currency as a means to access educational services, as part of disability assessment, and in the adoption-family reconciliation process.

> At the second visit, six months later, when Ana was already 14 months old, Isabella Bonilla reviewed Ana's developmental steps with an eye to the possibility of hyperprolinemia. Thus, when telling about Ana's difficulty transitioning to solid food, she noted, "We were not sure whether it was simply a delay where it would soon happen or there was something that is going on inside." Isabella had Ana tested at a service center focusing on developmental disabilities, and she was diagnosed as two to three months behind in her motor development and qualified for physical and occupational therapy. The hyperprolinemia diagnosis also had consequences in the adoption process. Social services had intervened because the children were generally neglected, but out of a variety of issues, the court focused on malnutrition and the lack of follow-up for positive newborn screening. Consequently, to show that she was qualified to parent, Isabella had to document that she took Ana's hyperprolinemia very seriously.

Such actions that prove the social relevance of hyperprolinemia created resistance to a biological redefinition of the condition as benign based on additional test results.

Some parents had to take a stance on whether the disease was real very early on. One local hospital routinely sent lactation consultants to young mothers to help them with breastfeeding. The mother of a Duarte galactosemia patient had to resist the normative message that "breast is best" as a nutritional source and mode of infant-bonding while still uncertain about the recommended treatment: "Then you have the lactation consultants coming in to me going, 'Are you okay with not nursing your baby?' And I said, 'Yeah. I want her to see, I want her to have kids. I don't want her liver to fail. I'll bond with her in some other way.' " This mother also had a difficult time locating formula in the hospital because of its strong pro-breastfeeding stance.

For mothers who *were* able to breastfeed, it often proved stressful due to the heightened emotions surrounding infant feeding in the context of metabolic disorders. One woman, whose son was suspected of having MCADD but was dismissed as a false positive when he was five months old, spoke of how the clinic's message about the importance of regular feedings amplified concerns about her son's feeding difficulties: "You know, every two hours, I was feeding him around the clock and trying to give him a little two ounce thing of milk. I was pumping incessantly, because he couldn't latch on. I was just physically tired and emotionally drained."

As we saw in the Baios' case, the possibility of disease could also shape the relationship between parents. The mother of a one-year-old with potential MCADD told us that she would like "to have a date every once in a while" with her husband. When we asked her why this was a problem, she explained that her husband "is just really untrusting of anybody who's not family. And plus I think he's just incredibly cautious about our first child. I think he's overly cautious. Yes, it's rough." Here, the uncertainty about the MCADD diagnosis—the child had elevated levels with one known mutation but a second had not been found—led to lingering concerns on the part of the father that something bad would happen to their son if they asked anyone else to care for him. This father did not even trust his own mother, and the couple had not gone out alone in more than a year.

Because metabolic disorders are genetic, even a potential or tentative diagnosis could lead to close scrutiny of the family tree to identify possibly affected but undiagnosed relatives. Thus, Lacey Tadwell, the mother of a four-year-old boy diagnosed with carnitine deficiency, reinterpreted her family's medical history: "My sister passed away at 31 from an enlarged heart. And the hospital could not detect, they had no idea what was wrong. But now that we know about Dimitri, I'm associating the two." Linking her son's results with the unanswered questions about her sister's death, Lacey worried about the dosage of carnitine supplements for her son. She also wondered whether carnitine was sufficient to hold off a premature death:

"It's difficult to grasp, but then you're telling us that something so simple as carnitine or this amino acid, but he's gonna be okay. And it makes us truly wonder if this is all that he needs." Lacey had herself tested for carnitine deficiency and questioned the normal results. She observed that she had become more tired, a possible symptom of carnitine deficiency, and decided to take carnitine supplements, despite not having a diagnosis.

Even if geneticists went out of their way to impress on parents that their children were basically normal, screening results spilled over into the lives of families. Through preventive measures and family-specific adaptations, diagnoses received traction beyond the recommended preventive measures. Several factors contributed to this course of action. Visiting an academic hospital at regular intervals, giving blood serum for laboratory tests, and meeting with geneticists were all actions associated with having a disease. Furthermore, parents were inclined to take their children's condition seriously because newborns are unable to articulate if anything is wrong, and metabolic patients are often unaware that they may have a condition: the symptoms are vague with few warning signs and potentially serious consequences.

Traction in the lives of families also created resistance to change. Each time a family acted on a patient-in-waiting as if the infant had a disease, they placed a "side bet," as sociologist Howard Becker explained in a classic paper on commitment. Becker elaborated the notion of side bet with an example from economics:

> Suppose that you are bargaining to buy a house; you offer sixteen thousand dollars, but the seller insists on twenty thousand. Now suppose that you offer your antagonist in the bargaining certified proof that you have bet a third party five thousand dollars that you will not pay more than sixteen thousand dollars for the house. Your opponent must admit defeat because you would lose money by raising your bid; you have committed yourself to pay no more than you originally offered.[16]

Becker argued that consistency in human behavior is a consequence of multiple side bets, which increase the cost of changing course. With every action informed by the possibility of disease and with every stance the family took on behalf of the infant as likely diseased, the patient-in-waiting status became entrenched in the family's social life and constituted the parents as parents of a patient-in-waiting.

Although continued vigilance was the primary reaction among families, our study contained some families who were not as vigilant as the staff would have preferred. Some of these families were too reassured that the condition was likely nothing to worry about, and, to the staff's dismay, were unresponsive to repeated requests for confirmatory testing.

*Once under Medical Supervision . . .*

Some families expected that inconclusive tests would lead to their dismissal from the clinic, but once they were under medical supervision, the geneticists monitored infants carefully. In addition to repeat testing, the other means of assessing infants with metabolic disorders was checking whether infants met developmental milestones or experienced any of the symptoms associated with the condition, although even then it was difficult to causally link generic developmental signs to a metabolic condition.

The power of the genetic gaze was apparent in the case of Kyle Stardust, who screened positive for GA1 at birth. All follow-up tests, including DNA testing, came back normal. At the eighth clinic visit, Nicole, Kyle's mother, told us that she expected to be dismissed from the clinic. Instead, Dr. Silverman announced: "We're going to start from scratch today." He asserted, "We might just do a general genetic screening, you know just to check his chromosomes." In Dr. Silverman's opinion, Kyle continued to have low muscle tone, an unusual appearance of almond-shaped eyes, a large head, and signs of developmental delay. These symptoms could suggest an underlying genetic condition.[17] Dr. Silverman explained that "it's interesting that macrocephaly or big head is one of the characteristics of glutaric acidemia." When Nicole did not react visibly to this news, Dr. Silverman remarked, "You're doing good with this issue." Nicole replied tersely, "Well, I thought there was no issue until today." She added that her other son had had low muscle tone as well, and that the large head was familial. Nicole worked in the entertainment industry and the child's father was a famous athlete with whom Nicole was no longer in a relationship. She asked the genetics team to check his picture online and see the familial resemblance for themselves. Not swayed, Dr. Silverman ordered a chromosome study and asked a neurologist who was already following Kyle to order an MRI. The neurologist refused because he did not consider an MRI indicated.

At the next visit, Dr. Silverman decided that the physical symptoms were less pronounced and abruptly reversed his opinion: "I wrote this note last time that said since his head was big should we think—continue to worry about GA1. But that's crazy. You know, we did the tests. My question is: Are you going to miss us? Because I don't see any purpose in coming back here."

A similar sequence of events occurred with Jacob Levinson. During one of the visits when Wendy expected Jacob to be dismissed from the clinic, Dr. Silverman raised the possibility that Jacob might also have biotinidase deficiency, a different metabolic disorder that can lead to serious complications such as behavioral problems, learning disabilities, and seizures. Wendy sighed: "We're back on the rollercoaster."

The impact of newborn screening may even transfer from one sibling to the next in spite of extensive precautionary measures and prenatal testing. This spillover effect was dramatically demonstrated in the situation of Sylvia and David McAllister, who had lost a daughter due to VLCADD about a year before their son Simon screened positive for VLCADD and was referred to our field site. The McAllister's daughter had been picked up by newborn screening in Nevada and was asymptomatic at birth. At 11 months of age, she developed flu-like symptoms, was hospitalized, deteriorated quickly, and died. When Sylvia became pregnant again, she underwent chorionic villus sampling (CVS) to test for VLCADD. The fetus was identified as a heterozygote carrying David's mutation. This prenatal genetic testing should have provided more conclusive information than the newborn screening, but when the newborn screen indicated a slight elevation for a secondary biomarker of VLCADD,[18] the state newborn screening medical director flagged the elevation and asked Dr. Silverman whether he wanted to follow up. After speaking with the couple's pediatrician and learning about their history, Dr. Silverman decided that it would be prudent to bring the child in for further testing to be completely sure that he was not affected.

The McAllisters' agony upon contemplating the possibility that their son Simon could have VLCADD after all was palpable in the examination room. Sylvia was teary-eyed throughout the consultation, holding Simon tightly. Dr. Silverman opened the conversation with strong reassurance: "I don't doubt for a minute that the baby is unaffected, that the amnio[19] is correct." Sylvia explained the grounds for her anxiety: "Well, we were told to be optimistic with our first child and we re— we tested her and everything. So we were, you know, we were trying to be optimistic and then got the bad news, you know. So now it's like—it's hard to be optimistic right now." Sylvia further articulated her worries: "So you don't think it's possible during [the CVS] test that they just missed my mutation, that they definitely identified it? That it's only [David's] mutation?" Dr. Silverman replied: "It's always possible but it's just not likely." Thinking aloud, he added that the CVS likely only checked for the two known mutations and that there was always a possibility of an unknown mutation. Dr. Silverman decided to repeat the mutation analysis and check the serum levels again. Still, the mutation analysis would only check for the two known mutations.

When we asked the McAllisters afterward whether they found the conversation reassuring, they expressed considerable concern. Sylvia answered: "I'm worried. I can't get those secondary test results back fast enough." David noted, "It was reassuring to come in and meet with him and hear him say that he's confident there's nothing to be concerned with." Then, he, too, qualified, "But at the same time, he talks about a degree of error that's involved in any testing. There's still some degree of inaccuracy." Sylvia continued, "I still just want those other test results as soon as possible. I just can't get them fast enough. It's hard to lose a child. Our other child, she was doing so good, too. Everyone thought that she had maybe a mild form of it. She was doing so well. It was just a shock to everyone." The follow-up test confirmed that Simon was only affected with one of the two known VLCADD mutations, and Dr. Silverman considered him a VLCADD carrier.

\* \* \*

In sum, after the shock of positive newborn screening results, the patient-in-waiting trajectory was structured by the fallout of ambiguous testing results. Because retesting did not provide the hoped-for closure, geneticists and parents erred on the side of caution and acted as if there was indeed a disease that was serious and required preventive measures. Diagnostic uncertainty was thus marshaled to emphasize the potential seriousness of the condition. For most families, these precautionary measures gradually became part of family routines and spilled over into other areas of life. Once the suspicion of a genetic disorder was raised, observable developmental signs could further fuel the possibility of disease. Consequently, the initial fear of a positive newborn screening result was channeled into caution and vigilance, and parents were inclined to treat the condition as if it was real even though the results increasingly called this evaluation into question.

## Fading Away

Precautionary practices, repeat testing, and regular consultations fostered a partnership between parents and genetic staff exemplified by close surveillance of the infant.[20] When, after time passed, the baby remained fine, clinicians sometimes had trouble getting the parents to tone down their level of vigilance. At this point, parents and physician were sometimes at odds about the appropriate course of action.

From the genetics team's perspective, diagnostic uncertainty faded in relevance when further testing was unlikely to clarify the diagnosis and the evidence suggested that the condition was unlikely to be serious. Thus, when reviewing the medication for an eight-year-old boy who was one of the first infants identified with MCADD during a pilot-screening program, Dr. Dati noted that the drug dosage was low: "That's probably underdosed and let me tell you: no one agrees whether it's a useful treatment or not. So, there's several ways to deal with this. One way is to just stop it, and measure it, and there is another way, which is just to leave him at the same doses, and then at some point in two years from now, it'll be so underdosed that then you'll be able to just stop it." Here, Dr. Dati resolved the dilemma of whether medication was indicated by gradually underdosing the patient on carnitine, as in a natural experiment. The fact that this boy was eight years old and had not displayed any symptoms favored downgrading the seriousness of the manifestation.

Elapsed time played a similar role in downgrading the severity of the condition in patients-in-waiting who had remained asymptomatic during the period of retesting. The persuasiveness of the message to relax vigilance, however, was undercut by lingering uncertainties and measures taken to keep the patient-in-waiting under medical supervision. The geneticists did not unequivocally state that the child was "disease-free." Dr. Silverman summarized one patient as "he is not sick but he's not normal," which must surely be the ultimate mixed message.

When the testing cycle ran its course, the condition faded away in spite of unresolved issues. In some cases, the infant continued to have elevated biochemical levels but did not seem to have a clinically relevant disorder. The best the geneticist could do was to offer a conditional assurance: most likely it was nothing. The emphasis was on probability. Dr. Silverman explained to the parents of a child whose screening values were suggestive of GA1: "So the question you can well ask is why is the baby continuing to test positively? And the answer is, if I know the answer I will be a rich man. We don't know the answer to that but there are people who do know. The thing that concerns us and must concern you as a parent: do I have an abnormal kid? My point would be that a lot of us have little abnormalities." After reviewing the preventive measures, Dr. Silverman continued:

DR. SILVERMAN: All of the children that we know, they really have much more significant abnormalities than this. They have a higher elevation of the blood. So
there's a good chance that it would be gone in a month. On the other side of the
coin, there are kids who are affected by this who have very slight elevations but
they are the minority. A much larger number are exactly like your boy. I obviously think it's probably nothing. Now we've been through this twenty times in
the last three years.

MOTHER: That many?

DR. SILVERMAN: Oh yeah, and in every case that has been positive, the abnormalities were higher than this and more persistent. And every case that turned out
to be nothing was like this. This doesn't mean a hundred percent to be nothing,
but it's ninety-five plus percent. It's a pretty good figure.

Here, even the information conveyed to parents that the testing had
reached a natural endpoint and that the disorder was not likely to be significant remained a statistical probability. All the evidence the geneticist
had—especially the repeated mild elevations—pointed to "nothing," but
he was not certain that it was nothing. The conclusion rested upon the vol-
ume of patients identified with such ambiguous test results.

The decision to dismiss a patient from the clinic was based on a collective assessment that the infant did not have a clinically relevant condition, even though there was no absolute evidence to definitively support this position. The broader field of genetics remained divided about
what to do with these patients. In a staff meeting where another baby who
screened positive for GA1 was discussed, Dr. Silverman reported that the
consensus at a professional conference he had recently attended was that
these babies could be "low excreters," meaning that they could be more
affected with the condition than their biochemical levels might suggest. In
the ensuing discussion, the geneticists admitted that it all came down to
how much risk one was willing to tolerate as a clinician. They stated that
their field tends to "overcall" (i.e., diagnose more than warranted) rare
metabolic conditions.

## Recalcitrant Traction

The majority of parents tended to obsess about the lingering dangers and
downplay the qualified reassurances. For them, the child was no different
than before, and without a critical time period defined in advance, it was
difficult to accept that the baby was now out of danger. The fact that the

child was doing well, according to parents, demonstrated that the preventive measures were working. Parents were therefore reluctant to stop preventive measures that they had incorporated into their lives. Here, Becker's notion of "side bets" points to the resistance to change. Parents had taken measures to offset the "real" disease such as waking up the child during the night for extra feedings, distributing copies of the emergency letter, limiting proteins, providing nutritional supplements or other foods, closely monitoring the child for developmental delays, accessing therapeutic services, routinely disinfecting eating surfaces, limiting play dates, and adjusting childcare arrangements. Taking the possibility of disease seriously could have far-reaching consequences for the parents' own lives such as postponing a return to work or a move to a less well medically serviced area, sticking with a job because of health insurance, and changing social activities. Often such changes were driven by fear: a survey of parents of children with urea cycle disorders showed that 50 percent of them thought daily about the possibility of their child's death and three-quarters thought of it at least weekly.[21]

Consequently, parents sometimes resisted changes to the treatment protocol. In the following conversation, Dr. Silverman tried to gently persuade Genevieve and Stephen Darlington, the parents of two children diagnosed with an MCADD mutation that, according to Dr. Silverman, "had never been associated with illness," to stop waking them up at night, referring to the lack of consensus in the field. He conceded that it might be okay to wake the infant as a precautionary measure, but he did not think waking up necessary for her four-year-old brother, Flavin.

GENEVIEVE: So nothing changes with the MCADD protocol?
DR. SILVERMAN: Well, you know there's still certain debates. Remember that we never recommended that you wake the kids at night to feed them, under normal circumstances. Well, there are people who would do that. But the world divides about half and half that way. And I think it has to do partially with confidence level. I've been around here for an awful long time. And I spend a lot of time at meetings.
GENEVIEVE: But you wouldn't have a little baby go, you know, long hours.
DR. SILVERMAN: No. But if a parent tells me that the baby goes eight hours by their own choice I would feel comfortable with that. Are you waking her during the night?
GENEVIEVE: It's about set at six or seven.
DR. SILVERMAN: That's okay, if you're happy. Are you waking her or is she waking you?

GENEVIEVE: No, she wakes me up. But I wouldn't feel comfortable having her go too long.

DR. SILVERMAN: No, but you have to do what makes you feel comfortable.

STEPHEN: We wake Flavin too.

DR. SILVERMAN: That I wouldn't do. You don't have to.

STEPHEN: Okay.

DR. SILVERMAN: I mean I think they would be in a complete consensus about that.

Interactions such as these in which family members expressed their reluctance to scale back preventive measures show how parents could mobilize diagnostic uncertainty as a resource to counter geneticists' recommendations. At a visit we observed for Lucia Schubert, a five-year-old girl with 3-MCC, Dr. Silverman would have liked to discontinue the supplements and the diet, but the parents were resistant. Dr. Silverman explained his rationale for "liberalizing" the diet: "All levels of scrutiny and vigilance can just be scaled back. We talked about this [in the past] but we were in a different place and different amount of knowledge. Most of the kids with this are going through life without any episode. Germany is not testing for this because they think that it is not in most instances a serious disorder. And certain US states are going to stop. Our level of concern is reduced." Nathan, Lucia's father, turned the tables on Dr. Silverman by citing an article Dr. Silverman had provided at a previous visit that stated that one should never relax the diet. Dr. Silverman dismissed it as the opinion of a single person and noted that a more recent expert consensus recommended against a special diet for 3-MCC. Nathan also insisted on taking further blood tests, but Dr. Silverman argued that the results would be difficult to interpret.

This exchange highlights the role of shifting understandings of ambiguous screening results as more clinical experience accumulated. Over a three-year period, we noticed how certain issues that initially stumped clinicians received increasingly authoritative answers. For example, Dr. Silverman's approach to 3-MCC reflected an increasing belief that most of the dietary interventions for this condition were likely unnecessary. As time passed, newly diagnosed patients were put on a regime of watchful waiting rather than dietary supplements.

Thus, while geneticists could be ready to let the condition fade away, family members could nevertheless perpetuate the medicalization of their child. The vigilance indicative of serious diseases might linger even after a family no longer visited the clinic. A mother whose child was dismissed early on in our research came back three years later because a new pediatrician recommended that she visit the clinic to make sure that her son was truly disease-free and did not require additional preventive measures. Here, the information in the medical file kept the condition viable in spite of an explicit dismissal from the clinic.

Diagnostic uncertainty for asymptomatic patients was difficult to resolve because part of this kind of fundamental disease-based ambiguity is that there was no conclusive endpoint. Consequently, in most situations families ended up taking the condition more seriously than geneticists. In our study were a number of families that were exceptions to this general rule. In two Spanish-speaking families, the geneticist took the condition more seriously than the parents. We suspect that in those families the doctor was unable to communicate the seriousness of the disorder because of language barriers in spite of interpreters, but other structural and cultural factors might have also played a role.[22] In addition, it is also possible that for some of these families—who were among the poorest in our study—interpretation of diseases and coping with uncertainty were luxuries they could not afford in light of their everyday struggles. A nonresponse then became a telling reaction.

In one non-Latino white family, the father questioned continued follow-up after the physician had decreased his level of concern because the father "felt part of an experiment" that risked turning him into a "hypochondriac." This father believed that the cascade of tests benefited medical science but was no longer of use to his daughter. He noted that even if the DNA test turned up an anomaly, he would be very skeptical about the results. The staff removed the patient from the clinic roster after the family failed to appear for three appointments. This was the only instance of overt resistance to newborn screening we encountered in our study.

## Living between Health and Disease

Newborn screening for biological entities with tenuous links to rare, poorly understood genetic conditions created a population of newborns with suspicious biological measures. Physicians and parents had to determine whether these abnormal levels indicated a biological quirk or an actual disease, and, if a disease, what kind of disease. The trajectory of patients-in-waiting was characterized by mixed and ambivalent messages that signaled either a biochemical anomaly or a very serious condition. The uncertainty petered out when the staff determined that the results were more

akin to a false positive after all, when sufficient time had passed without the emergence of symptoms, or when genetic markers or symptoms
appeared. Families sometimes ended up at odds with clinicians because
in their experience no clear benchmark of reassurance has been reached.

For patients-in-waiting, the waiting time for diagnostic resolution was
indeed much longer than for other patients in our study. In the 42 patients
we identified as patients-in-waiting, only two families received a confirmed diagnosis within three weeks. For an additional 17 families it took
up to three months; for 8 families it took up to six months; and for 9 families it took more than six months before the geneticists settled upon a diagnosis. (We were unable to determine the time until diagnostic confirmation for 6 families who enrolled in our study after a diagnosis was already
settled or who were lost to follow-up.) For the rest of our sample (non-
patients-in-waiting), all but 5 families whose children were flagged for a
positive newborn screen received a confirmed diagnosis in less than three
weeks. It is clear that the diagnostic experience of patients-in-waiting is
distinct from other positive newborn screening patients.

Our findings are consistent with preliminary follow-up data from the
15 California newborn screening centers. According to one published report, between July 2005 and April 2009:

> The median time between birth through case resolution (as having a disorder
> or not having a disorder) was 29 days. The median number of days to resolve
> disorders was 23 days, whereas the number of days taken to resolve those
> referrals who were found not to have a disorder was 30 days. The three dis-
> orders that took the least amount of time to resolve were citrullinemia—type I
> (median = 7 days, $n$ = 7); methylmalonic acidemia: mut0 (median = 8.5 days,
> $n$ = 12); and maple syrup urine disease (median = 10 days, $n$ = 14). This is in
> contrast to carnitine transporter deficiency (median = 91 days, $n$ = 27); methyl-
> malonic acidemia: mut— (median = 65 days, $n$ = 18); and short chain acyl-CoA
> dehydrogenase deficiency (median = 65 days, $n$ = 53), which took a much lon-
> ger time to resolve.[23]

When visiting the different metabolic referral centers, the authors of this
study found "that cases cannot always be clearly defined as either having
a confirmed diagnosis or not having a disorder. Rather, cases fall along a
'continuum of certainty.' "[24] This suggests that the time to resolve diagnoses was likely underestimated and that interpretations of diagnostic resolution may not have been shared by all clinicians and parents.

The geneticists in our study directly linked the emergence of diagnostic uncertainty to the recent expansion of newborn screening. Dr. De Vries explained the novelty of these uncertainties to the parents of Mike Honan: "So, that's the pluses and minuses of doing this newborn screening: it's good when you can find something and you're sure, but then, when you're kind of in this gray area, you're kind of just not sure. This is sort of the gray area that we're in, in terms of newborn screening and identifying whether this is really an affected patient or not." Expanded newborn screening identified more patients than anticipated, most of whom were asymptomatic, and required the production of new knowledge and testing to determine whether they were truly affected.

Patients-in-waiting were made in clinical interactions and did not strictly correlate with specific conditions. The ambiguity of geneticists' interactions with patients-in-waiting, however, reflected geneticists' understanding of how screening and test results corresponded to what they knew about conditions. As such, if the understanding of these conditions changed, some of the uncertainties might disappear. The contrast between patients-in-waiting and patients with established conditions was clearest in our observations of patients diagnosed with classic PKU via newborn screening. Parents whose children had PKU were also shocked by the results of newborn screening and came to the clinic with many questions. But when they visited the geneticist they received authoritative answers, a clear diagnostic picture, and an overview of the treatment options. Geneticists anticipated particular PKU-related concerns because they had been dealing with the same situations for 50 years. What was still an emergency for families had become a routine for clinicians.[25] This did not mean that families of children with PKU skipped happily out of the clinic, but physicians' communication took on a more authoritative tone.

Over the course of our study, we noticed that some clinical interactions with the families of newly diagnosed patients started to look more similar to the encounters with PKU patients. As time passed, the geneticists seemed to gain confidence in diagnosing and treating some patients with ambiguous screening results. In other cases, diagnostic uncertainty was no longer a surprise: it was something to work through. Geneticists warned families early on that it was possible they would never come to a conclusive answer. For still other conditions, some test results were increasingly viewed more definitively, as either true or false positives, while still others continued to perplex the geneticists.

This gradual and still tentative demonstration of confidence developed from personal clinical experiences and the accumulated wisdom of an international collective of geneticists facing similar diagnostic and treatment dilemmas. The clinic participated in the previously cited statewide follow-up study, but, according to the geneticists, such follow-up fell short of the kind of in-depth, prospective study required to evaluate health outcomes. Geneticists engaged in a collective learning process by exchanging experiences at conferences, state and regional meetings, on Listservs, and through e-mail and phone calls. As we work out in more detail in the next chapter, this collective learning process affected how clinicians approached ambiguities and understood the nature of the screened disorders. Tests that clinicians might have wavered over for several months were later done as a matter of course, even before the infant was referred to the clinic. Questions about diet or sleeping were answered with greater certainty and authority, even if the answers reflected opinions gleaned from a Listserv.

While accumulated experience allowed the clinical staff to answer patient concerns with greater confidence and certainty, diagnostic uncertainty did not undermine their authority. Rather than exposing clinicians as incompetent, diagnostic uncertainty posed a common challenge for the genetics team and the parents. By commenting on the uncertain characteristics of diagnosis and conveying that they would go out of their way to help resolve the ambiguity, clinicians laid the groundwork for trusting relationships. With few alternative sources of information and expertise available, parents had little choice but to rely upon the genetics team. Thus, rather than undermining authority, diagnostic uncertainty reinforced the healthcare team as professionals.

*     *     *

Despite the ongoing refinement of diagnostic uncertainty, patients-in-waiting are here to stay. Newborn screening will inevitably create a population of people who are caught betwixt and between health and pathology. Parents may receive a diagnostic label without a clear idea of whether and how the condition will affect their child. We can find patients-in-waiting in other settings, too. One hot spot lies around genetic susceptibility testing. People undergoing such tests and assessments are typically asymptomatic but may be at an increased risk for a condition. Another group includes those who suffer from what historian Charles Rosenberg called proto-disease states,[26] conditions such as elevated blood pressure, high cholesterol levels, or obesity that once indicated contributing factors or symptoms but now are treated as incipient diseases. Patients-in-waiting inhabit a liminal state between normality and pathology, imposed by medical screening and testing technologies, characterized by a lengthy process of medical surveillance to resolve diagnostic uncertainty, which might spill over into personal identity and other areas of social life.

Patients-in-waiting experience a declassification without reclassification:[27] no longer healthy but not really sick, they hover in an in-between state due to abnormal test results. Without illness experiences but with novel harbingers of disease, they experience the anticipation of a disease that they may never acquire. The social significance of diagnosis has always been its functionality: the ability to structure medical encounters, institute health policies, shape life strategies, even control deviance. In the case of patients-in-waiting, this social significance is extended to those living between health and disease. For newborns, this meant that they were launched soon after birth onto a diagnostic journey.

## CHAPTER THREE

# Shifting Disease Ontologies

D iseases change. They are not stable objects but are transformed based on the practices they become part of.[1] They change not simply within patient bodies and populations but also ontologically and epistemologically: what we understand as a specific disease and how we know about a disease. Historians have examined how signs and symptoms are grouped differently over time and place, rendering dissimilar physical and mental processes visible, shifting processes of causality, affecting novel patient populations, relating differently to professional practices and healthcare systems.[2] Key examples include the medicalization and demedicalization of homosexuality in psychiatry;[3] the radical shift in understanding of HIV/AIDS over a 20-year period from a fatal, mystery condition affecting heroin users, Haitians, hemophiliacs, and homosexuals to an equal opportunity chronic disease;[4] and the transformation of high blood pressure over the past century from a health indicator to a proto-disease linked to stroke and heart disease.[5] In fact, the notion that people suffer from a specific disease—rather than an imbalance between a person and the environment—is a historical achievement of medical thinking that dates back to the late eighteenth century.[6]

Ontological and epistemological changes in diseases matter for the actions they facilitate. A disease is a medically sanctioned opportunity for action: to diagnose, prevent, prognosticate, care, and cure, but also to commiserate, suffer, hope, fight, take stock, vindicate, surrender, and legitimate other actions. Among these actions is a resilient but underappreciated category of medical work: teasing out the altered disease parameters. Changes in the nature of diseases may occur gradually or be provoked by technological innovations. Technological catalysts include pharmaceuticals in search of a disease target,[7] the creation of new classification systems or guidelines for disease detection,[8] the development of diagnostic tools,[9] or, as we will illustrate in this chapter, the introduction of population-based screening programs. Such technological change agents are insufficient to consolidate new realities for diseases. Social scientists have noted that new disease categories require massive infrastructures needed to operationalize diseases as feasible clinical entities and link potential patients to diagnostic and treatment modalities.[10] Throughout this process the understanding of what the disease is—its natural history, severity, patient populations, treatment response—and its possibilities for action are also transformed.

We showed in the previous chapter how the genetics team managed diagnostic uncertainty for families whose infants with positive newborn screening results lingered in the borderland between true and false positives. As geneticists worked out what to tell these families, they faced a related set of uncertainties about the nature of screened conditions that transcended the immediacy of individual patients and families. As clinicians and public health researchers have learned from population screening for phenylketonuria (PKU),[11] sickle cell anemia,[12] cystic fibrosis,[13] cervical cancer,[14] and other conditions, once screening was implemented, diseases did not behave as expected based on previous scientific knowledge. Population screening produced anomalous findings in light of what clinicians thought they knew about the conditions. These unexpected findings encompass all clinically relevant aspects of prevention: disease incidence, severity, the distinction between pathological and benign variations, and response to treatment. These anomalies provoke the fundamental question: *what is the nature of the condition we are screening for?* As we will show, clinicians helped to bridge the ontological gap between pre- and postscreening knowledge.

We examine here a critical dimension of the work required to incorporate new medical technologies into work settings. This dimension of bridging work addresses the production of new knowledge about the nature of conditions included in newborn screening. Newly adopted screening technologies are supposed to detect well-known diseases but instead produce information that no longer fits the knowledge base. We refer to unexpected findings related to the knowledge properties of screened conditions as *anomalies* because these findings are unusual in light of the scientific knowledge base prior to the implementation of new technologies. These anomalies require identification and remedial work to incorporate the technology into work practices. Such work involves recognizing anomalous findings in light of the existing knowledge stock, collectively negotiating the parameters of the anomaly, and developing new operating procedures to manage the changed understanding of the disease.

Adjusting the knowledge properties of diseases unsettled by screening technologies involves the realm of translational research, or the process of linking the laboratory and the clinic. As others have pointed out, the relationship between the laboratory and clinic is bidirectional and requires frequent adjustment.[15] Science studies scholars Peter Keating and Albert Cambrosio's notion of a "biomedical platform," consisting of interconnected biomedical entities and a set of technologies, skills, and regulations necessary to move across the laboratory-clinical interface, highlights that new technologies are not automatically clinically relevant but require further work for standard clinical use.[16] Their example of immunophenotyping demonstrated that the introduction of a new technology to ascertain cell populations also required the creation of new reagents, a new nomenclature of biomarkers, and consequently, standards of equivalence between different reagents, new disease categories in light of these new markers, and new disease entities that could be tested in clinical trials. In turn, these innovations looped back, defining the utility and efficacy of the technological platform. This work thus revealed the reflexive and creative dimension of technology implementation: clinical relevance is earned.

In genetics, where most knowledge about disease susceptibility depends on specific laboratory tests, the ontological properties of diseases are established not only in the laboratory but also in the clinic. Rather than playing a secondary role in the era of evidence-based medicine, the clinic reemerges as a site of knowledge production. For rare genetic diseases, randomized clinical trial data are nonexistent and even clinical experience is in short supply. Sociologist Joanna Latimer and colleagues observed how genetic dysmorphologists actively generate, debate, and evaluate categories of genetic classification rather than apply externally produced molecular or cytogenetic laboratory knowledge.[17] Observations of dysmorphology and other perceptual clues may qualify genetic findings, especially because genetic tests are often inconclusive. Similarly, in oncology and psychiatric genetic clinics, the implementation of molecular medicine "far from reifying and simplifying pathological situations, expand[s] and recompose[s] them in different ways."[18] This continued role for the clinic in the production of genetic knowledge is not simply a temporary placeholder until technologies provide more definitive tests. Instead, the promise of each new test to resolve ambiguity remains "deferred" until clinicians determine how and when to use genetic knowledge.[19] The clinic thus remains a site of knowledge production where anomalous results need to be addressed for screening technologies to obtain intended goals.

Because we are interested in how expanded newborn screening changes the understanding of specific diseases, we have organized this chapter by disorder and focus on how clinicians shifted the knowledge properties of diseases over the course of our study. A caveat: the processes of knowledge production are ongoing in the clinic and the laboratory, and consensus about the nature of the conditions we discuss will continue to evolve. Rather than pinning down precisely what these conditions are, we draw attention to the clinical work that transformed knowledge properties for rare diseases.

## MCADD

Medium-chain acyl-coenzyme A dehydrogenase deficiency (MCADD), first identified in 1982, has repeatedly been presented as the prototype disease for the expansion of newborn screening. With little symptom development, the natural history of this condition was not well understood, but the prospect of death as an initial manifestation and an uncomplicated treatment made a compelling case for screening. During the expansion of newborn screening, advocates marshaled research suggesting that infant deaths attributed to sudden infant death syndrome (SIDS) might have been caused by undiagnosed MCADD, although the number of SIDS cases attributed to MCADD postmortem remained small.[20] Yet despite being the model for expanded newborn screening, even this most common of the fatty oxidation disorders was transformed with the expansion of screening.

What did geneticists know about MCADD prior to newborn screening? MCADD is caused by mutations in the ACADM gene that can cause shortages of medium-chain acyl-coenzyme A dehydrogenase, an enzyme required to metabolize medium-chain fatty acids. This enzymatic deficiency can result in the improper metabolism of medium-chain fatty acids and their accumulation in the blood, which in turn may be associated with lethargy, hypoglycemia, and liver and brain damage. The primary threat for such metabolic crises is a prolonged period of fasting, especially during an illness, which, if left untreated, may result in death. MCADD thus constitutes a predisposition to disease requiring a second trigger of metabolic stress to produce symptoms.

Prior to newborn screening, MCADD patients usually came to medical attention with an episode of severe lethargy or even coma due to hypoglycemia. Mortality rates during such episodes hovered around 25 percent, and another large minority of survivors suffered significant morbidity, including irreversible neurological impairments or developmental delays.[21] According to the prevailing wisdom prior to newborn screening, MCADD occurred due to a founder effect most common among non-Hispanic white populations of North-West European descent.

The treatment for MCADD is a low-fat diet and, above all, to avoid fasting and be particularly vigilant when the patient becomes ill and stops eating. Occasionally, clinicians prescribe additional dietary measures such as carnitine supplements or drinking a cornstarch solution—a slow-metabolizing carbohydrate—before bedtime or in the middle of the night. Geneticists recommend that parents take the child to an emergency department to receive intravenous glucose if the child vomits repeatedly and cannot keep food down. Most symptoms occur before age six, a period of rapid development, but adult onset remains a possibility.

## Diagnosis

In clinical consultations, we observed knowledge-in-the-making in tandem with a shifting biomedical literature: what had been viewed as a more or less homogeneous disease with little variation, newborn screening unsettled. The first contested issue was what qualified as an MCADD diagnosis. Tests working at different levels of analysis produced different possibilities for diagnosis, and these differences needed to be reconciled. In the recent past, patients identified with MCADD exhibited clinical signs and symptoms, which were then confirmed by biochemical testing. The combination of clinical symptoms and biochemical findings was sufficient to establish the diagnosis, but physicians could confirm the diagnosis with genetic mutation analysis. Before the introduction of population screening, about 80 percent of patients were homozygous and about 18 percent heterozygous for the c.985A>G mutation.[22] Since symptoms were already present and the child was obviously affected by the condition, genetic testing did not offer therapeutic value. MCADD was thus a disease in which physical symptoms signaled a biochemical abnormality that corresponded to a common genetic profile. A 2001 study identified a second mutation, c.199T>C, which the authors described as a "*mild* folding mutation that exhibits decreased levels of enzyme activity only under stringent condition."[23]

The consistency between symptoms, biochemistry, and genetics was undone by prospective population-based screening. With screening, the entry point for an MCADD diagnosis became a biochemical value, rather than phenotypic evidence. In our study, all newborn screening patients suspected of having MCADD were asymptomatic in the period just after birth. The main indication that an infant might have MCADD was an elevated C8-acylcarnitine level.[24] The anomaly requiring bridging work in the clinic was whether *all* abnormal biochemical levels constituted pathology in the absence of symptoms or whether *some* screening results reflected incidental findings without clinical implications. Here, genetic testing gained importance because the prevailing knowledge suggested that the c.199T>C mutation had "milder" pathogenic effects than the c.985A>G mutation. Screening thus separated symptoms from biochemical indicators and turned genetic information into the arbiter.

We observed the development of the increased reliance on genetic testing to determine the severity of MCADD when, early on in our research, Dr. Silverman urged Kim and Dan Martin to consent to DNA analysis for their daughter Molly. At the time, the newborn screening program did not cover the approximately $1,000 cost of genetic sequencing. Dr. Silverman's request was complicated by his acknowledgment that the results would not affect treatment since he considered Molly's biochemical levels sufficient to constitute an MCADD diagnosis. Regardless of the DNA results, he would recommend that the Martins feed Molly a low-fat diet and increase their vigilance during periods of fasting. After first declining the test, Kim and Dan consented, and the results showed that Molly was heterozygous for the c.985A>G and the c.199T> C mutation. Dr. Silverman presented this as "reassuring news" because "nobody who's had this [c.199T>C] mutation found on newborn screening has yet turned up to have an acute episode due to MCADD." He explained: "They're both affecting her but together the 199 is mild enough to generally protect her from the adverse consequences of the 985." He also referred to the c.199T>C mutation as an "optimistic" mutation. Perceptively, Dan interpreted the finding as "two wrongs can make it right."

From then on, Dr. Silverman urged his colleagues to conduct DNA analysis for MCADD routinely and not simply rely on biochemical levels. Genetic testing offered an added "good counseling" value because it allowed for a more precise prognosis about the disease trajectory. This strategy seemed to pay off when the c.199T>C mutation was identified in a large number of patients with elevated C8 levels. Because of these experiences, Dr. Silverman and others successfully advocated for state re-imbursement of mutation analysis for the common MCADD mutations.

Genetic testing for MCADD was only helpful in making a diagnosis when the results confirmed the two common mutations. Initial DNA analysis specifically targeted these mutations, but following population screening, DNA testing also identified previously unknown variants. About a year into our study, Dr. Flores ordered a test for the two common MCADD mutations for a patient that screened positive at birth. The results came back negative. Dr. Flores was prepared to dismiss the patient as a likely carrier when, at Monica's insistence, he sequenced the full gene. He found that the patient was homozygous for a mutation that was at that point unknown. Unknown genetic information did not clarify the clinical significance of the biochemical elevations.

When Dr. Flores found that the daughter of Brigitte Berns and Alain Bonniau had a known and an unknown mutation, he ordered mutation analysis for both parents to see whether the person who had passed on the unknown mutation showed phenotypic signs of MCADD. He explained his rationale: "But we don't know for sure [that the mutation causes MCADD]. So how do we find out—how do we get additional evidence to strengthen our suspicion that this might actually cause MCADD? One way is to test both of you. How do we do that? Well, we just get a teaspoon of blood from you, a teaspoon of blood from you, get the genetic material, and do the same thing. Who carried what, because these mutations came from either one of you. Did both of them come from one of you, or did one come from Dad and one come from Mom, we don't know that. To find that out we'll check one of you, each one of you. Let's say one of you carries this change that we really don't understand. If we compare that to your blood and see what your fatty acids look like, if your fatty acids look abnormal then we know that the mutation causes the condition. Does that make sense so far?"

The test results indicated that Alain had a single copy of the unknown mutation but no elevated C8 levels. This information had limited value because it failed to confirm that biochemical elevations could occur with the unknown mutation. Dr. Flores explained the still ambivalent status of MCADD diagnosis to the couple: "Newborn screening has opened up a whole new era of research on the molecular basis of this condition because now the original test just measures the fats, right? So now we're finding that we cannot sometimes just diagnose the condition just based on that. So we have to go to the DNA test, which is what we did in your case. And when we do that, we find all sorts of new mutations that have never been seen before because the cases are probably milder, and so we never saw them before."

Thus, MCADD was transformed from a disease with consistency between symptoms, metabolic levels, and genetic mutations, into a condition for which these levels no longer correlated and clinical consequences had been cast into doubt. Genetic testing, long believed to be the definitive indicator of clinical significance, could now aggravate uncertainty when the mutations had unknown clinical significance. Geneticists' efforts to overcome these uncertainties relied upon the general modus operandi of medical professionals faced with a situation lacking a scientifically agreed-upon course of action: repeat testing and checking with colleagues.

## Severity and Incidence

"DNA sequencing," Dr. Malvern explained to a family, "can either tell us a lot of information or not give us conclusive information." An increased reliance on genetic testing to interpret the meaning of biochemical elevations in asymptomatic patients required geneticists to revise their knowledge of the severity and incidence of MCADD. At a 2010 staff meeting, Dr. Silverman mentioned an article that had taken stock of five years of gene sequencing at the Mayo Clinic. The authors noted that newborn screening revealed several "ACADM variants of unknown significance for which it is not clear whether the DNA variants are rare polymorphisms or pathogenic mutations."[25] MCADD broke down into "carrier-like," "intermediate," and "severe" variants.[26] "Carrier-like" meant that an individual inherited a genetic trait but did not exhibit symptoms associated with the mutation. The intermediate level implied "a degree of functional deficiency" that required treatment and clinical follow-up although the "clinical risk" remained unclear, while the severe form suggested a higher clinical risk.[27] To distinguish between these three types, the authors correlated 75 genetic mutations—many of which had not been previously documented—with a broad array of biochemical findings including the concentration of C8 in blood plasma, the ratio of $C8/C2$, the ratio of $C8/C10$, and the excretion of hexanoylglycine (HG) in urine.[28] The geneticists in our study treated this article as a new tool to deal with the problem of genotypic variants with unknown clinical significance. Dr. Silverman mentioned the research in a consultation with a family to explain why the condition needed to be taken seriously: "Well, it's a paper from the Mayo Clinic, in which they do a lot of the sequencing, and they're also experts on this whole business of testing. What the object of the paper was, and this sounds a little bit pedantic, what the object of this testing is, is to say, can you guess from unknown mutations, how likely they are to be serious?" Dr. Silverman continued, "They took people who were known [to have] serious mutations, and both of these mutations may be serious, but they're not well known, which is okay. One of them is known, and one of them can be inferred to be pretty serious. . . . So anyway, they have this algorithm." Dr. Silverman then proceeded to discuss the patient's hexanoylglycine level, which we had not heard him do before in an MCADD case. Bringing the scientific literature to bear on the experience of clinical uncertainty resulted in an expanded set of biochemical criteria for defining MCADD, and a stronger sense that this patient's MCADD was serious.

What qualified as "common" MCADD also needed revision. Prior to newborn screening, researchers estimated that 80–90 percent of MCADD patients had the c.985A>G mutation, but following the implementation of screening programs in Germany, Australia, and the United States, the incidence was downgraded to about 50 percent.[29] The same newborn screening experiences also suggested that while the c.985A>G mutation is more common among Northern Europeans, other population groups may have different mutations and the worldwide incidence of the condition is approximately twice as high as previously thought.[30] One couple in our study was hopeful that their child might not have MCADD because the father was Eastern European and the mother Mexican, and they had read on the Internet that, as they told us, "this is mostly a Northern European trait." However, Dr. De Vries explained that such information was quickly becoming outdated. Indeed, when the Mayo study became available, we e-mailed Dr. Flores the article to see whether it could help clarify the situation of a patient we saw in the clinic. Dr. Flores replied and copied the entire genetics team:

> Stefan forwarded me the article that [Dr. Silverman] mentioned at clinic conference in which they classify the severity of mutations identified to date in MCADD patients. This was very helpful. For [Osiel Gamboa], whom we saw this past Monday, he is homozygous (due to consanguinity) for the c.443G>A variant. Turns out that according to the paper "the c.443G>A variant is frequent among individuals with Latin American ancestry and is a biochemically intermediate mutation. In vitro fatty acid ß-oxidation flux analysis of fibroblasts from one subject homozygous for the c.443G>A mutation demonstrated

a phenotype consistent with intermediate MCAD deficiency (C8 = 0.165 lmol/g protein)."[31] This mutation will become more and more relevant as our patient population is relatively skewed towards "Latin American ancestry" and this mutation may be over-represented in future cases.

Beyond expanding the patient populations previously associated with MCADD, this discussion shows one way in which ethnicity may become salient in genetics. Some social scientists have regarded causal connections between race and genetic variants with suspicion, fearing that the conflation of racial categories with biomedical classifications may reify race as a biological construct.[32] One concern is that population differences could be used to classify people in biomedically similar groups, in which race would function as a placeholder for disease risks. For example, geneticists might screen only people of "Latin American ancestry" for the c443G>A variant rather than the entire population. We did not observe this occurring in the discussion of Osiel Gamboa. Dr. Flores picked up on the link between MCADD and ancestry after the MCADD variant had been found. Here, Osiel's heritage did not suggest a particular genetic risk. Rather, an indeterminate variant became meaningful in light of his ethnic background. Thus, Dr. Flores did not rely on race to screen for genetic variants but located an individual variant in a racially congruent context.[33]

Due to newborn screening, MCADD proliferates. There are more asymptomatic cases of MCADD, but more variants of the condition exist alongside each other. Inevitably, such heterogeneity provokes important questions about which variants constitute "real" cases of disease or whether MCADD is too diverse to be considered a singular disease. Here, proliferation did not lead to ontological disintegration because the geneticists worked to maintain a common identity across the MCADD variants. Clinicians reclassified and ranked the patients and corresponding MCADD variants along a continuum of severity based upon their genetic and metabolic profiles.

*Treatment*

The ontological transformation and expansion of the MCADD category did not affect treatment protocols. Geneticists erred on the side of safety by sticking to the treatment protocol developed prior to screening, despite postscreening MCADD differentiation. The standardized treatment protocol helped to maintain a singular identity for MCADD and indirectly addressed some of the confusion about the changing nature of MCADD following the implementation of screening. This uniform treatment regimen worked for MCADD because the treatment was noninvasive; it consisted of vigilance during periods of vomiting and reduced food intake, regular feedings with a low-fat diet, and, occasionally, dietary supplements. The geneticist instructed the parents to go to the closest emergency department if the child became ill and could not eat, and issued an emergency letter for parents to share with hospital staff. The genetics staff strategically deployed the universal treatment protocol in spite of MCADD variation to address the parental distress caused by newborn screening results. Here, universal treatment suggested that clinicians were knowledgeable about treatment in spite of the wide range of MCADD variations discovered via newborn screening.

When Molly Martin's test results showed a heterozygous mutation, Dr. Silverman warned the Martins that they should not get "cocky" with the results because Molly was not disease-free: "Obviously, if she pukes her guts out one day, you really want to take more precautions than you would take for the child who didn't have this." Regardless of the severity of the condition, Dr. Silverman reminded Kim and Dan not to let Molly fast for more than four to eight hours and to be especially vigilant if she was ill, and more particularly, vomiting. Dr. Silverman summarized the knowledge about treatment: "It turns out that the only thing that we know for sure prevents the adverse consequences of this is not letting the kids fast for a long time. All the other [treatments] appear to be window dressing."

With this treatment regimen in place, geneticists adapted other, less critical interventions to a changing consensus in the field. For example, the number of hours that MCADD patients were advised to go without food evolved over the course of our study. Initially, geneticists instructed parents of MCADD patients to feed their newborn every two to three hours and to keep up this regime until the sixth month. Informed by an international Listserv, the geneticists changed their recommendation, adding one extra hour for each month since the infant's birth. Thus, a four-month-old could sleep for four hours uninterrupted and a six-month-old for six hours. The limit of uninterrupted sleep was set at eight hours. We observed other preventive measures being relaxed over the course of our study, again regardless of the severity of the mutation. Some of the parents whose children were diagnosed with MCADD soon after newborn screening was implemented had been instructed to feed their children a solution of water mixed with cornstarch, a slow-metabolizing carbohydrate, before bedtime to avoid prolonged fasting.

The geneticists used the ambiguity in treatment regimens strategically: they erred on the side of caution but also adjusted less critical preventive measures in response to parents' concerns. In some cases, the geneticist negotiated the number of hours the child could sleep, responding to parents' reluctance to wake a sleeping baby. Dr. Flores told the parents of a four-month-old boy whom the parents preferred to let sleep: "We just have to reach a compromise. I'm happy to reach a medium of five [hours of sleep] but not more than that." The compromise showed responsiveness to parental desires and conveyed that MCADD should not be taken too lightly. The number of hours of sleep was a negotiable preventive treatment: geneticists realized that the time limit of one hour extra for each month since the infant's birth was chosen largely for its heuristic and mnemonic value. Some parents preferred to hold to stricter preventive measures to strengthen their child's safety net.

The uniform treatment regimen indirectly addressed some of the anomalies in the knowledge base revealed by expanded newborn screening. The geneticists' actions conveyed that despite uncertainties about whether every mutation and biochemical abnormality was pathological, the treatment was straightforward and effective. Bridging work in the treatment area thus involved maintaining prescreening knowledge in spite of changed MCADD ontology.

*Outcomes*

An early literature review on MCADD health outcomes after newborn screening concluded: "There is very little risk of death after diagnosis" and "The risk of intellectual deficit or other morbidities in survivors is small."[34] The geneticists in our study initially echoed this message to reassure anxious parents, whose experiences seemed to confirm a growing consensus about the nature of MCADD. Several patients went to the emergency department during an illness episode, but none suffered lasting consequences. One patient, Kari Buchanan, required a hospitalization after contracting swine flu, but she also stabilized quickly when the emergency department staff administered glucose intravenously, which provided further evidence for the genetic staff's opinion that MCADD could be treated effectively. The proliferation of "carrier-like" and "intermediate" MCADD in the clinic increasingly seemed to suggest that most of the MCADD cases revealed by expanded newborn screening lay at the "milder" end of the spectrum.

In September 2010, however, the genetics team became aware of a study showing that some infants have died from MCADD even after newborn screening diagnosis and close medical surveillance.[35] Monica, who forwarded us the article, described it as "scary stuff," and indicated that she wanted to call the parents of all of her MCADD patients to tell them to be very cautious, especially when the child vomited. This article modified the MCADD knowledge base once again and encouraged the genetics staff to impress on families with even more urgency to seek medical care at the first signs of illness. The article may also prompt adjustments for a different set of anomalies. Rather than employing uncertainties to reassure, the staff may deploy the same uncertainties to alert families to unpredictable dangers. Bridging work, then, consisted of continuously working out unexpected results in the clinic, as they emerged in real time.

\* \* \*

MCADD as a singular and distinct disease category survived the incorporation of anomalous findings produced by expanded newborn screening. The prescreening spectrum from "mild" to "severe" MCADD combined with a noninvasive treatment proved sufficiently flexible to integrate MCADD infants that differed from prescreening patients. MCADD diversified along multiple dimensions, but it remained the same broad category of disease.

## Hyperprolinemia

Hyperprolinemia, in contrast, was weakened by its encounter with expanded newborn screening, raising the question of whether the condition was a true disease and a viable screening target. Hyperprolinemia was not included on the ACMG's recommended uniform screening panel, but the state of California still reported elevated proline levels and mandated follow-up treatment because public health officials had decided that the program had an ethical obligation to report all abnormal screening results.[36] Here, we revisit the case of Ana Lancerio, introduced in the previous chapter, to focus on how Ana's case affected the ontological status of hyperprolinemia.

When Dr. Dati discovered that he had a baby with hyperprolinemia on his schedule, he went online and checked the NIH Genetics home reference page[37] to read up on the condition, which he was unfamiliar with, despite his expertise in metabolic disorders. He read online that there are two kinds of hyperprolinemia. Type 1, generally considered benign, is associated with proline levels 3 to 10 times above the normal level and mutations in the PRODH gene. Type 2 involves levels 10 to 15 times higher than normal and is associated with mutations in the ALDH4A1 gene. The prevalence of the condition was unknown, and it had been linked to mental retardation and schizophrenia. There was currently no treatment indicated for type 1 or type 2 hyperprolinemia, except for treating seizures with anticonvulsants.

Dr. Dati could not determine the relevance of Ana's proline levels with any certainty. Ana's proline levels were 1,300 μmol/L, while the normal range is 100–250 μmol/L. She was on the cusp between type 1 and type 2, and only a genetic test could provide a conclusive answer. At the time of Ana's visit, however, commercial testing for the genetic mutations was unavailable. Other uncertainties related to the discrepancy between normal cutoff points and much higher levels indicative of pathology, the question of whether hyperprolinemia was an abnormal biochemical variant or a disease with clinical implications, as well as the symptoms indicative of hyperprolinemia, their timing of onset, and the required course of action. Without a differential diagnosis protocol to adjudicate the seriousness of the condition, Dr. Dati had to determine what constituted an appropriate level of follow-up and vigilance.

Falling back on the routine of additional testing, his first step was to gather more data through urinalysis, to check his hunch that the elevated level could be an artifact of the initial screen that would disappear upon retesting. The follow-up test showed a proline level of 25 in the urine, while anything under 100–250 is normal. "In other words," Dr. Dati explained at Ana's next clinic visit, "in the urine the proline is normal. Now, what does it mean? Well, it's uncommon for kids to have high proline in the blood and not high in the urine. What is possible is that everything has gone away. So I would like to do another test in the blood to see. I am just wondering whether it was not something transient because the urine was so normal and usually if the proline is high in the blood, it is high in the urine." Dr. Dati interpreted the discrepancy between the two data points as either a testing artifact or an indication that the initial elevated level had stabilized within the normal range. When Isabella, Ana's foster mother, asked Dr. Dati how the proline level in the urine could be low but high in the blood, he answered that he did not know. He added: "My read of it is that it is going to end up as a biochemical finding. I can't prove it right now but it looks like type 1 hyperprolinemia which is almost a serendipitous finding and there is almost no symptoms." Still, he wanted to see them back in six months to make sure that everything was progressing appropriately.

The repeat blood test indicated a blood proline level of 329, close to the normal range. For Dr. Dati, the evidence pointed strongly to a clinically insignificant biochemical finding. Yet, just in case symptoms developed later on, he decided to follow Ana once per year. In the end, the data strategy left questions unanswered. Dr. Dati did not know for sure whether the initially elevated levels for hyperprolinemia indicated a biochemical artifact. But he was confident that with repeated levels in the blood plasma and the urine close to the normal range, he had sufficient information *in this case* to follow the patient only annually.

The ambiguous nature of hyperprolinemia became apparent when Isabella asked Dr. Dati whether Ana's older brother should also be tested for hyperprolinemia because he was born prior to the implementation of newborn screening. Because hyperprolinemia is an autosomal recessive disorder, Ana's brother had a 25 percent chance of also being affected. Dr. Dati demurred, "I am not for testing to burden kids. There is an ethical issue here. Sort of medicalizing. Let's say we find that proline is high. Then there will be a totally different look on this kid, whether you want it or not. I would rather not." This answer was striking because, of course, the same medicalization was now in full force in Ana's case.

In the end, the knowledge produced in this one patient was pooled with other similar patients and led to a different screening cutoff point. Dr. Silverman and other metabolic specialists requested that the state raise the cutoff points for hyperprolinemia because symptomatic individuals typically had levels multiple times higher. They prevailed, and the cutoff point was raised to 1,000, making hyperprolinemia a very rare disorder.

The inclusion of hyperprolinemia in expanded newborn screening led to a short-lived expansion of its patient base. The visibility that expanded newborn screening brought to the condition also brought its ontological properties into sharp relief and led to tinkering with cutoff points. Without genetic testing or any available treatment, the condition settled more as a biochemical artifact than a bona fide disease entity. Indeed, when, 18 months after the first hyperprolinemia patient, a second patient with elevated proline levels was referred to the clinic, Dr. Malvern's first reaction was: "I thought we decided this was a nondisease." The trajectory of this patient was very different from Ana's: the patient was dismissed after an initial visit to explain the nonsignificance of the findings.

## Maternal Diagnosis in Carnitine Transporter Deficiency

> Dr. Dati entered the examination room of Clara Miner, a two-month-old baby, saying to her mother, Sybil: "Hi, good to see you." After Sybil answered, "Good to see you," Dr. Dati turned to Clara: "Hi baby." Sybil volunteered: "We didn't know if we were supposed to get her back dressed." Standing next to Clara, Dr. Dati answered: "This baby looks great. She's chunky." Sybil added: "Twelve pounds. She just measured." Dr. Dati began to examine the baby apologizing: "My hands are cold. They are cold. I'm mean. I'm sorry." His examination showed nothing remarkable. Then Dr. Dati caught himself and turned to Clara: "In fact, you know, I don't think she's supposed to be the patient today, right?" Sybil answered: "I didn't think so." Dr. Dati then added, "You're supposed to be the patient." Sybil replied, "Yes."

Dr. Dati's confusion over the patient role was understandable in this case. An undressed, weighed, and measured infant had appeared in a pediatric genetics clinic for a newborn screening consult. Yet the baby was not the patient. The mother was. This was Sybil and Clara's second visit for carnitine deficiency. Clara was identified with low carnitine levels on newborn screening. Her initial levels were 5 μmol/L while the normal levels are between 28 and 59 μmol/L.

A review article published in 2006 summarizes the state of knowledge about carnitine deficiencies prior to newborn screening.[38] Carnitine is an amino acid, produced in the kidneys and liver and derived from meat and dairy products in the diet. Carnitine is involved in the transfer of long-chain fatty acids into the mitochondria for beta-oxidation. Carnitine deficiency is a metabolic state in which carnitine concentrations in blood plasma and tissues are less than the levels required for normal function of the organism. Low carnitine levels may imply several issues. They may indicate a dietary side effect—that is, low levels may be due to a vegetarian or vegan diet. Low levels may also be a secondary indication of other metabolic conditions such as fatty acid oxidation disorders and organic acidemias. This is why some patients with MCADD in our study took carnitine supplements. Finally, low levels may also indicate a stand-alone condition called carnitine transporter deficiency. The disorder was identified in 1975,[39] and the inherited mutations in the SLC22A5 gene that encodes the carnitine transporter were cloned in 1998 and linked to chromosome 5q31 in 1998.[40] The condition weakens muscles and may cause cardiomyopathy and skeletal muscle weakness by age two to four, and also affects the central nervous system. Carnitine transporter deficiency can be treated with carnitine supplements, which raise plasma carnitine levels to normal but muscle carnitine concentrations to only 5–10 percent of normal. Still, these low levels seem sufficient for affected patients. Because some patients died after stopping treatment, carnitine supplementation is lifelong.[41]

In the case of carnitine transporter deficiency, the main ontological dilemma brought up by newborn screening was not only the nature of the disease but also the nature of the patient: screening may lead to the diagnosis of the mother, rather than the infant.[42] Some infants had low carnitine levels at newborn screening due to low maternal carnitine levels. Once fed formula, however, these infants did fine. In spite of initial low carnitine levels, the infants "improved briskly."[43] "Truly" affected infants would need a longer period of carnitine supplements to normalize levels and even then might never attain normal rates. Follow-up testing showed the reason for this anomalous recovery: their mothers had low plasma carnitine levels, consistent with carnitine transporter deficiency. The infants had low levels at birth because of carnitine transferred from the placenta to the fetus during gestation, and later, to the infant through breast-feeding. Maternal diagnosis via expanded newborn screening was an issue not only for carnitine transporter deficiency but also for glutaric acidemia type 1,[44] cobalamin C deficiency,[45] homocystinuria and methylmalonic acidemia,[46] 3-MCC,[47] and most recently, for MCADD.[48]

If an infant recovered quickly from anomalous metabolic levels, geneticists might have categorized the positive newborn screening value as a false positive result. Why, then, did the geneticists turn to mothers? Dr. Silverman recalled a chance hallway conversation at a conference in which the topic of maternal carnitine deficiency was raised. Mulling it over, he thought that they had a patient who also recovered unexpectedly rapidly from a carnitine deficiency. When they tested the mother, they found carnitine levels below the normal levels. Reflecting back on the discovery pattern, Dr. Silverman wondered why they had not thought of maternal mutations earlier. Geneticists knew of several precedents from population-based PKU screening in the 1970s.

When Dr. Silverman's patient was pooled with five mothers from other parts of the country, a set of anomalies emerged similar to those encountered in MCADD after newborn screening. Genetic testing indicated the presence of several known but also some unknown mutations implicated in carnitine transporter deficiency. In addition, while the consensus about the disorder was a "life-threatening inborn error of metabolism,"[49] three of these mothers had been asymptomatic, two had only experienced symptoms of fatigue, and one had experienced cardiac problems not necessarily linked to carnitine deficiency. The lack of symptoms was a puzzling finding because the conventional wisdom in genetics circles prior to expanded newborn screening was that carnitine deficiency was a serious condition that would lead to muscle weakness and neurological problems if untreated. Here were mothers with low levels of carnitine and corresponding genetic mutations and they had been doing well for decades. The authors also noted that the incidence of this condition should be revised. Based on screened cases, they estimated an incidence of 1/40,000 with 1 percent of the population as carriers, but cautioned that this was likely an underestimation because asymptomatic males were not identified through newborn screening, and, unaware of this maternal-infant link, some geneticists would have interpreted the rapidly stabilizing carnitine levels of infants as false positives.

Dr. Silverman drew two lessons from the discovery of maternal carnitine transporter deficiency. First, the experience required a revision of what was known about carnitine deficiency: the condition was not always "severe" and genetic mutations did not predict symptom developments. Second, these findings established, according to Dr. Silverman, "a new principle" that one could use newborn screening to pick up maternal disease.

We met the patient from the original article early on in our study. Ruth Chen was a Chinese immigrant with two children. At the time of the visit, she was pregnant with a third child. According to the article, her free carnitine level was 4 μmol/L and her son's level was 8 μmol/L and rose to 37 μmol/L on carnitine supplements. Dr. Silverman revealed during the visit: "Your levels were so low that we were scared to death." Ruth countered that she used to practice gymnastics in her youth. Prior to Dr. Silverman's arrival, she told us that she was more worried about taking supplements than about a condition that was supposed to be very serious but that did not seem to have affected her. She confided that according to her health beliefs, adjusting energy with medication was not necessarily beneficial: "Even though [the doctors] say [the supplement]'s like pure, natural, whatever. But any medicine to the Chinese is some poison. So I don't know. Because I was fine until they found out. Of course, it gives me some energy but a lot of stuff could give you energy." She agreed that she needed extra energy because she had young children but didn't consider supplements necessary after they grew up. Her family in China advised her to avoid doctors because "they just finding trouble for you."

Ruth's skepticism about the role of supplements was reinforced by her impression that "probably they don't know too much about [carnitine deficiency]" and that it was "probably not as bad as they say." When Dr. Silverman came to see her, he might have inadvertently confirmed her suspicions of ignorance when he stated, "Remember this is a new discovery. We're only finding women like you because we're testing your babies so we don't have very much experience with this. We think that you might have done fine without treatment but the treatment is protective." When Ruth asked whether adults with carnitine deficiency did badly, he answered, "We don't know that, for all we know, untreated you could drop dead at 50. We don't know. We don't know. It is a new discovery." Dr. Silverman expressed the consensus position among geneticists: that although maternal carnitine transporter deficiency is not well understood, the condition is sufficiently serious and the treatment sufficiently benign that lifelong treatment with carnitine is recommended. For someone who believes that taking pharmaceuticals has negative implications, his honest acknowledgment might have reinforced the conclusion that it was best not to take the carnitine long-term.

Our study contained four mothers who came to the geneticist's attention for carnitine transporter deficiency and two infants with the condition. In the former cases, the child's newborn screening results revealed that the mothers might have had carnitine transporter deficiency for their entire lives. Kayla Vennick asked incredulously, "So this is something, let's say, that you're born with. So technically if I have it I've had it for 30 years and I'm fine?" Dr. Flores responded, "That's correct. And in many cases, mothers are actually [fine]." Similarly, Sybil asked Dr. Dati, "That would mean that I've already had this my whole life, right?" Tina Schaffer found it hard to believe that she could have carnitine deficiency: she had been running marathons and worked out four to five times a week before the birth of her baby. Still, she noted that when she ran out of the carnitine supplement, her calve muscles seemed to cramp faster but, she qualified, the cramps could be due to dehydration. For Kayla and Sybil, the symptom of fatigue fit, but how many mothers of newborns would not admit to experiencing fatigue? Dr. Dati also asked whether Sybil experienced shortness of breath. Sybil answered that once in a while she indeed experienced shortness of breath, but she had attributed it to asthma. What she thought might have been asthma now became a possible symptom of carnitine transporter deficiency. Yet because Sybil's DNA analysis did not reveal any mutations involved in carnitine transporter deficiency, Dr. Dati thought it likely that she was a carrier of the deficiency whose carnitine levels were affected due to pregnancy. From a metabolic viewpoint, pregnancy is a "metabolically challenging state as energy consumption significantly increases."[50]

"Carnitine transporter deficiency," Dr. Flores explained to one mother during a clinic visit, "does not have a cure or a treatment." When the transporter is deficient, insufficient carnitine is absorbed into cells to turn nutrients into fats and sugar and remove toxins out of the body. Geneticists prescribed a supplement of carnitine in order to "shock" the system. One mother reported that the carnitine supplement gave her more energy but another noted no effects. Dr. Silverman replied that she was not supposed to feel a difference. He noted that an oversupply of carnitine would be excreted in the urine, but Dr. Dati told a mother of an infant that it was important to provide the right amount of carnitine because too much carnitine could cause problems as well. Geneticists described carnitine supplements as "neutral" and equivalent to a "protein shake," but the side effect was that the patient could develop diarrhea and a "fishy smell." (One woman's husband quipped that he did not "want to sleep with a fish.")

The question of who was the patient did not end with the mother. Mothers wondered whether their current and future children, their siblings and *their* children, and their parents were at risk for carnitine transporter deficiency. Carnitine deficiency is an autosomal recessive disorder, and therefore, the patient's siblings would have a 25 percent chance of being affected as well. The geneticists encouraged some of the mothers to discuss the possibility of carnitine deficiency with other family members, but they did not insist on testing even close relatives. For example, the geneticists checked mothers, but they did not check fathers for carnitine deficiency. This was partly because the infant's initial low carnitive levels could be attributed to the gestational environment and breastfeeding. Still, the fathers provided half of the genetic material and, especially in the two infants whose carnitine deficiency had been confirmed with mutation analysis, might also have been affected with the disorder. When we asked Dr. Silverman about the rationale for testing mothers but not fathers, he admitted that logically speaking fathers should be tested. He joked, "Nobody cares about fathers." Dr. Dati offered Sybil's husband the possibility of being tested, but because Clara had only moderately low carnitine levels and was likely only a carrier, the possibility that Sybil's husband was affected was low. The offer was not picked up.[51]

Although the treatment protocol called for lifelong carnitine supplementation and earlier experience had shown that asymptomatic patients could die suddenly, the geneticists were not adamant about following up with mothers diagnosed with carnitine deficiency. In part, this was because the clinic specialized in pediatric patients and the geneticists gave more leeway to adults in making decisions about their own health. Yet the uncertainty about the seriousness of the condition also made it more difficult to take a hard line. Another issue complicating care was that not all of these mothers had health insurance and easy access to follow-up visits and dietary supplements.

## Knowledge Ecologies

Newborn screening shifted the knowledge base of rare genetic conditions: geneticists found more and different diseases than they had anticipated. The genetics team worked to reassemble what newborn screening undid. The ontological component of bridging work implies several interrelated tasks: the recognition of unexpected outcomes; collectively negotiating the parameters of the anomaly, including seeking more refined genetic tests and checking observations with colleagues worldwide; and developing new operating procedures to manage the changed understanding of diseases. The continuous tinkering with disease categories affected their ontological and epistemological status: some diseases split into variants; others disappeared after being redefined as biochemical oddities without clinical implications. In the case of MCADD, geneticists were able to retain a common disease identity in spite of the emergence of disease variations. The geneticists relied on a double move of, first, creating a nuanced and diverse understanding of MCADD for diagnostic purposes, and second, holding on to the traditional treatment regime calibrated for the most serious variant. At worst, the error being made was harmless overtreatment. Hyperprolinemia was unmasked as a clinically irrelevant condition. Maternal diagnosis further underscored the widespread nature of these metabolic conditions and called into question who the patient was and whether the patient always needed therapy.

The knowledge work in the clinic took place in a knowledge ecology,[52] a broad open-ended environment consisting of interdependent institutions and cultural attitudes facilitating the production of knowledge. Each geneticist discussed individual patients at the weekly clinic meetings to receive feedback on the planned course of action. The geneticists further drew upon an international community of experts and their contacts in state laboratories to double-check action plans and stimulate scientific knowledge production. They communicated via Listservs and other digital communication, discussed unusual patients and findings at conferences, and wrote case reports in the biomedical literature. The knowledge produced in the clinic was only loosely connected to other domains affected by such information. Thus, the testimonies that parents were likely to encounter online before they spoke to the genetics staff reflected prescreening MCADD morbidity and mortality. Parents also felt judged as overreacting when they brought their infants to an emergency department after a prolonged episode of vomiting. Their pediatricians often knew little about rare metabolic conditions. In those instances, parents need to bridge a new set of knowledge gaps aimed less at changing the nature of disease than at educating healthcare providers about what these conditions have become.

Geneticists' actions suggested a mixed attitude toward fixing the knowledge gaps revealed by expanded newborn screening. On the upside, the anomalous findings offered some of the more intellectually stimulating instances of genetics clinic work. During clinic meetings, geneticists spoke excitedly about these puzzling patient findings and how to resolve them. The geneticist presenting such a patient would introduce these issues with: "This was an interesting case."[53] Geneticists facing anxious parents also felt little choice but to work out the anomalous findings because the screening results suggested that a child could be at risk for a preventable metabolic crisis. At the same time, there was also an implicit recognition that the ad hoc tinkering in the clinic fell short of the scientific opportunity that expanded newborn screening offered. Although the clinic participated in a follow-up study,[54] Dr. Silverman noted repeatedly that what they really should do is follow newborn screening patients prospectively in a rigorously designed multisited study aimed at examining their long-term health outcomes.

The ad hoc remedial work in the clinic to fit new knowledge properties in with the existing knowledge stock had a conservative effect. By resolving anomalies and gradually accommodating changes in disease conceptualization, the geneticists prevented a credibility crisis about the feasibility of newborn screening from emerging. In the first chapter, we saw that screening programs are justified based on incidence figures, severity, preventability, and treatment possibilities. Here, we showed that many of the original assumptions that helped to institute expanded newborn screening looked different over time. Yet the remedial fixes in the clinic buffered the surfacing of anomalies at a broader policy level. Solving the immediate practical clinical demands of individual patients results turned expanded newborn screening into what historian Thomas Kuhn has called a normal science project: geneticists became a community of scientific practice developing a consensus to make the screening program work, rather than a community torn apart by competing explanations for anomalies.[55] Thus, in spite of the fact that the MCADD discovered was not the MCADD anticipated, the screening program trundled along.

At the same time, expanded newborn screening has prompted a tremendous knowledge explosion about rare metabolic conditions. The screening program has generated new diseases or at least reconfigured current conditions to such an extent that they can plausibly be considered entirely different conditions. A large number of people have likely been walking around with what we now understand as MCADD or carnitine transporter deficiency, when prior to screening we had no way to find out who they were or what they had. Newborn screening enabled the discussion, assessment, diagnostic testing, and management of these diseases. Yet the screening program did not create neatly finished disease categories. Geneticists made them fit the practical situation at hand.

The emergence of patients-in-waiting and shifts in disease categories demonstrate the interactive quality of diagnostic classification, as explored by Ian Hacking. With the implementation of expanded newborn screening, new opportunities to classify patients into genetic disease categories drastically change how parents view their infants, and because of the far-reaching repercussions for the future of the child, may lead some to question the fit between diagnostic categories and the situation at hand. Anomalies and misfits result in a revision not only of the disease category but also of who qualifies as a patient. Over time, we observed how both the grounds for patient identities and the essence of diseases continued to evolve, propelled forward by anomalous findings and abductive double-fitting of all of the parts of the classification system.

This gradual process was difficult for clinicians in the midst of screening to appreciate because once a disorder changed, the "new" disorder overshadowed its past incarnations by offering a different conceptualization of the *true* nature of disease. Families who did not experience the process of ontological adjustment across different patients, informal professional contacts, and the biomedical literature might resist the idea that diseases are thrown in flux or evolve. This explains why over the years of visits with the same families, geneticists might have trouble convincing parents to qualify earlier understanding of diseases and treatment recommendations. The child had changed, but so had the disease. It also explains why rather than dismissing patients from the clinic completely, geneticists recommended that they visit once per year to receive an update of what geneticists had learned about conditions. Expanded newborn screening thus detected, protected, *and* created metabolic disease.

## CHAPTER FOUR

# Is My Baby Normal?

In the last chapters, we showed that follow-up testing for abnormal new-born screening results could continue for as long as one year after a child's birth, and that uncertainty about the nature of screened conditions could linger even longer. Despite such prolonged uncertainties, however, follow-up testing eventually petered out, and parents and genetics staff had to determine how the child's health—and incipient disorder—would be managed long-term. In this chapter, we focus on the medical consultation as a site where uncertainties regarding children's ambiguous health status were worked out collectively as the child grew. One of the most pressing questions facing parents of newborn screening patients was: is my baby normal? While these babies might have appeared to look like any other baby, uncertainties about their health and development could remain for many months, even years. As we will show, it was within the confines of mundane clinical encounters and routinized developmental assessments that geneticists attempted to scale back the initial anxieties prompted by the shock of a positive newborn screen and to provide reassurance about a child's uncertain future.

Despite the high-tech infrastructure of expanded newborn screening and genetic testing protocols, once the possibility of further genetic testing was ruled out, newborn screening follow-up visits adhered to a familiar format. Typically, they mirrored the structure of well-child visits, with the geneticists focused on carefully monitoring children's growth and developmental progress. The geneticists fired off rounds of questions about physical and cognitive development and carefully tracked measurements of weight, height, and head circumference. Just as missing developmental milestones often provide the first indication of a childhood medical disorder,[1] the timely attainment of developmental milestones reassured parents and clinicians about a child's uncertain health.

Growth is a particularly important domain of assessment for children with metabolic disorders because enzymatic deficiencies and attendant dietary restrictions can lead to growth impairments. Consequently, normal development supported an optimistic view of what abnormal newborn screening results might mean for a particular child. At the same time, the possibility of disease sparked by abnormal results attuned parents and geneticists to the likelihood of problems. Thus, ordinary signs of slower development could transform quite easily into putative symptoms. Whether a child with developmental delays was simply developing slowly or affected by a serious metabolic disorder had important consequences for the type of future that parents could envision for their children.[2]

The question of whether a baby was "normal" was one that faced all of the parents in our study. Indeed, one might argue that *all* parents ask themselves this question at one point or another—although the stakes are obviously higher for parents whose children have been identified with a genetic disorder. In the great majority of cases we witnessed, geneticists aimed from the outset to assuage parental concerns and to provide reassurance that a newborn screening patient would indeed grow up to be a normal child. This strategy occasionally produced ambiguous assessments such as: "He turns out to be totally normal. Except for if he gets sick." Generally speaking, however, the clinic staff emphasized that newborn screening patients should be treated like normal children most of the time. As Dr. Flores explained to one family, "So, if she is sick, you must make sure that if she's not eating and she is vomiting, you must take her to the hospital so that she receives calories. Apart from that, the rest of the time you should treat her as a normal baby. She doesn't need a special diet or anything like it." Likewise, Dr. Malvern told a couple that if their baby became ill and did not want to eat, "it's just a matter of making sure she gets some sugar. But otherwise you can treat her like a normal kid."[3] In contrast, for the small but significant number of children who had already been symptomatic, geneticists sought instead to subtly alert parents to the likelihood of future dangers. Geneticists' routine developmental assessments thus offered parents a window onto their children's normality, enabling them to realign discrepancies between the shocking news of a child's newborn screening results, the child's present health, and future expectations. By calibrating parental expectations in key prognostic domains, geneticists made judgments not only about the nature of disease but also about the idea of the normal child.

In what follows, after situating the concept of the "normal child" in historical perspective, we provide an overview of the structure of clinic appointments. Next, we turn to a series of clinical conversations about growth and development to consider two dimensions of the normalization process. First, we illustrate how normalization occurred through the implementation of *objective developmental standards*. Here, normalization refers to the social processes by which individuals and populations are subjected to regulation via statistical norms.[4] Geneticists, like other pediatric specialists, routinely employed three normalization techniques to foster a sense of objective normality: parental reports about developmental milestones, infant growth charts, and the physical examination. Drawing on key work in the history of science,[5] we show how each of these normalizing techniques corresponds with a different type of objectivity.

If the techniques of normalizing objectivity were designed to illuminate children's current health status in light of the past shocking news of positive newborn screening results, the second dimension of normalization that we explore concerns its capacity to convey prognostic information about the child's *future* in light of present indicators. From this perspective, normalization relayed moral assessments about the kind of life a child might be expected to lead, and thus performed important foreshadowing work. Normalization in this sense was not only part of a scientific clinical practice but also part of an everyday strategy of making sense of uncertainty.

## The Very Idea of the Normal Child[6]

Notwithstanding a number of important conceptual challenges from disability scholars, contemporary popular wisdom suggests that every parent, regardless of culture or national background, desires a "normal" child.[7] Despite its implied universality and normative power, however, the concept of the normal child has emerged only relatively recently. In a carefully researched work, philosopher James Wong traced the appearance of the concept of the normal child to a series of cultural and historical transformations beginning in the late nineteenth century that established childhood as a privileged period of human existence.[8] Social and economic changes in the United States and Europe during this time increasingly rendered children a distinctive demographic group with unique needs (e.g., nutrition, schooling, restriction from work), thereby transforming their societal position. At the same time, the field of statistics emerged as a means of organizing kinds of people within a comparative social framework.[9] Together, these developments constituted the conditions of possibility for a new social category: the normal child.

In late nineteenth-century industrializing countries, increasing public awareness of high infant mortality rates accompanied a growing societal emphasis on the protection of the child.[10] With children's health a mounting social concern, new forms of knowledge about children began to appear. Anthropometric studies during the 1870s and 1880s had already provided a great deal of information about children's height and weight. In tandem with public health efforts toward primary disease prevention and the emergence of pediatrics as a specialized field of medicine, the growth chart became the key apparatus for tracking infants in the early twentieth century. During this time, public health interventions provided new opportunities for monitoring populations. For example, historians have observed how milk depots set up to distribute milk to mothers in urban areas served multiple purposes: they supplied infants with necessary nutrition while also providing a venue for medical exams, regular weigh-ins, and education.[11] The introduction of compulsory schooling similarly fueled the growing trend toward surveillance by gathering children in a single geographic location to monitor their growth and competencies.[12] Such public health measures expanded the domain of growth charts beyond the physician's office and put all children, healthy or sick, under the medical gaze.[13] As a normalization technique, this surveillance enabled the initial establishment of a set of standards for child growth and development. Thus, as the eminent philosopher of science Georges Canguilhem has argued, norms follow normalization.[14]

Sociologist Nikolas Rose has observed that before the twentieth century, "it was by no means self-evident that a systematic knowledge of childhood should be grounded in the notion that their attributes should be linked along the dimension of time in a unified sequence."[15] The infant growth chart posited an explicit link between growth and temporality. This link was concretized in the disciplinary dogma of developmental psychology, which views human growth and psychological development as linear processes that unfold through specific, progressive phases.[16] Furthermore, the notion of "age-appropriateness" suggests that such phases ideally occur at specific ages.[17] Normality is thus mapped through time, with children expected to attain certain capacities at appropriate intervals. The stage model of human development has generated a spate of popular literature—from Dr. Spock's baby books to *What to Expect When You're Expecting*—that has played an important role in American culture and shaped many of its cultural schemas for childrearing.

Some scholars view normalization as an insidious process that pathologizes children who do not conform to standardized models.[18] Such critiques recognize that concepts such as age-appropriateness are informed by specific knowledge practices that reduce a complex process like human development to simple outcomes.[19] Biological anthropologists have likewise observed that growth curves are rather poor indicators of infant health.[20] Growth charts may provoke unnecessary anxiety when children quite literally do not measure up. Moreover, as we will show, the practice of growth monitoring enlists mothers to perform the work of surveillance, rendering them morally accountable when children fall short of developmental standards.[21]

Yet beyond providing repressive mechanisms of social control, normalization offers a new kind of social order that is rife with opportunities as well as challenges. Normalization performs a greater social function than objectification and measurement. Ian Hacking and others have observed that beyond its statistical connotations, the idea of normality is frequently used to close the gap between "is" and "ought," and hence contains a moral quality.[22] Therefore, it enables crucial interpretive work about children's possible futures and provides a semiotic framework for addressing questions of social difference and exclusion. From this perspective, normalization is a site that affords creative possibilities in addition to regulatory constraints.

It is against this historical backdrop that we must begin to understand the experience of families with children who are "genetically abnormal." Of course, as Nikolas Rose has suggested, at the genomic level, none of us are normal: there is no "normal genome," only a complex array of risk statistics that aggregated, mean very little.[23] Like Rose, we recognize that the concept of genetic normality is elusive. But even elusive concepts can have significant social effects. Thus, we are not convinced that his articulation of a "pathology without normality" in which "variation *is* the norm"[24] claims much explanatory purchase with families dealing with the ramifications of genetic disorders in their day-to-day lives.[25] Rose's assessment seems to characterize molecular knowledge of the human species more appropriately than it does people diagnosed with genetic conditions, for whom the specificity of genetic variation matters greatly. The moral imperative to have a normal child lives on within Western society's cultural imaginary,[26] even if the molecular gaze of genetic technologies has complicated what, precisely, it means to be normal.

We will demonstrate in this chapter that parents of newborn screening patients were preoccupied with, and perplexed by, the issue of normality.

Once a positive newborn screen raised suspicion of a metabolic disorder, multiple aspects of a growing infant's life offered a window onto his or her normality. As we will show, the geneticists relied upon normalization to arbitrate biomedical uncertainty. In doing so, they reinforced the cultural significance attached to the very idea of the normal child. Rather than simply locking children into constraining models of ideal growth, however, the category of the normal child also enabled certain actions and opportunities, preparing families for many unknowns.

## Coming to the Genetics Clinic

Parents of newborn screening patients anticipated their children's return visits to the genetics clinic with a sense of benign resignation, at best. Many admitted to us that they actively dreaded coming to the clinic. The geneticists often ran behind schedule, leaving families sitting for long periods in a crowded waiting room full of screaming children. The waiting room, a borderland space between the clinic and the outside world, was fraught with palpable tension,[27] and the fact that families had been referred to a prestigious academic medical center made the child's medical situation seem all the more grave. Looking around while they waited, surrounded by patients who suffered more visible signs of disease, the parents of newborn screening patients were often unsure what to expect for their own children—whether they, too, might be wheelchair bound one day, or rely upon the assistance of a nursing aide. As one father told us, "You're so concerned with your child and you go and you have to see what the outcome might be and it is completely devastating."

Eventually, a nurse would call the family into a room where the patient's vital signs and height and weight measurements were collected. Then, the nurse would lead them into a tiny consultation room to wait for the doctor. Although air-conditioned, these rooms became stuffy when crowded with several family members—often toting strollers, diaper bags, and older siblings—and the genetics staff, with their entourage of medical students and fellows, not to mention nosy ethnographers, who did their best to take up as little space, and air, as possible.

After asking for an update on any illnesses or significant events that had occurred since the last meeting, the geneticists engaged in three forms of developmental assessment. First, they typically began clinical consultations by asking parents to report on what the child could do. For example:

Can she hold up her head? Does he roll over? The informal, conversational tone of this line of questioning helped to establish rapport by demonstrating the geneticist's interest in matters that were not, on the surface, strictly clinical, while also providing a window onto the child's typical activities and behavior.

Next, the geneticists plotted the child's weight, height, and head circumference on the standardized infant growth charts that are widely available in pediatric clinics. While monitoring growth is important in any pediatric setting, it is particularly critical for children with metabolic disorders, who often experience stunted growth due to the challenge of getting essential dietary nutrients. Like routine questions about developmental progress, growth charts helped to construct children's normality by aligning individual children with standardized norms. Finally, the third form of assessment consisted of a general pediatric physical examination, during which the geneticists checked major organs and assessed the child's cognitive and motor development.

The visit would conclude with a discussion of any changes to the treatment plan. If no problems were apparent, interactions with geneticists at follow-up appointments were often quite brief. After the geneticist left the room, the dietitian counseled families about any special dietary measures, and when necessary, a staff social worker offered assistance with reimbursement from state insurance agencies and connected families to social services that they might qualify for as a result of their child's health issues. The appointment would typically end with a visit to the hospital laboratory for a blood draw, where the family would often encounter another long wait. Upon leaving the hospital, the family was almost certain to encounter terrible rush hour traffic, since patients were only seen in the afternoon hours, and rush hour began soon after lunch. Some patients traveled from many hours away to attend the clinic, due to the rarity of metabolic disorders, including some families from as far away as Arizona, Hawaii, or Nevada, where fewer genetic specialists were available.

Because the actual time spent with the geneticist was rather short, particularly in relation to the time spent traveling to the clinic and waiting once there, some parents found their clinic visits to be frustrating. This was particularly the case when checkups elicited a positive report. One mother told us that she could just as easily call in with her daughter's height and weight measurements and receive the same benefit. Another couple, whose daughter with MCADD was discharged from the clinic when she was two years old, reported that their appointments had been a waste of time.

Paradoxically, however, it was the mundane, business-as-usual nature of these pediatric interactions that helped to persuade parents to relinquish their anxieties about the alarming screening results. The sense that the genetics visits were unnecessary demonstrated the genetics staff's ability to establish a sense of normalcy through subtle repertoires of reassurance. Growth monitoring and developmental assessments marked an important starting point for accomplishing such reassurances and portraying newborn screening patients as "normal" babies. Yet there was a point of diminishing returns for liberal reassurances. Some degree of caution was necessary to motivate parents to return to the clinic consistently and to ensure that they followed clinical recommendations. The geneticists had to maintain a delicate balance between reassuring parents and encouraging vigilance.[28] As we will show, the balanced tipped toward fostering awareness of potential problems as clinical concern escalated for the children deemed to be most at risk.

## Normalizing Babies through Standardized Norms

When parents brought their children to the genetics clinic for a newborn screening follow-up appointment, there was always a possibility of learning that something was seriously wrong with the child. In this setting, then, normalization carried profound urgency. Developmental standards helped physicians to anchor their assessments of children relative to their peers and evaluate how they were doing under conditions of considerable uncertainty. We identified three principal arenas for such evaluations: responding to parental reports about children's capabilities, plotting the child's measurements on an infant growth chart, and conducting a physical examination. Here, we show how normalization functioned in each of these domains. In all three of these areas, normalization was an objectifying process that operated through the application of scientific judgment. Children were normal if they conformed to established developmental standards. Each normal assessment also contained a negative corollary: saying a child was normal suggested that there was no pathology. Conversely, the identification of developmental differences suggested that the child was *not* normal, and that pathology was possible.

In what follows, we show how each domain of clinical assessment—parental report, growth chart, and physical examination—corresponded with a different normalization technique and associated form of objectivity, defined broadly as "the ability to know things as they really are."[29] We consider these each in turn: narrative objectivity, mechanical objectivity, and disciplinary objectivity.

## Narrative Objectivity: Parental Report

Medical history-taking typically involves a set of standardized questions designed to elicit background information as quickly and efficiently as possible.[30] The first type of normalizing technique flowed from such routinized questions about children's physical and cognitive abilities during the history-taking period. The opening question was often pitched broadly, such as, what can she do? But this open-ended approach hinged upon a shared stock of institutional knowledge about the type of information that such a question was designed to elicit. In the excerpt below, Dr. Silverman inquires broadly about nine-month-old Nina Campos's capacities and obtains a specific, detailed response.

DR. SILVERMAN: She's a year old now?
MOTHER: No, gonna be nine months.
DR. SILVERMAN: Oh nine months. So what does she do? Does she pull to standing?
MOTHER: She's tried to stand on everything. She crawls.
FATHER: Yes.
DR. SILVERMAN: Yes.
MOTHER: She's eating her baby food. She's teething.
DR. SILVERMAN: She holds her bottle?
MOTHER: Uh huh, she holds her bottle.
DR. SILVERMAN: So she's normal.
MOTHER: Uh huh.

Dr. Silverman's broad line of inquiry elicited a simple narrative about the child's abilities. Not only could she pull to standing, but she also stood on "everything" and crawled. Moreover, not only was she eating, but she was also teething and holding her bottle on her own. After mentally comparing Nina's progress to age-graded developmental standards,[31] Dr. Silverman concluded that she was "normal." In this case, then, normalizing objectivity assumed a narrative form: Nina was rendered normal by evaluating her developmental trajectory against a standardized account of what events should happen by certain points in time. The moral thrust of this assessment, as we will explore in more detail later in the chapter, was for Nina's parents to have high expectations for her future.

Narrative objectivity afforded some flexibility if children did not follow developmental timelines perfectly. For example, Dr. Silverman minimized incipient concerns about language delays in Darren Holt, a 21-month-old boy who had been diagnosed with citrullinemia yet remained asymptomatic. When the Holts expressed concerns that their son was developing language more slowly than his three-year-old sister, Dr. Silverman downplayed the possibility that Darren's citrullinemia was responsible for this delay by emphasizing that boys tend to speak later than girls.

DR. SILVERMAN: You did tell about, you know, the fact that he speaks a little more slowly than she despite the same bilingual exposure. But you know boys tend to speak later than girls. So that may or may not be anything significant. I mean, do you have any reason to think that there's a hearing deficit?

FATHER: No, he seems to respond to the sounds.

DR. SILVERMAN: Yes. So I wouldn't worry about that. And I'm gonna suspect—I mean, you know he's at risk. He has a metabolic disorder. But he also is a boy and boys speak later. He's up to normal level in every other area. He climbs; he runs.

Although Dr. Silverman acknowledged that Darren was at risk because of his metabolic disorder, he emphasized that the language delay could also be attributed to his sex, since boys tend to begin speaking later than girls. The fact that Darren was "up to normal in every other area"—that is, normal vis-à-vis other developmental standards—bolstered Dr. Silverman's favorable assessment. Thus, Dr. Silverman produced a good-enough narrative to explain why Darren's speech development had been slow.[32]

Of the three normalizing techniques, narrative objectivity was most accessible to parents, who showcased their developmental expertise by evaluating children against culturally shared developmental standards. For example, Gary Thompson offered an assessment of his daughter Sherise's development that foregrounded her potential abnormality.

GARY: Well, let me ask you a question. As far as her physical part with everything. I was mentioning to Carolyn that to me, she seems to be on her very own time schedule.

DR. SILVERMAN: She is.

GARY: So I don't want to judge it by what the months say or what.

DR. SILVERMAN: Yes.

Here, Gary's reference to Sherise's "time schedule" demonstrates his understanding of child development as governed by cultural schemas about age-appropriate competencies. Gary's speculation about his daughter's developmental differences reflects the ease with which parents leveraged narrative objectivity to make judgments about their children's development. As Joanna Latimer observed in a different pediatric context, parents make active contributions to normalization by employing professional discourses and inserting knowledge of standardized norms:

> Some parents are thus not just engaged in surveying and assessing their child but also in measuring specific aspects of their child against technologies of what Foucault has called "normalizing judgment." In doing this, they seem to be performing a different kind of parent to the one who is tired and up all night with a hyperactive child or the one who is attempting to encourage and support the child's socialization and development through practice of control and stimulation. These parents are consumers of expert and scientific discourses, willing and able to talk the talk of the clinic.[33]

What Latimer referred to as "normalizing judgment" is evident in the following excerpt, in which Tina Schaffer responds to a routine question from Dr. Dati about her five-month-old daughter by introducing her knowledge of developmental norms.

DR. DATI: Can she roll over?
TINA: Yeah, she has trouble rolling back over, but as far as the book says she's okay.
DR. DATI: Okay. She looks fine.

With her reference to "the book," Tina foregrounded her familiarity with the popular developmental literature that provides an indication of children's expected abilities relative to age. Such savvy with respect to developmental norms reveals a wealth of cultural knowledge and is an important form of what sociologist Janet Shim has called *cultural health capital*: tacit or deliberate cognitive, behavioral, and sociocultural resources that predispose patients to optimal healthcare encounters. By referencing such widespread, shared norms in her developmental report, Tina enhanced the clinical significance of intimate personal knowledge and helped to foster narrative objectivity.

The value of narrative objectivity was thus its accessibility to parents and clinicians alike, since it depended on common stocks of cultural knowledge rather than professional expertise. In addition, because physicians depended on parental reports, and because parents asked for verification of their own assessments, there was more of an interactional component than in the two subsequent forms of objectivity. However, as we will show later in the chapter, disciplinary authority could quickly overrule the democratic character of narrative objectivity.

## Mechanical Objectivity: Growth Charts

Infant growth charts offer the sort of objectivity that historians of science have referred to as *mechanical objectivity*, the reliance upon mechanical rules, procedures, and numbers as a source of expert authority.[34] As instruments of mechanical objectivity, infant growth charts serve as material artifacts of the normalization process. By depicting children's positioning with respect to age-graded standardized norms, growth charts define children as normal through graphic representation. Today, growth charts are routinely shared with parents in pediatric visits and used to help anchor discussions.[35] Consequently, the perception of a favorable growth plot left many parents in our study with the sense of passing an important developmental test.

At each appointment, the geneticist plotted the child's growth measurements in each of three domains: weight, length (height), and head circumference. The growth chart displayed the child's age in months along the $x$ axis and the measurement (in kg or cm) along the $y$ axis. The chart also depicted a series of percentile curves that represent the growth measurements of a normal (i.e., statistically average) population (see figure 3).[36] By comparing the infant's growth plots over time to these normal curves, the geneticist could see how the infant compared to other children her age, as the following excerpt demonstrates.

GENETICIST: So she's growing really well. Here is when she was born, and here she is now. This is her weight. So she's still like at the—almost the ninetieth percentile.

MOTHER: So that means she's bigger than ninety percent?

GENETICIST: She's taller and weighs more than ninety percent of the kids her age.

MOTHER: Oh wow.

GENETICIST: And this is her head, same with her head.

MOTHER: Okay.

GENETICIST: So that's good.

Here, the geneticist explained that the child's growth plots, which aligned closely with the 90th percentile curve, revealed that she was taller and

**Birth to 36 months: Girls**
**Length-for-age and Weight-for-age percentiles**

NAME _____

RECORD # _____

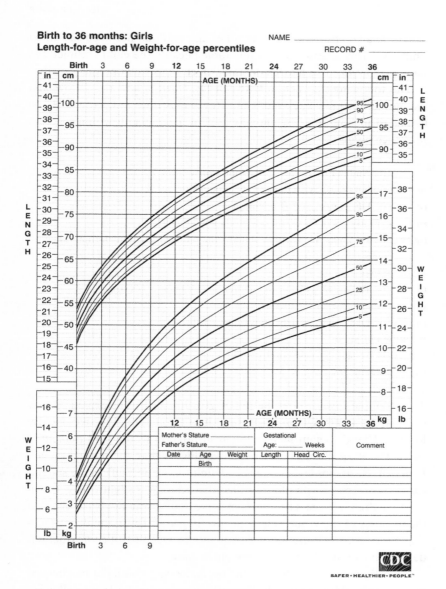

FIGURE 3. Infant growth chart, courtesy of the Centers for Disease Control and Prevention. *Source:* http://www.cdc.gov/growthcharts/clinical_charts.htm#Set1, accessed February 8, 2011.

heavier than 90 percent of children her age, and that her head size rated similarly.[37] This assessment was favorable because the child occupied the same percentile curve in each domain, which suggested optimal growth.

The following interaction between Dr. Nazif, a genetics fellow, and the mother of three-week-old Kiara Reyes illustrates how growth charts helped to anchor otherwise ambiguous clinical judgments within concrete reference points.

DR. NAZIF: And her height is . . . fifty-four. Pretty good.

MOTHER: What does—what does really good mean?

DR. NAZIF: Uh, pretty good. (Laughing)

MOTHER: Pretty good. Or what does pretty good mean?

DR. NAZIF: It's good. She's within actually the—higher than the normal range. So the mean.

MOTHER: Okay.

DR. NAZIF: The mean is like most children in her age are this size.

MOTHER: Okay.

DR. NAZIF: Okay, so she's right above that a little bit.

MOTHER: Oh, good.

DR. NAZIF: So she's growing pretty well.

MOTHER: Okay, great.

This example reveals how the infant growth chart transformed "pretty good" from an ambiguous assessment into a concrete objective one. By locating Kiara's height measurement in relation to the 50th percentile curve, Dr. Nazif illustrated that she was "higher than the normal range." Here, Dr. Nazif employed a specific definition of "normal" as the statistical average. The growth plot revealed that Kiara was slightly bigger than most children her age. Using evidence created in situ, Dr. Nazif clarified the meaning of the vague judgment "pretty good." This normalizing technique thus provided the mother with a more meaningful contextual understanding of the child's developmental status.

As with narrative objectivity, the normalizing potential of mechanical objectivity could signal problems as well as reassurances. In the following example, the dietitian has plotted a child's measurements and observed a slowed rate of growth.

DIETITIAN: So she is nine kilos right now. A month ago she was here. Eight point seven. So she's progressing, but she's still on the low side—fifth percentile. And in height she is growing a little bit too.

MOTHER: How is her height?
DIETITIAN: Seventy-six centimeters.

As the dietitian noted, the child only grew .3 kilos since the last visit. The child ranked near the fifth percentile for height, which the dietitian deemed "on the low side," revealing a measure of concern.

Similar concerns could also arise at the opposite end of the growth spectrum.

DR. SILVERMAN: So twenty-six months and ninety-one centimeters. He's above the fiftieth. Weight of fourteen point five kilos. He's big enough. I don't want him any bigger.
MOTHER: He's a little chub chub. He drinks a lot of milk.

In this case, Dr. Silverman determined that the child, Jacob Levinson, was above the 50th percentile curve for height at 26 months of age, and advised Wendy, Jacob's mother, that he did not want Jacob to gain any more weight—a preference that likely had more to do with general pediatric guidelines than with Jacob's metabolic condition, hyperphenylalaninemia. Thus, we can see that the growth chart functioned as a normalizing technology that created difference as well as normality by providing a concrete frame of reference for otherwise subjective clinical assessments.

Growth chart assessment presupposed that parents and geneticists would take certain corrective actions if children's growth raised concerns. Consequently, growth plotting foreshadowed the possibility of developmental problems and entailed considerable future work. In the next chapter, we further explore how stunted growth required parents and genetics staff to modify the diet, a complicated endeavor for patients with metabolic disorders.

### Disciplinary Objectivity: The Physical Examination

Although the geneticists elicited parental input when conducting developmental assessments, their own specialized knowledge played a preeminent role. This professional knowledge was most evident in the physical examination, which requires specialized training in a particular way of seeing the patient. As philosopher Michel Foucault has demonstrated, medical practice has hinged upon specific professionalized forms of perception since the nineteenth century.[38] Consequently, the physical examination provides a platform for *disciplinary objectivity*: the specialized evaluative knowledge that emanates from expert communities.[39]

The geneticists in our study, who trained in pediatrics as well as in medical genetics, leveraged disciplinary objectivity in each clinical consultation when they conducted a physical examination. They palpated the child's major internal organs, assessed basic bodily processes such as vision and reflexes, and held and lifted newborns to check their muscle tone. The medical gaze was thus manifested not only in the application of a specific professional vision, *the disciplinary eye*, but also through tactile engagement with the child.[40] The geneticists also asked toddlers and older children to walk, run, or count to 10 to check gait and cognitive function. Thus, even everyday activities such as walking in the hallway were transformed into objective developmental indicators when incorporated into the physical examination. The following excerpt relays Dr. Silverman's evaluation of week-old Jason Arnold after examining him at his first clinic visit.

DR. SILVERMAN: Good head control for a one-week-old child. I look at all of the things, but remember this is a general pediatric exam that I'm doing and all I'm really observing is how active Jason is and how he moved about. But all of those indications are just very excellent. Moves like a normal kid.
FATHER: And, have you checked everything from head to toe?
DR. SILVERMAN: That's fine.

While it is worth noting that Dr. Silverman stated that Jason "moves *like* a normal kid" (our emphasis), an assessment that preserved a measure of ambiguity, Dr. Silverman nevertheless offered an overwhelmingly reassuring assessment. He observed Jason's bodily movements, and all of the signs were "excellent." In this case, objectivity was generated through Dr. Silverman's specialized perceptual reasoning: the medical gaze produced a normal judgment.

The importance of medical perception as a normalizing technique was further underscored by the father's orientation to Dr. Silverman as a source of authoritative knowledge. The father explicitly enlisted the expert gaze by asking Dr. Silverman to verify that he had "checked everything." For parents, then, the value of disciplinary objectivity resided in its ability to provide reassurance about the newborn's uncertain health status. This feature of disciplinary objectivity was particularly important in the context of newborn screening, since the numerical indicators provided by laboratory readings often proved equivocal during screening and follow-up testing, as we described in the last chapter. In other words, disciplinary objectivity was for parents an attractive form of normalizing judgment because lingering ambiguities in testing results could erode some of their trust in numbers.

Moreover, while it is true that mechanical objectivity has increasingly prevailed over physicians' interpretations of clinical signs in contemporary biomedical practice, even mechanical objectivity demands an implicit faith in expert knowledge. As historian of science Ted Porter pointed out, "There is an element of unarticulated expertise built into every attempt to solve problems according to explicit rules." Furthermore, "it requires institutional or personal credibility even to produce impersonal numbers."[41] In the following discussion of Kyle Stardust, whom we first introduced in chapter 2, we see that mechanical objectivity cannot stand on its own entirely: clinicians depend on disciplinary expertise for the interpretation of numerical readings.

DR. SILVERMAN: You know what strikes me here is his unusual appearance. Kind of almond-shaped eyes, hypotonia, the high forehead. May or may not be significant but it's a good head size. Do we have the head size?

MONICA: Forty-eight point five. I didn't plot the head size but I plotted the um—

DR. SILVERMAN: How many months is he?

MOTHER: Nine.

DR. SILVERMAN: Oh, wait.

MONICA: Forty-eight point five.

DR. SILVERMAN: You got it.

MONICA: Oh, yes.

DR. SILVERMAN: You know it's interesting that that macrocephaly, or big head, is one of the characteristics of glutaric acidemia type 1.

Here, we see Dr. Silverman's concern about some unusual features of Kyle's physical appearance: his large head and high forehead, almond-shaped eyes, and hypotonia (low muscle tone). Although Monica had already measured Kyle's head circumference, Dr. Silverman could tell that Kyle was macrocephalic simply from looking at him. Disciplinary objectivity and mechanical objectivity converged on a troubling interpretation of Kyle's growth trajectory. However, although Kyle's head circumference might have suggested a problem on its own, Dr. Silverman's disciplinary knowledge was necessary to frame Kyle's growth measurements within a broader developmental context and link them to other signs of GA1, such as hypotonia.

In Kyle's case, these signs were particularly perplexing because Dr. Silverman had already ordered a skin biopsy to test Kyle for GA1, and the test results had been negative. Nevertheless, the clinical signs were alarming enough to prompt Dr. Silverman to reconsider the findings. As he remarked later in the visit: "We're going to follow through on this. There are things that bother me, and the big head is one of the signs of glutaric acidemia type 1, even though we did what we thought was a definitive study. So I don't think we can drop that. This just comes as sort of a surprise to me." In this case, then, the disciplinary eye overruled previous applications of mechanical objectivity.[42]

In the next excerpt, we see Dr. Flores wield a similar form of disciplinary objectivity in relaying his concern about a flat spot on the back of 10-month-old Reynaldo Gonzales's head.

DR. FLORES: So, Mom, the only thing that I'm noticing is that the back of his head is kind of flat.
MOTHER: Uh huh.
DR. FLORES: Have you noticed that? Right here.
MOTHER: Oh, the back? Right here?
DR. FLORES: Yes. Yes.
MOTHER: Yes.
DR. FLORES: So, I think we should send him to (*indecipherable content*) because he's uh, his soft spot is going away.
MOTHER: Uh huh.
DR. FLORES: And if we wait too long, I mean, I just want to see if maybe we can help with position changes and stuff. If we can—
MOTHER: Oh. Fix that.
DR. FLORES: Fix that.
MOTHER: Yes.
DR. FLORES: So I'm going to try to send him to the craniofacial clinic?
MOTHER: Okay.

The flat spot that Dr. Flores described is an anomaly that has sometimes been linked to developmental delays.[43] This finding provoked enough concern that Dr. Flores referred Reynaldo for an evaluation in the craniofacial clinic, which shifted the domain of disciplinary objectivity. In this example, as in the previous one, the normalizing gaze was mobilized in the pursuit of additional pathology rather than to reassure the mother that her son was normal. Whether normalizing objectivity was disturbing or reassuring thus depended on the conclusions drawn from it, not on the normalizing technique itself.

## Normalization as a Moral Project

To this point, we have illustrated how the genetics staff normalized—or inversely, pathologized—children by aligning them with standardized developmental norms. Comparing favorably with standardized norms provided a child's family with a measure of reassurance that served as a counterweight to the lingering concerns generated by newborn screening. As Kelly Lopez, whose son Anton had been diagnosed with carnitine transporter deficiency disorder, told us, "We were more worried in the beginning but seeing how he's developing and how alert he is, I don't worry." Dr. Malvern expressed a similar sentiment when she told the parents of Kiara Reyes, an infant with SCADD who had hit all of her developmental milestones, "I wish I could tell you very concretely but, you know, I have kids who have this disorder who've never had a crisis, and then I have kids who from the minute they were born had trouble. Obviously she's one of those people who is very mild."

But normalization is more than a form of objective assessment. It is also a way of projecting normality, as the comments cited above indicate, by anticipating and illuminating moral assessments about the kind of future that a child might have. For heuristic purposes, we have separated these two dimensions of normalization in our discussion thus far. However, they frequently overlapped within the clinical encounter. We begin to make this point by returning to the growth chart, a domain in which the "is" and "ought" of normal assessments necessarily converge.

On the surface, growth charts might appear to provide a purely objective assessment of children's development: they indicate children's positioning relative to age-graded standardized norms. Yet it is not always clear from scrutinizing a growth chart what should be considered ideal. Surveys indicate that American parents prefer children's growth chart curves to lie at higher percentiles, even though there is little evidence that this offers a health advantage.[44] As one geneticist told a parent, "The important thing, from our perspective, is that she stays along a curve." This comment suggests that it is most important that children's growth maintains constancy over time, without sharp increases or decreases. Yet insofar as parents might judge their ability to nurture and care for their children based on their growth chart locations, growth charts are morally charged. For many parents in our study, "normal" was not the ideal, as we can see in the following interaction between Dr. Silverman and Samantha Buchanan regarding Samantha's daughter Kari.

DR. SILVERMAN: Her height, she's obviously normal.

SAMANTHA: She's huge. She's more than normal. (Laughing)

DR. SILVERMAN: Only a parent worries about more than normal. Doctors worry about normal.

In this exchange, Dr. Silverman and Samantha drew on different dimensions of normality in their evaluations of Kari. For Dr. Silverman, Kari's height was statistically average, which suggested that her growth was not a medical concern and that she was normal. Yet Samantha, who focused on the moral dimensions of normality, rejected the normal label because she proudly perceived her daughter's size as bigger (and implicitly, better) than average. Thus, for Dr. Silverman, normality was a desirable attribute, whereas it carried worrisome implications for Samantha, who wanted her daughter to be *better* than normal.

Children's positioning on growth charts was of central importance to parents in no small part because of the ways in which growth chart assessments implicated parental—and often, specifically maternal—responsibility. As Dr. Flores told one mother, "Well, Mom, you're doing a good job because she's grown literally. So she was below—she wasn't doing very well in terms of her length, but she's now back in the normal range." This comment suggests that the child's accomplishment of growth could be attributed solely to her mother's effortful work. Of course, such remarks also imply their inverse: that mothers might be held accountable when their children fall short of ideal growth. When children were smaller than average, their mothers could harbor considerable anxiety about growth charts, as the following interview report from Leah Mabini, a Filipino woman in our study, demonstrates:

LEAH: Think about it, those scales that they put you through is for a, you know, an average American child. What is that? (Laughing) You know what I mean?

MARA: Yes.

LEAH: So it's like, you're arranging that from like so many different cultures, you know. (Laughing)

MARA: Yes. Exactly.

LEAH: To be honest, as a first-time mother, I was very paranoid about it, because I was like, "She's not on the charts. Why is she not on the chart?"

Such comments point to how infant growth charts promote a popular bias toward larger body size. Isabella Bonilla proudly noted the moment at which Ana, who was born with a low birth weight and diagnosed with failure to thrive, finally grew large enough to reach the lowest percentile represented on the charts. She told us, "And she just made it onto the weight and height charts. Last doctor, her one-year-old visit, she made it onto the charts." At the same appointment, Dr. Dati observed Ana's progress.

DR. DATI: So she's between the tenth and the twenty-fifth for height.
ISABELLA: Yay.
DR. DATI: That's good. And she's between the fifth and tenth for weight. So she's skinny.
ISABELLA: Yes. She is skinny. She is. (Laughter) We celebrate each pound.
DR. DATI: That's just fine.

Notably, Dr. Dati's assessment of Ana as "skinny" positioned her on the low end of normal, as opposed to being sick. In relation to her low birth weight, thinness was something to "celebrate" rather than a source of concern. In this case, then, due to her particular biography, Ana's growth chart location between the 5th and 10th percentile for height carried a very different meaning from what it might convey in a purely objective context. This example reveals how mechanical objectivity could be leveraged to normalize—in the moral sense of the term—a child with a rather precarious beginning of life. Ana was by no means statistically normal, yet her entry onto the growth chart suggested that she might be able to live a "normal" life.

This second dimension of normalization, in which normal assessments communicated moral claims about the future in addition to statistical measurements, was most apparent in interactions with families of children who were perceived to be at the greatest risk due to the severity of their prognosis. As Dr. Silverman told one couple at their daughter's first appointment: "You have a child at risk. It's difficult but it's the reality and my job is to talk with you sincerely about its seriousness." For these patients, normalization was far less concerned with standardized norms than with more general questions about how to prepare parents for an uncertain future and what kind of life the child might lead.

## Normalization as Foreshadowing Work

Thus far, we have focused primarily on the positive side of normalization, in both its objective and moral dimensions. But the negative corollary of normalization is the production of difference. Such difference is generated in two primary ways: through a gradual movement away from the norm, and through a shifting of the norm itself. As we will show, children from the most high-risk group of patients were increasingly compared to children with disease rather than to healthy norms. In this section, we explore the tension between normality and difference with respect to the developmental assessment strategies employed with this group of patients. For these patients, developmental assessments focused on prognostic claims about the children's futures more than evaluations of children's current status.

Anthropologist Rayna Rapp has argued that parents of children with Down syndrome engage in a "doubled discourse of both difference and normalization," which both recognizes and normalizes their children's differences.[45] As Rapp explains it, parents of children with Down syndrome must come to terms with having a baby whose developmental trajectory and cognitive abilities remain uncertain. In this sense, their children are undeniably different from their peers. On the other hand, however, parents love and accept their children with Down syndrome, and even come to appreciate certain differences. Furthermore, Rapp suggests, when given the right resources, parents come to aspire for their children's success. Parents thus embrace their children's *differences* even as they assert that they are *just like other children*. Hence, the "doubled discourse."

When dealing with the families of high-risk patients, the geneticists in our study engaged in a doubled discourse much like the one that Rapp describes. On the one hand, they tried to reassure parents about their children's uncertain health and offer them hope for the future. At the same time, they also attempted to warn parents about the potentially difficult pathways ahead. The purpose of the doubled discourse was thus to convey two possible trajectories within the same breath: a child might be doing better than expected based on developmental parameters, but that would not guarantee a future free from disease. For this group of patients, the geneticists attempted to balance between normalization and difference in their developmental assessments, yet future expectations were shaped by a gradual deviation from the norm. As we will see shortly, however, the balance increasingly tipped in favor of difference. In what follows, we employ Rapp's characterization of normalization as a process of applying moral claims about children's futures.

### Precarious Normality

Sherise Thompson was one patient for whom Dr. Silverman offered only qualified reassurances. Sherise was born prematurely at 35 weeks, after her mother developed preeclampsia. Following her birth, Sherise was kept in the hospital for several days due to an irregular heartbeat. While in the neonatal intensive care unit (NICU), she began to have trouble feeding and became extremely lethargic. On day six, she was transferred to the NICU at the academic hospital where our research was based, where she was diagnosed with propionic acidemia.

After this initial metabolic crisis, Sherise remained healthy for her first 10 months, and Dr. Silverman tried to reassure her parents about her delayed developmental trajectory. Over time, however, he scaled back his attempts to assuage her family's concerns. Below, we revisit an excerpt from Sherise's five-month appointment quoted earlier in the chapter. Here, Sherise's father Gary inquires about her developmental milestones and what he perceived as a physical delay. It is important to note that Gary's uncertainty may have partially resulted from Sherise's premature birth, since premature babies are expected to display some developmental delays.

DR. SILVERMAN: Okay. Well fortunately she looks terrific.

GARY: Well, let me ask you a question. As far as her physical part with everything. I was mentioning to Carolyn that to me she seems to be on her very own time schedule.

DR. SILVERMAN: She is.

GARY: So I don't want judge it by what the months say or what.

DR. SILVERMAN: Yes.

GARY: As far as development, is there—should it be more like the rolling over, the reaching? She's just starting.

DR. SILVERMAN: Well, uh, look at what we're doing. She's perfectly normal for getting physical therapy, which means she's not getting it to make up for any deficit.

GARY: Uh huh.

DR. SILVERMAN: She's getting it just as a protection, as a precaution. But let me give you a picture of what the jeopardy is for her. When children are born with these inborn errors, there's often a honeymoon period in the first six or nine months or year. And the reason is, they're growing so rapidly that any extra of the amino acids and stuff they're using up for growth. As the growth rate slows down and as they get out with other kids, so they get sick more, they may—she may have periods when she's hospitalized for several days. And when she really goes out. So what you're really looking for and have to expect is going to happen is that there may be ups and downs that are coming in the future. And that the idea is not to get too discouraged because that's expected to happen. Now we may get lucky and it doesn't happen.

Previously, we described Gary's tentative assessment as an example of
narrative objectivity: Sherise seemed to be "on her very own time schedule," lagging behind in development. In response to Gary's query, Dr. Silverman first offered a positive assessment aimed to reassure Gary about his
daughter's progress. He suggested that Sherise's physical therapy had been
started prophylactically, rather than in response to an observed deficit, and
characterized Sherise as "perfectly normal." Here, rather than citing standardized norms, he drew upon a gestalt sense of normality that highlights
its moral dimensions. But Dr. Silverman undermined these opening reassurances with the cautionary note appended to his normal assessment:
although Sherise was "perfectly normal," her parents should expect for
things to get worse. By invoking "child born with inborn errors," Dr. Silverman introduced a new benchmark for her development. Rather than compare Sherise to other "normal" children, she should be compared to other
children who are sick. Here, then, normalization gave way to the identification of difference. Even though Sherise might have appeared "perfectly
normal," her diagnosis rendered her normal status contingent. In this way,
Dr. Silverman leveraged disciplinary expertise to subtly foreshadow a potentially problematic future. In doing so, he recalibrated Gary's concerns
about his daughter's development with grave expectations for unforeseen
threats. Normality, from this perspective, is always a precarious normality.

Despite the role of expertise, disciplinary judgment functioned differently in this context than it did in normalizing objectivity. Here, disciplinary authority is more diffuse, less dependent on specific perceptual experiences (observing, feeling, and listening to the child) than on a more
general sense of what the child's life might be like. At the family's next appointment in the genetics clinic, 10 weeks later, the specter of danger was
raised once again when Carolyn Broderick, Sherise's mother, inquired
about her daughter's ability to take swimming lessons.

CAROLYN: Do you think she'll ever be able to have like swim lessons and things
    like that?
DR. SILVERMAN: Well, if we get very lucky, she'll be a perfectly normal girl. If you
    wanted to take her now for swim lessons, like go to a pool, you should go.
CAROLYN: Germs.
DR. SILVERMAN: What?
CAROLYN: I'm scared of germs.
DR. SILVERMAN: Yes, I know.
CAROLYN: (Laughs)

DR. SILVERMAN: Uh, you know this brings up something else I was going to mention. And that is that this next year may not be as good as this first year in
terms of not getting infections or anything like that, or not getting ill. And the
reason I'm saying this is not so much to scare you but to make you feel comfortable with the fact that if things change, it's not because thing have gone
to hell in a handbasket. What happens after six months of age is that the rate
of growth diminishes the ability to soak up extra amino acids—diminishes
because they're not growing so fast. So we may have to make some adjustments. I don't want you to get panicky if it happens. And as far as germs go, you
really have to decide whether or not you're going to raise this child in a bubble
or you're going to try to help her to develop her resistance. And we don't know
what she can tolerate. You may end up protecting her and then discovering that
she really didn't need protection.

Once again, Dr. Silverman offered an explanation for Sherise's "honeymoon period" similar to the account offered at the previous appointment.
The rapid rate of growth during the first year of life protects the infant
with propionic acidemia from the buildup of amino acids in the blood. As
the growth rate slows, amino acids are depleted less quickly, and metabolic crisis can occur. Structurally, this example is similar to the previous
one: Dr. Silverman moved from a relatively optimistic assessment of Sherise's normality to a somber warning about potential complications on the
horizon. In the second appointment, however, Dr. Silverman's assessment
was increasingly guarded. Although he alluded again to the possibility of
Sherise being a "perfectly normal" girl, her normal status was now even
more contingent. This shift diminished the family's expectations for a normal childhood, which had now been relegated to the realm of luck. The
doubled discourse thus swayed in favor of difference.

We call the type of developmental assessment that Dr. Silverman offered above *normalizing subjunctivity* to highlight three specific characteristics of this normalization strategy that distinguish it from normalizing objectivity: its uncertain epistemic status, its future orientation, and its
fundamentally moral nature. In grammatical terms, the subjunctive refers
to a verb mood used to express a hypothetical or imaginary thought. It
may relay a hope, wish, or desire, or other possibilities or actions that have
not yet occurred. Dr. Silverman's statement "if we get very lucky, she'll be
a perfectly normal girl" is expressed in the subjunctive mood. Thus, if objective normalizing assessments describe things as they are, subjunctive
normalizing assessments describe things as we wish they might be.

Anthropologists Byron Good and Mary-Jo DelVecchio Good have used the concept of subjunctivity to describe the contingent nature of the illness narratives of Turkish epilepsy patients. Drawing on narrative analysis, Good and Good highlight the "subjunctivizing" elements of epilepsy narratives that help to construct illness experience as "open to mystery, potency, and change" and "allow sufferers and their families to justify continued care-seeking and to maintain hope for positive, even 'miraculous,' outcomes."[46] Quoting narrative theorist Jerome Bruner, they write, "To be in the subjunctive mode . . . is to be trafficking in human possibilities rather than in settled certainties."[47] Good and Good argue that illness stories contain subjunctivizing elements not only because of the desire for narrators to produce an empathic response in the listener but also because of the strong commitment of narrators to portray a world in which healing is possible. In a similar way, Dr. Silverman demonstrated a strong commitment to maintaining parents' hope for children to have a "normal" future, in the moral sense of the term. In this clinical context, as other social scientists have observed, uncertainty and contingency were valued resources because they enabled parents to preserve a measure of hope with respect to their children's health and future normality.[48]

By Sherise's 14-month appointment, she had already been hospitalized for another metabolic crisis. She was still not walking, and her father inquired about her shakiness in the trunk area. Dr. Silverman explained that it was probably indicative of delayed development due to the disorder. When Gary expressed surprise, Dr. Silverman acknowledged, "Yeah, she's not on track," adding: "We can't predict how she's going to do at school. She'll likely be able to walk and talk and be able to function in those respects. A little dangerous to predict, but it's pretty encouraging." Thus, even here, when Dr. Silverman finally admitted that Sherise had fallen behind with respect to standardized norms, he remained cautiously hopeful, attempting to optimize her uncertain future despite obvious abnormalities. In other words, the subjunctive dimensions of normalization prevailed over objective assessments of increasing differentiation.

We witnessed a similar tension between normalization and difference in Dr. Silverman's interactions with the family of Dionna Walker, a patient with methylmalonic acidemia (MMA). Like Sherise, Dionna developed signs of a metabolic crisis shortly after birth, after which a gastrostomy tube was implanted in her navel to assist with feedings in the event of another metabolic crisis—a common practice for patients with MMA. Following her initial hospitalization, Dionna remained healthy for many months. In the following transcript excerpted from Dionna's four-month appointment, Dr. Silverman attempted to reassure Rachael Johnston, Dionna's mother, about her daughter's uncertain future by asserting that "nobody would distinguish her from a normal kid."

DR. SILVERMAN: I think she seems developmentally okay.

RACHAEL: Yes.

DR. SILVERMAN: It's hard to say you know. It's a difficult period.

RACHAEL: Mm.

DR. SILVERMAN: But all things considered, nobody would distinguish her from a normal kid.

RACHAEL: Right.

DR. SILVERMAN: So, of course she has the tubes sticking out of her stomach.

RACHAEL: Yes.

DR. SILVERMAN: (Laughing) Little thing like that.

RACHAEL: Okay, but no one really knows about that either.

DR. SILVERMAN: That's right. And so she's not going to be good in a bikini. (Laughing)

RACHAEL: Not with that, no.

DR. SILVERMAN: Few of our patients won't get into bikinis after we get done with them.

RACHAEL: (Laughs)

Here, Dr. Silverman displays the three defining features of normalizing subjunctivity. His hedging ("it's hard to say") reveals the *uncertain epistemic status* of his developmental assessments, while the subjunctive construction ("nobody would distinguish her from a normal kid") and prognostic foreshadowing ("she's not going to be good in a bikini") reveal his *future orientation*. Overall, in this context, being "normal" conveyed a *moral claim* about the kind of life Dionna might be expected to lead, as well as a set of gendered assumptions about typical girlhood. If her biggest problem was her ability to wear a bikini, Dr. Silverman implied, there was little cause for concern. Still, the use of the verb "distinguish" suggests a weak form of normality in which Dionna's differences were only partially hidden.

Over time, Dr. Silverman increasingly tempered his normalizing assessments, just as he did with Sherise. By the time she was six months old, Dionna stopped gaining weight in proportion to her height, an important sign of developmental problems in children with metabolic disorders. At

Dionna's eight-month visit, when Dionna's mother and grandmother inquired about Dionna's low body weight, Dr. Silverman offered a somber prognosis.

DR. SILVERMAN: Well, but, but, look. This disorder is a pretty serious disorder and so far we've dodged the bullet.

GRANDMOTHER: Mm hm.

DR. SILVERMAN: And the weight is the last thing I'll worry about.

GRANDMOTHER: Mm hm.

DR. SILVERMAN: I mean, one of the issues is with many kids, even those who do well with this disorder, end up with kidney problems at ten or fifteen. And she may eventually need a kidney transplant. So for me, weight is the least of my concerns.

GRANDMOTHER: It's just that helps her being healthy and [helps her] bones.

DR. SILVERMAN: The brain.

GRANDMOTHER: The brain.

DR. SILVERMAN: That's our big risk here.

In this excerpt, Dr. Silverman tells Dionna's mother and grandmother rather pointedly that their mundane worries about body size have missed the mark—they should worry instead about kidney failure and brain damage. Significantly, growth, the same domain of assessment used in other cases to assess normality, was here framed as inconsequential. Dr. Silverman thus recast Dionna from a normal child—for whom height and weight were typical concerns—to a patient with a serious metabolic disorder, inclined to face graver trepidations. As we saw with Sherise Thompson, that Dionna had done so well thus far could only be attributed to luck. Once again, the balance tipped from normalization to difference.

By her 15-month visit, Dionna's weight had escalated to a more pronounced concern. Below, we see the growth chart return as a focal concern and normalizing apparatus.

DR. SILVERMAN: Let's see what her height is. Oh, seventy-four point five. So the height's doing fine.

RACHAEL: That's good, yes.

DR. SILVERMAN: And the head circumference is going to be okay.

MONICA: Has she been eating well?

RACHAEL: Yes.

MONICA: She has?

RACHAEL: Mm-hm. That's why I don't know. But she's very active. I don't know if that's—

DR. SILVERMAN: Look. Here's—the head circumference is fine. The height is fine. And the weight is low. Weight is the least of the issues. But I think we should try to get more calories into her.

RACHAEL: Yes.

DR. SILVERMAN: But for concern, it's the head, obviously it's the brain. Excuse me. And it's growing fine. Now it doesn't mean—normal size head doesn't mean normal function. But a small head often means abnormal function. And the height—in malnutrition, it's always the weight that goes first, height second, and head third. So she's maintained height and weight—height and head. So even if she's getting too few calories, so far she's showed up only weight. So I think we really obviously have to get more calories into her.

RACHAEL: Okay.

DR. SILVERMAN: I think we can do that when we meet with the dietitian today.

Where earlier Dr. Silverman had dismissed Dionna's low weight as a serious problem, here he admitted its relevance to her metabolic disorder, since it appeared that her malnourishment had been caused by her restricted diet. Still, although he determined that they needed to feed her more calories, he nevertheless continued to minimize the importance of her weight problem by declaring it "the least of the issues." In this case, Dr. Silverman's limited concern for Dionna's growth chart position portended the likelihood of more serious problems in the future. Mechanical objectivity and Dr. Silverman's disciplinary judgment thus converged on the pathologization of difference.

\*　\*　\*

Although Rapp's original use of "doubled discourses" focused on parents, it is worth noting that when cloaked behind the mask of disciplinary expertise, doubled discourses are all the more effective at conveying seemingly contradictory messages simultaneously. Yet while apparent contradictions in clinical assessments can perplex and befuddle anxious parents, the parents of symptomatic patients exhibited considerably less outward anxiety than those of patients who were ostensibly more "normal." This was the case, in part, because there was little ambiguity for the parents of the symptomatic group that the child was, to some extent, affected by the disease. At the same time, the ambiguities inherent in doubled discourses preserved a measure of subjunctivity with respect to children's futures. This subjunctivity was valuable to families coping with the day-to-day challenges of raising a child with precarious health. The doubled discourse conveyed to parents that children could be ill yet still be normal, in some sense of the term.

We have shown how Dr. Silverman relied on a doubled discourse of normalization and difference to finesse clinical judgments and offer reassurance. Over time, however, clinical assessments of symptomatic patients increasingly emphasized difference more than normality, and parents were left to wonder what kinds of lives their children might lead. Would they be placed in mainstream classrooms and make friends when they came of school age? Would they grow up to hold jobs and find partners?

If the parents of patients-in-waiting were preoccupied with the question, is my baby normal?, the question was framed slightly differently for the parents of babies who had already displayed symptoms. For them, normality was not a categorical question. Instead, they wondered, "*How* normal will my baby be?" By framing the question this way, parents engaged in their own subjunctive normalization techniques. Anthropologists Kelly Raspberry and Debra Skinner have observed that parents of children with genetic disorders "were involved in a process of renorming the 'normal,' a recalibrating based on an idiosyncratic state of health that can not be averaged because it is based on a population of one, their own child."[49] Although parents might share with biomedical evaluative frameworks a concern for the "normal," they redefined what this might mean in relation to their own individual child. For symptomatic newborn screening patients, normality was thus precarious both because their health status was fragile and because the meaning of being "normal" was itself unstable.

## Creativity in Normalization

Regardless of the prognosis or the nature of the metabolic disorder, parents of newborn screening patients were confronted with persistent uncertainties about their children's health. We have seen that follow-up visits for newborn screening were motivated by an implicit, unspoken question: is my baby normal? Overwhelmingly, geneticists attempted to answer this question with an emphatic yes. In some cases, however, the desire to reassure the parents of newborn screening patients came up hard against a competing demand: to prepare parents for a potentially difficult road ahead.

Owing to a dominant Foucauldian legacy, some social scientists have assumed that normalization is necessarily insidious and repressive.[50] Yet, as we have shown, the types of normal assessments entailed by developmental standards enable a wider range of normalizing judgments than is often assumed. Normalization in the genetics clinic contained two overlapping dimensions: the implementation of standardized norms for infant growth and development, and the application of moral judgments about children's future lives. We have argued that normalization afforded new forms of knowledge, judgments, and practical activities that helped parents to prepare for many unknowns. By providing guideposts about children's development, normalization techniques permitted physicians to visualize problems that might not otherwise be apparent, to facilitate corrective action. Moreover, the uncertainty produced through normalizing subjunctivity could be a creative resource used to instill and preserve hope. Consequently, we have suggested that normalization strategies are not inherently constraining but rather offer the potential for increased understanding and therapeutic possibilities.

It may come as a surprise to find creativity in normalization because normalization implies standardization and the reduction of idiosyncrasy, which seem by definition to be anticreative. However, the process of measuring individuals against norms entails a creative dimension because of its combined objective and moral subjunctive aspects. Fitting a norm when clinicians expect no fit, or falling out of the statistical normal range, offers a situated moment of friction that asks for reconciliation. Similar to the knowledge ecologies resulting in shifting disease epistemologies and ontologies and the emergence of patients-in-waiting, normalization reveals abductive reasoning in daily clinical work. Developmental assessments in pediatric encounters are guided by objectivizing norms. Yet when such norms no longer offered clear prognostic value, as in the case of symptomatic newborn screening patients, clinicians engaged in creative abduction to recalibrate future expectations in light of present unknowns.

Overall, we have seen how for the patients most seriously affected by metabolic disorders, normalizing techniques served to reduce geneticists' reassurances over time so that parents could prepare to meet their children's needs, yet without completely abandoning hope. While the futures of these babies were no more certain, expectations for normality were substantially diminished. In the next chapter, we describe their families' experiences.

CHAPTER FIVE

# The Limits of Prevention

The rationale for newborn screening, as with most population screening programs, is one of secondary prevention, which aims for early
diagnosis in order to begin treatment before significant morbidity has
occurred. While there is no cure for metabolic disorders, the logic of secondary prevention suggests that early detection and intervention can help
to avert the most serious consequences of disease. As we demonstrated in
the last chapter, however, preventive measures cannot insulate all newborn
screening patients from the threat of metabolic crisis. Metabolic disorders
remain unpredictable, and inevitably, some patients diagnosed through
newborn screening will develop symptoms and experience serious, life-
threatening metabolic events.

This chapter speaks to the limits of prevention by focusing on the
care of children who developed symptoms for metabolic disorders despite screening and early diagnosis. Newborn screening was designed to
serve these symptomatic patients, and as such, they should constitute the
best-case scenario for screening outcomes. These were the patients whom
screening advocates had in mind when they lobbied policymakers for expansion, sharing tragic testimonies from families whose children were not
fortunate enough to have had newborn screening. These were also the patients with whom the geneticists were most familiar, since symptomatic
patients formed the bulk of clinical caseloads prior to newborn screening.
As a result, their disease trajectories more closely reflected the knowledge base of medical genetics than their asymptomatic counterparts. And
yet, as we will illustrate in this chapter, early detection and clinical expertise were not always sufficient to prevent serious morbidity. Many of the
newborns discussed here exhibited signs of disease before their newborn
screening results were even delivered. Others experienced metabolic cri-

ses within the first year of life. Consequently, the families of this subset of patients experienced a very different sort of healthcare trajectory from that of the asymptomatic patients whom we introduced in chapter 2. For the patients explored in this chapter, uncertainty crystallized around prognostic claims rather than the diagnostic process. In what follows, we consider this patient trajectory more closely as we turn to the families who spent much of their children's first years of life in and out of the hospital.

Urban hospitals in the United States increasingly operate in what anthropologist Cheryl Mattingly has called *border zones*: hybrid spaces in which multiple languages, nationalities, and race, class, and religious identifications intersect, leading to palpable tensions and misunderstandings.[1] For several reasons, these problems were accentuated among the families that form the focus of this chapter. As we noted in the introduction, the families that participated in our study reflect the demographics of California, a state that is celebrated for its ethnic diversity as much as it is maligned for its discomfiting juxtaposition of profound wealth with extreme poverty. When compared to our overall sample, the symptomatic patients in our study were more likely to come from lower income minority families. Of the 11 patients whom we turn to shortly, 7 had parents who were first-generation immigrants, and 5 of these came from families who spoke only Spanish. In addition to the 6 patients who came from Latino backgrounds, there were two children of recent Asian immigrants, and two from African-American families; the remaining patient was European-American. Only three of the families could be described as middle-class. Due to the size of our sample, we can only speculate as to whether differences between the symptomatic and asymptomatic patients might reflect a correlation between social inequalities and biogenetic outcomes.[2] Whatever the cause of such differences, it is clear that the interactional risks that these families encountered in the genetics clinic were substantially higher: they had relatively fewer social and economic resources and their children were demonstrably more ill. As Mattingly cautions, "Failures of communication are magnified to intense proportions in situations characterized by both perceptions of difference and high stakes."[3]

Yet border zones offer the possibility of care and collaboration in addition to skepticism and mistrust, and despite the heightened stakes and extensive uncertainties faced by the families of symptomatic patients, most persevered to develop trusting relationships with the genetics staff. In this chapter, we begin to tease apart the layers of care and suspicion that confronted families and clinicians in the long-term management of children's metabolic disorders. We begin with the case of Reynaldo Gonzales, a patient whose story lays the groundwork for the analysis that follows. Then, we identify and describe two phases of the symptomatic patient's trajectory: a precarious neonatal period followed by the stabilization and routinization of care. We conclude by discussing the treatment options for metabolic disorders in children and considering some of the common problems that emerged during the course of treatment.

## Fragile Beginnings: Reynaldo Gonzales

Vanessa Ramos brought her son Reynaldo to the emergency room soon after he was born, when the first signs of trouble appeared. According to Vanessa, her pregnancy and delivery had gone smoothly. She received routine prenatal care, "and everything came out good." Vanessa had a vaginal delivery, and Reynaldo appeared healthy at birth. Soon after, however, "He just didn't want to wake up at all," Vanessa recounted. "He took maybe two ounces that whole day. And he was sleeping. He just didn't want to wake up at all. He was crying. And didn't want to eat at all. And I figured obviously something else was wrong." The emergency department physician ordered intravenous fluids because Reynaldo appeared to be dehydrated, but instead of getting better, Vanessa recalled, "he was actually getting worse." Soon, Reynaldo was transferred from the small community hospital where he was born to the academic hospital, 30 minutes away, where our research was based. There, he underwent dialysis, and Vanessa received her son's diagnosis: "And, about an hour later, they took us in a room. And that's when they told me he was diagnosed with maple syrup urine disease. And that's—that's where it all started."

Noticeably absent from Vanessa's account was any mention of newborn screening. In fact, it is unclear from her report whether a clinical diagnosis predated the delivery of screening results. For patients like Reynaldo, the preventive orientation of screening was beside the point. Reynaldo's physicians were already dealing with a very sick baby. Later, when we pressed Vanessa further about Reynaldo's newborn screening results, she explained: "I didn't get the notice until afterwards. So I remember that. That was another little headache that I remember I had. . . . And then that's when I was already in the care of the genetics clinic. So, I just let them tell me exactly what was going on. But, with the newborn screening, I didn't really get much out of them until he was already sick.

And they told me some tests came back, you know, a little rare. And just to come back and have those tests done again. I don't remember exactly what it was. But I was already in the care of genetics."

Reynaldo remained in the hospital for three and a half months, with many ups and downs along the way.[4] He spent most of the time in the neonatal intensive care unit (NICU), where he received six blood transfusions and was fed through a nasogastric tube. "I remember him trying to cry," Vanessa told us. "And you couldn't even hear anything because of his breathing tube. All I saw was his face expressions . . . just asking for help. . . . I've never felt like that ever in my life."

Reynaldo's hospitalization was a trying time for Vanessa. Her own mother had died of stomach cancer just a week before Reynaldo was born. Soon after, Vanessa's grieving father and her two younger siblings departed for a six-week trip to El Salvador—the country that Vanessa's parents had emigrated from—to make peace with the loss of their wife and mother. Vanessa had been living with Reynaldo's father, her boyfriend, but they had begun arguing before the baby was born. She explained, "We tried staying together while he was in the hospital. But it was just too much stress. He was in and out of the hospital. He didn't really want to be there. He'd say he was at work. And he wasn't." Thus, for much of Reynaldo's hospitalization, Vanessa, who was in her early twenties, was on her own. She moved back to her father's apartment, where she came to crash in between long hours at the hospital. Unable to work, she stopped eating, relying only on the five-dollar coupons for hospital cafeteria food that she received from the hospital social worker. She said, "Sometimes I think I went maybe a week without even showering. Because I just wanted to be there. I didn't want to move myself from him. . . . I wanted to know what was going on."

Eventually, Reynaldo was released from the hospital. But Vanessa was told they would be back. Maple syrup urine disease (MSUD) babies get sick often, the genetics staff explained to her. "So, that's why I only go out when I really have to go out," she said. "Other than that, I really just keep him [at home]. Just try to make him as safe as possible, for him not to get sick." In addition to his MSUD, Reynaldo suffered from laryngomalacia, a narrowing of the airway that causes difficulty breathing. He made regular visits to the genetics and hematology clinics, and Dr. Flores, his geneticist, referred him to the ear, nose, and throat clinic several times during the course of our study because of his persistent drooling. Over his first three years of life, Reynaldo was hospitalized several times with pneumonia, high fevers, and seizures. Vanessa recalled Reynaldo's first seizure with palpable trepidation. "I always thought a seizure, you know, you shake. But he didn't shake," she said. "I was holding him. And he was crying just out of nowhere. I thought maybe he was just hungry. I think he was about four or five months. I had just brought him home. And I was trying to feed him. And he was just crying, crying. And out of nowhere, he just stopped crying. And he just put his eyes up, like he was just looking at the ceiling. He was—like he got stuck. And he put his arms up, you know, made them into a fist. And stretched out his legs. And he was just like that, holding it really tight. He stopped crying. He stopped breathing. He wasn't even breathing. And he just stood there for maybe about five, six, seven seconds."

Vanessa tried to avert hospitalizations by giving Reynaldo Gatorade and Tylenol. Although bringing Reynaldo to the hospital made Vanessa feel safe, it also created more problems. Once, when a physician inserted a central line, Reynaldo developed a clot in his artery and had to be put on anticoagulants. After this experience, Vanessa did what she could to try to control Reynaldo's illnesses on her own. "But once that Motrin, Tylenol doesn't help anymore, that's when I start getting worried. That's when I know it's time to get to the hospital," she said.

Until Reynaldo was 21 months old, Vanessa maintained a full-time job as an office receptionist, leaving Reynaldo to be watched by a neighbor in her apartment building. Eventually, however, Vanessa found it too difficult to maintain a job while caring for her son. Vanessa rationalized her decision to stop working: "I'd been working since he got out of the hospital. But I was just starting to get stressed. . . . You're just feeling like *everything* on you. I worked at an office. And it makes me feel good to know at least I'm doing something good. Even though the economy's not as good right now. But, I mean, if I'm home with him, I think that's pretty much all that matters. As long as he's doing better. I don't really care, to tell you the truth. As long as he's doing better. And trying to stay out of those hospitals. Just going for his checkups to see how he's doing." Although she had trust in Reynaldo's caregiver, Vanessa nevertheless felt "like I can maybe do a little bit better job and maybe he won't get sick so much." Vanessa indicated that she was "a lot happier" since she had made the transition to being a stay-at-home mother. With Reynaldo's Social Security payments and provisions from the federal Women, Infants, and Children program, Vanessa was able to support her small family, and eventually, following a terrible argument, moved out of her father's place and into her own apartment.

Reynaldo's father, Ricky, was "out of the picture" until Reynaldo was seven months old. After Reynaldo was discharged from his first hospitalization, Vanessa called her ex and begged him to try to work things out for the sake of their son. But she did not hear back from Ricky until several months later, when she received a notice in the mail that Ricky was suing her for custody of Reynaldo. Vanessa appeared in court on the appointed day, but Ricky failed to show up. "He kind of dug his own hole, is how they say it," Vanessa reflected. "And they ended up giving me full custody of my son. And they put child support on him. And I never even wanted to do that. Because I always told him, whatever happens between me and you, I don't—I don't want to be having problems, like child support and all that. I was like, if I have him, I'm just going to try my best to just take care of him by myself. And if you don't want to be in the picture. But, yeah, he ended up taking me to court. He didn't show up. They gave me full custody. And they gave him child support." Despite Ricky's failure to appear in court, Vanessa tried not to "close the door" on him because she did not want to foreclose the opportunity for Reynaldo to have a relationship with his father. By the time of his first birthday, Ricky was visiting a few times per month and paying child support when he had a job, which was not consistent. Vanessa indicated that they could get along "as friends."

Reynaldo's MSUD was treated primarily through dietary management. Vanessa said that Reynaldo followed "a very strict diet." She continued, "Not much of proteins, like a lot of meat, you know, chicken. Stuff that has dairy. Just—I'm really scared to give him any of that. Because I know that contains a lot of proteins in them. And with him having high protein in him, he gets sick." Vanessa tried to keep track of Reynaldo's protein intake by writing down everything he ate. Still, she admitted that sometimes she slipped, explaining, "It's a little hard." Reynaldo also drank a special formula that she mixed into his milk, and juice as he got older.

In addition to a special diet, Reynaldo was followed by a local Regional Center, the California agency that provides services for individuals with developmental disabilities. Vanessa began taking Reynaldo to the Regional Center when he was 21 months old, at the urging of Denise Moskowitz, the genetics clinic social worker. Vanessa was shocked to discover that her son was evaluated as having an 8- to 10-month developmental delay. Around this time, Vanessa told us, "I mean, I already knew he was going to be a little delayed because of his MSUD. But I didn't think it would be this much. Just taking it day by day. Seeing what he can do and can't. And just try to help him out." Vanessa vacillated between expressing concerns about Reynaldo's uncertain future and resolving not to look too far ahead. Reflecting on his attending school one day, she worried about whether his classmates would tease him about his special diet, a possibility she said would "break [her] heart." Other questions emerged, too. "Because of his delay, is he going to be in special classes? Or is he going to be with normal kids?" she wondered. In the face of such unknowns, she told us that she did not want to push Reynaldo too hard. "I just want to take it little by little," she said.

Vanessa was enthusiastic about the support she received from the genetics clinic. While she valued the care that they provided to her son, they were also attentive to Vanessa's own precarious social situation. Denise acknowledged the stress of being a single mother and assured Vanessa that she was doing a good job. She also counseled Vanessa to ask her Regional Center liaison for respite care, which would provide several hours a month of paid childcare and enable her to take a much needed break. Of Dr. Flores, Vanessa said, "Every time we see him, he always seems to have a smile on his face. And saying I'm doing good. So, that makes me feel good, too." Over time, Vanessa explained, she had established a rapport with the clinicians who had followed Reynaldo since his birth. "I've known them for a while already. And they know my son. And they're always there. I can always dial their cell phone and call them. Or they'll call me just to check up on him, how he's doing." She concluded: "The doctors are really, really nice."

## Newborn Screening and the Symptomatic Trajectory

The case of Reynaldo Gonzales introduces many of the salient themes expressed by the families of symptomatic newborn screening patients: a traumatic birth followed by frequent hospitalizations, the important role of dietary regulation in the management of metabolic disorders, the gendering of care for young children with special medical needs, and the crucial role of trusting relationships with the genetics clinic staff. Reynaldo was one of 11 patients in our study who developed signs of a metabolic disorder shortly after birth. In these cases, newborn screening follow-up procedures helped to confirm the presence of a serious, well-established metabolic disorder. Children in this group were liable to suffer metabolic crises with the potential for devastating consequences, often with little warning. Like the parents of other medically fragile children, their families grappled with considerable uncertainty regarding their children's futures.[5] However, whereas the patients-in-waiting faced diagnostic uncertainty, the symptomatic patients dealt primarily with *prognostic* uncertainty: their symptoms were familiar to the genetics staff, but their disease courses remained quite unpredictable.[6]

The symptomatic patient's trajectory consisted of two distinct phases: (1) a precarious neonatal period marked by an onslaught of medical interventions and a sense that the child's life was in serious jeopardy, (2) followed by a demanding adjustment period during which family life adapted to accommodate care for a chronically ill child. Medical surveillance for this group could be expected to continue indefinitely, and both parents and clinicians acknowledged the real threats of brain damage, coma, and even sudden death.

## Precarious Beginnings

Most of the parents of symptomatic patients told stories about the beginning of their child's life that were reminiscent of Vanessa Ramos's story, if not quite as dramatic. Typically, children in this group became sick soon after birth and displayed symptoms prior to receiving a diagnosis. Monica said, "All of them have been pretty much like, we get the result back and we found out the kid's already in the hospital."

Dionna Walker was rushed to the NICU minutes after her delivery because she was not breathing. Her mother, Rachael Johnston, recalled: "And then I started to get a little nervous after they had gotten her out. And then they were—everybody was kind of, seemed like they were kind of frantic. But, you know, they don't want to let you know. But I was listening to their conversation and I guess she wasn't breathing. So they were telling me, like after minutes were going by, they were like, 'Okay, it's been two minutes and she hasn't been breathing.' And I can hear that. I don't know if they knew that I could hear that but I was listening. And I, of course, you don't hear your baby crying, so." On the third day, hospital staff told Rachael that Dionna had an infection and would be started on an antibiotic. Later that day, however, the newborn screening results were returned. "But then they told me on the third day of us staying there but they had done the newborn screening and that she had come up with something that this hospital didn't really understand, so were like, 'We're going to have to fly her away to the academic hospital.'"

The early NICU days were particularly heart-wrenching for two couples in our study who had lost an older child—presumably to the same metabolic disorder, though neither child had been diagnosed. Lena and Ricardo Sanchez, whose son Diego was diagnosed with glutaric acidemia type 1 (GA1) through newborn screening, had a daughter who died suddenly at eight months for reasons that were not understood at the time. Likewise, Marcella and Louis Torres lost a daughter four days after her birth, 15 years before their daughter Claribel was born and diagnosed with methylmalonic acidemia (MMA) through newborn screening. Marcella told us, "When I looked at her, you know, the memories came back to 15 years ago, how I saw my daughter when she was dying, and we didn't know what to do. Even the doctors couldn't tell what was going on with my daughter."

After Dionna was transferred to a more specialized hospital, Rachael Johnston remained in the community hospital where she had given birth another five days with a uterine infection. When she was finally well enough to travel to the university hospital, an hour and a half away from her home, Rachael met Dr. Silverman: "He's like, 'This could happen. She could have a mental disability, she might develop like you think a normal baby would, she could have these complications.' And he went through all of it. He was like, 'I'm not going to sugarcoat it for you because in the long run that would make it worse.'" Beatriz Hidalgo, whose daughter Marisa was also diagnosed with MMA through newborn screening, recalled her first interaction with the genetics team similarly: "The first time, yes, they said it was very serious, that we had to baptize her. Because the same day they had another child with her same condition and that child died. They said, most likely, the same thing is going to happen to her. Because they are small babies and the blood is not good at all." Likewise, Dr. Silverman told Clarice Muños at her daughter Linda's first appointment, "She could be mentally retarded, she could have abnormalities in her body, in the most extreme situation, she could die. I don't think she's so much at risk, but I have to be really honest with you."

The initial uncertainty was even more pronounced for Spanish-speaking families like the Hidalgos and the Muños, whose diagnostic understanding was more likely to be hampered by communication barriers. In most cases, a hospital interpreter was present for clinical consultations with Spanish-speaking families. Yet communicating through interpreters is mired in interactional difficulties,[7] and in some cases, when an interpreter was not available, Dr. Silverman communicated with families in his own broken Spanish, which families found difficult to understand. As Lena Sanchez told us, "In reality they did not explain to me. Since the doctor does not speak Spanish well and since I never was into this, he would always say that we had to wait so that he doesn't get worse, and that there could be a miracle. And I would ask him what was it that my son would not be able to do. What limitations he was going to have?" According to Lena, the emergency letter she was given, which was written in English, was neither translated nor explained. Beatriz Hidalgo similarly recalled, "The first time she was in the hospital at the emergency room with the other baby and the babies, no one said anything. They would say the baby is sick, her blood is this way, but we didn't understand. I didn't understand exactly what it was." Fortunately, Dr. Flores, Marisa's physician, was able to explain her genetic condition to the Hidalgos in Spanish. But as Beatriz pointed out, "that was later on."

Although Rachael Johnston received Dionna's screening results relatively quickly, several parents suggested that their children had suffered needless setbacks during the neonatal period because the news had been delivered too slowly. Marcella Torres reported that a friend who worked in the hospital where Claribel was born had told her that Claribel's newborn screening bloodspot had not been collected until her fourth day of life, when she was already ill. Marcella recalled, "So I was upset. I didn't know. Well, I'm lucky, I have somebody here who was telling me, 'Hey, they didn't bring the blood here on time.' I was like, 'What? They should do that.' And I was reading about the baby screening program and within 24 hours they have to." While Marcella's reference to a 24-hour time limit was not quite accurate—state policy stipulated that hospital staff had six days for collection, and a later collection time was preferable for children remaining in the hospital because screening results would be more accurate—her suspicion highlights the frustrations felt by parents for whom neonatal diagnosis could not come soon enough.

Carolyn Broderick, for example, noted that Sherise had been given a spinal tap that might have been averted if her screening results were delivered more quickly. She said, "I might carry some of Gary's [her partner's] frustration about somebody dropping the ball somewhere. He thinks that someone dropped the ball as far as, you know, the hospital not getting those tests, or not even trying to get those tests when things started to go wrong." Gary related his own frustration with the false reassurance provided immediately after Sherise's birth, before the screening results were delivered. "Don't tell me everything is fine," he said. "Tell me everything except *this* has come back."

Such dissatisfaction, mild though it may be, is striking insofar as it high-

lights how expanded newborn screening may generate unrealistic expectations for swift diagnostic delivery. Marcella, Carolyn, and Gary had
bought into the paradigm of prevention through screening and ended up
somewhat disappointed by the outcome, even though newborn screening returned results remarkably quickly. Even Monica acknowledged that
while newborn screening helped physicians arrive at a diagnosis more
quickly, in most cases, the appropriate treatment had already been initiated by the time the diagnosis was made. She said, "You know, one kid,
they had already found out that the ammonia was high. I think they had
already, you know, hydrated the kid or started dialysis or something. And
then we got the result back." In fact, this was the case for half of the symptomatic patients in our study. Julie Lee screened positive for MMA, but
the results were delivered late, and Julie was already ill within 10 days
of birth. Carmen Rodriguez learned of her daughter Lupita's abnormal
screening results only after bringing her to the emergency room 8 days
after birth. Although Lupita was diagnosed with citrullinemia during this
hospitalization, she soon fell into a coma that lasted for several days, during which she sustained permanent brain damage. Marisa Hidalgo and
Linda Muños were already hospitalized in the NICU when their results
were delivered, and even Vanessa Ramos lamented that she had not received the phone call about Reynaldo's newborn screening results several
days earlier, when he first became ill. These cases suggest that newborn
screening may not come early enough for the families whose children are
at the greatest risk. In fact, between July 2005 and April 2009, 62 screen
positive infants died in California before follow-up care could be started
in a metabolic center.[8] Naturally, many of the families in our study whose
children became symptomatic prior to the return of newborn screening results wondered why their children's results had not been delivered
more quickly, and whether earlier intervention might have made a crucial
difference to their children's long-term health.[9]

At the same time, for four of the symptomatic patients in our study,
treatment was initiated *prior* to a significant metabolic episode. For children like Kari Buchanan, a newborn screening diagnosis was invaluable.
Kari had MCADD and suffered several metabolic crises. Because these
crises were treated appropriately in a timely fashion, newborn screening
very likely saved her life. Dionna Walker escaped from her initial NICU
stay relatively unscathed due to the prompt delivery of her results, and
Diego Sanchez began a special diet for GA1 prior to any hospitalization.

Furthermore, for all of the symptomatic patients, screening results, when they did become available, helped physicians to settle on a metabolic diagnosis much more efficiently than would have been possible in the absence of screening. Despite some initial delays, then, newborn screening enabled the families of symptomatic children to avert the diagnostic odyssey. For this, parents were extremely grateful. When asked directly about their attitudes toward screening, these parents, like all parents in our study, gave unabashed support for the preventive aims of screening. As Rachael Johnston put it, "He told me that it was something they had just started doing within the last five years. And I was so thankful for that. . . . Otherwise, you know . . . nobody would have really known what was wrong with her."

Still, although the diagnostic odyssey might have been averted, diagnosis marked a singular event at the beginning of a long journey. How these families found out ultimately mattered less than the content of the diagnostic news. In light of their children's fragile health status and early hospitalizations, newborn screening did not always register as a salient aspect of the healthcare experiences of symptomatic patients and their families.

## Stabilization and Routinization of Care

After an initial period of distress and confusion, the families of symptomatic patients settled into routines for managing their children's metabolic disorders.[10] While this care work was by no means easy, and still required an intense commitment from families, it did over time become part of the fabric of everyday family life. Some families were fortunate enough to receive in-home nursing support that was paid for by a state agency, as Marcella Torres did for a brief period when Claribel was first released from the NICU. For the most part, however, the burden of everyday care fell to the families.

An extensive literature has documented that caregiving responsibilities for children with special healthcare needs fall primarily to their mothers.[11] Results from large-scale surveys indicate that the presence of one or more children with a disability has a negative influence on the paid labor force participation of both single and married mothers.[12] Low-income families, in particular, face multiple resource constraints in caring for children with special healthcare needs.[13] Our findings reflect these general trends.

Some mothers, like Vanessa Ramos, quickly discovered that paid employment outside of the home was too taxing in light of their new caregiving responsibilities. Lena Sanchez attempted to find a day care suitable for her son Diego, who had sustained brain damage as an infant following an uncontrolled metabolic crisis, so that she could return to her factory job. Lena postponed her return to work, however, because she found it too difficult to find someone willing to care for an infant "like this," as she put it—a child with disabilities. Following Diego's birth, Lena's family gave up the health insurance she had received through her employer and instead had to rely on the income that her husband, Ricardo, earned as a migrant farm laborer.[14] Likewise, Carolyn Broderick decided not to return to her job as a childcare provider after Sherise's birth.[15] She reported that one of the doctors had instructed her, "No day care. None. Not right now, because you don't want her to catch any germs."

Not all mothers had the option to stay home with their children, however. Some, like Rachael Johnston, Carmen Rodriguez, and Beatriz Hidalgo, arranged for their mother or mother-in-law to care for their children so that they could continue to work in the paid labor force—Rachael as a nursing student, Carmen as a "nanny" for a boy with autism, and Beatriz as warehouse employee. The irony of Carmen's arrangement—leaving her daughter Lupita in the care of her own mother, Rosario Velazquez, so that Carmen herself could be free to care for someone else's child—was not lost on Rosario, who told us, "She babysits another baby and leaves her baby. But, like I tell her, you have to work, right? You can't live without money."[16] Rosario noted that her daughter called home from work "all the time" to check on Lupita, asking, "Is she okay? Is she playing? Is she eating?"

Rosario had prolonged what had initially begun as a short visit from El Salvador to help Carmen care for Lupita more permanently following Lupita's diagnosis with citrullinemia. Rosario's help became invaluable when Carmen separated from Fernando, her husband and Lupita's father, when Lupita was still an infant. Following the separation, Carmen became extremely reluctant to leave Lupita in Fernando's care. She reported to Dr. Silverman that Fernando had taken Lupita to Carl's Jr. and allowed her to eat chicken nuggets, which were prohibited on her diet, because she had cried and begged for them. Although Dr. Silverman encouraged Carmen to send Fernando to the genetics clinic so that he could educate Fernando about Lupita's metabolic disorder, Carmen remained extremely protective of her daughter and skeptical of Fernando's ability to follow the recommended restricted diet. Similarly, Rachael Johnston, who was also separated from her daughter's father, said that the only person whom she would trust to stay with Dionna while she was at work was her mother. Thus, even though some mothers continued to work outside of the home, the burden of care remained deeply gendered.

In interviews, mothers described the ways that they incorporated the care of their child with special medical needs into everyday family life. Lena Sanchez, who, in addition to Diego had an older daughter with cerebral palsy, enlisted assistance from her five healthy children to deal with the other children's limitations. The elder children accompanied Lena to physical and occupational therapy sessions and assisted her with Diego's care. "Like here they put a blanket, and they put him there, and they touch his head and his face, and they pull him from one side to the next or his little hands so that he can pick up the toys, and they give him things that he can touch," Lena explained. "And they put him in his little chair and with his toys. And we put beans or rice and a container so he can stick his hand in to grab it. So things like that." Carolyn Broderick noted how her 7- and 16-year-old sons adjusted their after-school routines once their sister Sherise was born: "They know they can't come and pick her up for me without washing their hands and changing their clothes after school." To prevent her sons from spreading germs to their sister, Carolyn "quarantined" them when they were sick.

Even in the face of stabilizing routines, families stressed that their daily lives were marked by substantial uncertainty due to the unpredictability of metabolic disorders. Rosario Velazquez said, "There are days that she only wants me to hold her, for me to be sitting, to lie down with her. So, there are days I spend the day with her. But, now there are days she's fine, like this." Rosario attributed this inconsistency to Lupita's variable metabolic state: "Days she's good, days she's bad, days she's like, very sad. But, you know the doctor has explained to us that that's the way it has to be." Beatriz Hidalgo noted similarly, "The thing with her—with that condition [is that] she gets sick very often. Yes, anything. Not like any other child. Her immune system is not strong, so she gets sick." When sick, Beatriz said, Marisa would stop wanting to eat, and quickly become dehydrated: "When she is sick, all she does is sleep."

Frequent hospitalizations threw established routines into disarray. Carolyn Broderick never left her daughter's side when Sherise was in the hospital. Once, when we asked if she had stayed in the hospital the entire time during one of Sherise's first four-day hospitalizations, Carolyn replied, "Where else am I going to go?" Carolyn was extremely blessed, she told us, to have Gary at home with her boys. Not all mothers were as fortunate. Those who worked were not always able to take time off when their children fell ill. In such cases, families relied upon their extended kin networks to ensure that a family member accompanied the hospitalized child and domestic responsibilities were fulfilled.

In interviews, mothers wavered between struggling to imagine an uncertain future and enjoying the present moment, wherever their children were. When we asked Marcella Torres what she thought Claribel's future would be like, she wavered between dogged optimism—"I'm expecting her to be just a normal kid"—and a more cautious outlook: "Whatever's going to happen to my daughter I just hope she will be normal, she won't have brain damage." Marcella hoped to find suitable benchmarks for developmental expectations in other children with MMA. She explained, "I usually ask questions to people where they are more exposed to children who have MMA. And I keep asking questions like, 'Oh, how old is that boy? How old is he?' For me to know, how are they behaving?" Still, she had many unresolved questions. For example, she wondered how her daughter's physical appearance would change as she grew. "Will their face change, like a Down's syndrome kind of people, you know? Will you actually . . . look at their eyes and tell that, oh, this boy or this girl has MMA?"[17] Despite lingering uncertainties about her daughter's future, Marcella assured us, "I am not in a hurry." She continued: "I'm not putting pressure on her to be like, 'Oh, hey, do this, and do that, and be a normal baby.' I will wait till she has this, you know, developmental skills, and everything. . . . I will wait till she will catch up on her age. But then I am really hoping she will be normal." Marcella's testimony captures the tension between accepting Claribel wherever she is developmentally and hoping for her to "catch up" and be normal.

In the face of substantial uncertainty about how the metabolic disorder would progress, parents stressed the importance of forming strong relationships with the genetics clinic staff as they developed new caregiving routines. Rachael Johnston recalled how Dr. Silverman had told her, "'I'm going to be a part of your life for the rest of *her* life.' So I was like, 'Okay, well, Uncle Mark is what I guess we'll have to call you.'" Rosario Velasquez said of Dr. Silverman, "He's an excellent person. My God. I ask God to give him plenty of life, so he can keep treating Lupita." Later, Rosario elaborated on how the genetics staff had been like a second family to her and her daughter: "I give so many thanks to the doctors and all the people that keep an eye on her and call us, that keep in touch, that call us and we call them, and they assist us fast. Anything about her food, anything she has, always. Always, all the time it's been like that, always. The communication that—well, at the end, I feel like they're the other family we have, oh yes. Like they're the other family, that any little thing we call, they know us, we know each other and because we're—they're interested and we turn to them when we don't know something. And yes, thank God they have never left our side because they're always there."

The genetics staff also viewed care as a joint endeavor to be taken on collectively with families.[18] While the staff encouraged parents to take responsibility for their children's health and to refine their judgment regarding the incipient signs of a metabolic crisis, they also made it clear that they were always available for consultation and support. Events that were overwhelming crises for parents were a matter of daily routine for the clinicians,[19] who worked carefully to address this disparity. One of the geneticists was always "on call" in the event of an emergency, and Monica spent a significant portion of her time fielding phone calls and answering questions from anxious parents. Denise helped to connect families with local resources and services that would enhance children's development, and the dietitian communicated frequently with families and procured free samples of formula and low-protein medical foods for families in need.

But the shared burden of care stretched beyond such instrumental concerns. As Dr. Silverman told Carolyn Broderick at one of Sherise's first appointments, "And if something goes wrong, you're not gonna carry that burden yourself. We'll share that burden with you." He added, "So I mean psychologically. We're obviously not coming to the house and babysitting." In good humor, Carolyn teased, "We'll come out to the golf course." As this light banter suggests, although the burden of care was to a certain extent shared, the brunt of the day-to-day labor inevitably fell to the parents.

In general, the geneticists were reflexive about the limits of medical knowledge and admitted when there was no clear consensus in the genetics community about the best course of clinical action. Minimizing their expertise helped to sustain caring relationships by putting them on more equal social footing with the families they were treating.[20] To maintain a nonhierarchical stance, the geneticists typically sought input from families in making clinical decisions. For example, when Vanessa Ramos brought Reynaldo to a routine clinic appointment with a high fever, Dr. Flores debated the options with Vanessa. He was nervous to send them home in case Reynaldo took a turn for the worse, but he did not want to send Vanessa to the emergency department unless she was prepared for the inevitable long wait. Together, Vanessa and Dr. Flores decided that Vanessa would take Reynaldo to the emergency department.

In another case, however, a collaborative approach had less favorable consequences. At another routine clinic visit, Dr. Silverman noticed that Dionna Walker's heart was beating abnormally fast. Although a fast heartbeat might suggest something as innocuous as "white coat" induced anxiety, it also raised the question of whether Dionna could be entering a metabolic crisis. Dr. Silverman indicated that he would feel more comfortable if he could order a blood test and asked the family not to leave the hospital until the results were delivered. When the family became impatient, however, he told them that they could drive home. About an hour later, the results confirmed that Dionna was indeed entering a crisis, and Dr. Silverman called the family, still in the car on their way home, and instructed them to go to the emergency department in their hometown. In the end, Dr. Silverman suggested that Dionna would have had better care had she remained at the academic hospital.[21]

In light of the clinic staff's care and sensitivity, families of symptomatic patients were generally extremely satisfied with their children's treatment in the genetics clinic. While the parents of asymptomatic patients expressed occasional skepticism about the utility of routine clinic visits and questioned whose needs these visits were serving, the parents of the symptomatic patients were uniformly grateful for the close partnerships that they developed with the genetics staff. As we will show in the next section, however, these partnerships required a great deal of effort to maintain and sometimes resulted in doubt and suspicion.

## Treating Metabolic Disorders

In this section, we discuss the primary treatments for children with metabolic disorders: dietary management, developmental therapies, and liver transplant. We describe the rationale of these therapeutic approaches and identify some of the interactional problems that emerged in relation to treatment negotiation. Rather than adopt medical guidelines as an unquestioned point of departure, social scientists have long observed that clinical judgments of "noncompliance" as rooted in perceptions of patients' knowledge, beliefs, and behavior[22] often obscure the broader institutional and political economic contexts of chronic illness management. In other words, providers may misattribute patient noncompliance to a lack of knowledge or failure of the will when they neglect to consider the practical constraints on patients' lives that make it difficult—or even impossible—for patients to follow medical advice absolutely, regardless of their intentions.[23] Here, we elucidate how the intertwining of structural factors and interpersonal dynamics can complicate the preventive aims of newborn screening.

## Dietary Management of Metabolic Disorders

Dietary regulation is the single most important component of metabolic disease management. Every day, children with metabolic disorders must balance between getting too much protein and fat, which results in metabolic instability, and getting too little, which impedes normal growth and development and promotes tissue breakdown. This metabolic tightrope, which Dr. Flores termed "the Goldilocks syndrome," presented a persistent challenge for the families and geneticists in our study. The clinic staff spent considerable time tweaking dietary regimens in an effort to optimize nutritional intake, while caregivers spent a good portion of their days counting, measuring, and monitoring their children's diets.

Dietary regulation for patients with metabolic disorders involves two types of preventive measures: restricting certain biochemical substances found in protein and fats that can lead to metabolic problems when they accumulate in the blood, and supplementing specific nutrients that are deficient in people with these disorders. Each diagnosis was associated with a particular dietary regimen that was adjusted specifically to the patient's weight. The clinic dietitian spent most of her time outside the clinic fielding phone calls from families, answering questions, and checking on the child's progress. After the results of blood tests were delivered, she adjusted the patient's dietary regimen based on new laboratory readings and called the family to explain the new plan. These long-distance interactions required a careful rapport that hinged upon relatively brief clinical face time. Although the dietitian officially occupied a part-time position, it was widely recognized by the genetics staff that keeping track of all of the patients could easily become a full-time job. All three of the dietitians who worked in the clinic during our study put in many more hours than they were officially compensated for.

Several factors complicate the dietary management of metabolic disorders in children. After formulating a dietary plan appropriate for the child's age, weight, and diagnostic condition, clinic staff must communicate the regimen to caregivers. Often, dietary regimens are quite complex, and language barriers can hinder comprehension.

Dietary prescriptions may interfere with cultural preferences for particular foods, such as beans or avocados among Latino families, forcing parents to choose between medical advice and long-held beliefs about childrearing. This poses particular challenges when children do not appear to be sick. Moreover, special formulas and low-protein medical foods were not always covered by private insurance, creating gaps in coverage for families that were not eligible to receive support from state agencies.[24]

Once a dietary regimen is established, it must be fine-tuned frequently as the child grows. Often, staff must gauge whether a child is receiving adequate nutrition by evaluating his or her interim growth. Failure to gain weight is a serious problem for metabolic patients, since children cannot attain key developmental milestones without proper growth and nutrition. Dr. Silverman often told families that when it comes to dietary regulation, "one of the rules in metabolic disease [is that] too much is better than too little." Despite these warnings, six of the symptomatic patients stopped gaining weight between appointments at some point during their first three years, prompting careful examination of their diets.

Finally, although parents and clinicians exercise more control over children's dietary intake the younger children are, even at the earliest stages, dietary regulation requires the child's cooperation. Metabolic insufficiency can inhibit the appetite leaving patients uninterested in food. Many families had to resort to feeding children through a gastric feeding tube, a device used to provide nutrition through a surgical incision in the abdomen. Not surprisingly, such "g-tubes" create a new set of problems for care and maintenance: they have to be kept clean, making bathing difficult, and children find them uncomfortable and sometimes pull them out.[25]

As children grew older, a different set of concerns emerged around dietary regulation. Formula consumption was relatively easy to regulate, but dietary regimens became increasingly complex with the introduction of solid foods. Later, as children became more aware of what they and others were eating, parents had to explain dietary restrictions to children and discourage them from sharing food at school or at day care. Colleen Roddick, the mother of a three-year-old boy with phenylketonuria (PKU), recalled explaining to her son Tobias why he could not eat a hardboiled egg like his mother: "And I went to take a bite of the egg. I'm like, 'Well, Mommy's having an egg.' He's like, 'But does it taste good?' And it just broke my heart." Mothers like Colleen lamented how dietary restrictions marked their children as different at a crucial developmental moment.

*Dietary Negotiation*

Dietary management was the most frequent arena for strained relations between families and genetics staff. To a certain extent, the staff recognized, and tried to address, the institutional and economic factors that made it difficult for families to follow the prescribed diet. Some of these barriers derived from the social organization of the clinic and the broader healthcare system. Following a complex dietary regimen was contingent upon acquiring the necessary dietary supplements, as well as formula for infants and special medical foods for older children. This required substantial bureaucratic legwork. Monica reported that over the years, even the most responsive families tended to run out of formula or medical foods at some point, requiring her assistance with a last-minute shipping of an emergency supply. One reason for this is that California Children's Services prescription authorizations last up to six months, after which they must be renewed. Often, however, families lose track of how much time is remaining on their prescription. Monica and the clinic dietitian routinely instructed parents to contact their pharmacy two days before they ran out of formula, but that did not permit time to process a new prescription if the six-month period had expired.

In addition to these practical hurdles, there were several institutional constraints on dietary planning. Dietary regimens for metabolic disorders demand a working knowledge of the nutritional composition of many different foods, which required that the dietitian educate families. Yet unlike another hospital in the area, the genetics clinic had no conference room space for dietary counseling, and the dietitian had to limit her face time with families to the last few minutes of the geneticist's examination. When institutional resources were lacking, clinic staff attempted to tailor dietary advice to the needs of individual families. As one dietitian we interviewed explained, "You have to take each family as an individual. And see where they're at and kind of pick up on the cues with that particular family and how you approach it." Later, she elaborated on how she approached this individualization: "Some of our families, you know, they work in the fields, and some of them don't write or read. So educational level is very tough. We have one family—I basically drew pictures for her, because she kept getting the formula wrong. And then, this last time, I took pictures, I printed up pictures of the cans. I put together this little thing to show her: this is what you use. Because she would never get it right."

As these remarks suggest, some families received a wealth of nutritional information while others were instructed with a few basic principles. The parents of children with PKU might be taught how to measure phenylalanine in their children's food to avoid exceeding a designated daily limit, while others might be instructed to simply avoid feeding the child a limited amount of protein at all. The darker side of such individualization was a therapeutic differentiation along the axis of "educational level" (i.e., social class).[26] Families who "work in the fields," the dietitian's gloss for lower social class, lack cultural health capital.[27] Cultural health capital is constrained by institutionalized inequalities that lead to the systematic privileging of well-educated, middle-class patients in US healthcare delivery. It includes, among other things, medical knowledge, interpersonal and communicative skills, a proactive disposition toward one's future, and crucially, "the ability to communicate social privilege and resources that can act as cues of favorable social and economic status and consumer savvy."[28] The concept of cultural health capital reminds us that, despite the best of intentions, characterizing families' education level may be bound up in stereotypes that act implicitly to generate or reinforce healthcare disparities.[29]

Patients that the genetics staff perceived as noncompliant typically came from low-income minority families. One clinic dietitian explained, "Most of our families that are fairly, well, middle-class, well-to-do, seem to be—I hate to say this, but . . . I can't think of anybody that's really outwardly noncompliant like that." The dietitian's hesitation to generalize about class reflects a clinical sensitivity to stigmatizing stereotypes. As Mattingly has observed in her research with chronically ill African-American children, "Explicit racial designations are rarely used, but there is a common taxonomy of 'difficult clients' that is often attached to low-income minorities, a language so polite that its stigmatizing influences are largely undetected by clinicians."[30] As in Mattingly's study, clinicians treaded carefully around allegations of "noncompliance." Families were rarely accused directly of failing to follow a child's diet, and education level was leveraged as an explanation for noncompliance as much as culture or ethnicity. When one geneticist suspected an immigrant family of noncompliance, he suggested to the dietitian that she ask the mother to fill out a diet diary, a record of the child's dietary consumption over a specific period of time.[31] He reasoned, "She has no clue about [the diet], so let's just get an idea of what she's giving her, and then when she sends it to us, we'll go over it." Modifications were generally proposed within the frame of making things easier for the family, and the staff was cautious when problems emerged.

In the most extreme example we observed, the team contemplated reporting a family to Child Protective Services (CPS) because the father, an Eastern European immigrant, had indicated on numerous occasions that he was ashamed of his son's PKU and did not want him to bear the stigma of a special diet. However, the geneticist resisted the suggestion to report the family because he suspected that such an action would virtually ensure that the family would not return to the clinic, and the child would not remain under his care.[32] His opinion remained controversial, however, because the staff also realized that they had a limited window of opportunity before cognitive deficits would set in.

On one occasion, a parent in our study was reported to CPS, though not by the genetics staff. In this case, Rachael Johnston ran out of formula for her daughter Dionna, prompting a metabolic crisis and an emergency department visit. During the ensuing hospitalization, a social worker at the family's local hospital reported Rachael to CPS for child neglect, because she had run out of formula. The claim was eventually dropped, but it left Rachael and the genetics staff, who had great respect for Rachael's dedication to her daughter, shaken.

One of the most prolonged struggles that we observed over dietary regulation involved the family of Marisa Hidalgo. Tensions emerged between the clinic staff and the Hidalgos early on, when they refused to provide consent to give Marisa a g-tube. As Esteban Hidalgo, her father, later explained in an interview, "I did not agree. [My wife] was convinced but I disagreed because the baby eats everything when she is not sick." Esteban's remarks reveal his doubts about the necessity of an invasive procedure, given that Marisa ate well most of the time. More importantly, however, they illustrate that clinical suspicions can cut both ways: Esteban questioned the physicians' motives (in this case, the gastroenterologist's in addition to the geneticist's) for requesting a g-tube just as they questioned his reasons for refusing.

Relations between the Hidalgos and the clinic staff became even more strained when concerns surfaced that Beatriz, Marisa's mother, was not following the diet recommended for Marisa. When Marisa was six months old, she was admitted to the hospital for monitoring because she stopped gaining weight. There, it became clear that Beatriz had not been administering Marisa's formula correctly. Three months later, after an educational intervention, Dr. Flores was dismayed to learn that Beatriz was still not mixing the formula correctly, and moreover, that she had been feeding Marisa chicken soup. Dr. Flores instructed Beatriz once again not to give

Marisa any protein, including chicken and other meat. Six months later, Beatriz reported feeding Marisa yogurt and beans. In the team meeting later that afternoon, Dr. Flores said that Beatriz had "no clue" how to mix the formula. With regard to feeding Marisa beans, however, he was decidedly less sympathetic. "She knew what she was doing," he said. "She confessed. She knew the label and noted that it had 21 grams of protein. She told me that it has a lot of protein but [Marisa] loves it." When the other geneticists asked Dr. Flores what he planned to do, he presented Monica and Lucy Chin, the dietitian, as the "true heroes of the story." Monica stated their plan: "We are going to educate her. We gave her foods to avoid. We are trying to do our best."

When Marisa returned the next month for another hospitalization, the genetics fellow, Dr. De Vries, set up a meeting with Beatriz, Esteban, a hospital social worker, and a hospital interpreter. Reporting on this meeting to the rest of the team, Dr. De Vries said that the parents "lacked a sophisticated understanding" of Marisa's disorder and that she was uncertain about their literacy skills. She predicted that Marisa would become ill again, requiring a subsequent hospitalization, which would provide another opportunity for education. Dr. De Vries suggested that perhaps they might understand more then. In the meantime, she agreed to work on a list of approved foods and dietary limits.[33]

Marisa's case bears a striking resemblance to the tragic story of Lia Lee, a Hmong immigrant child with severe epilepsy whom Anne Fadiman memorialized in her critically acclaimed book *The Spirit Catches You and You Fall Down*.[34] For Lia's family, the logic of preventive treatment for seizures was not only counterintuitive but also deeply dangerous from the perspective of their cultural worldview. As a well-trodden social scientific critique has made clear,[35] clinical notions of "noncompliance" may gloss over the complex processes through which multiple forms of expertise must be reconciled in order to negotiate treatment. Clashes between forms of cultural knowledge—biomedical and familial—raise important questions about whose expertise counts in the care for the chronically ill. Although the family's expertise may become part of the problem with respect to dietary management, it is also the family's labors that keep the child alive.

Moreover, while Marisa Hidalgo's frequent hospitalizations provide a relatively clear-cut example of the problems posed by poor dietary management, there was not always a straightforward relationship between dietary regulation and the patient's health status. Dr. Silverman described

Carolyn Broderick as a model parent in her management of Sherise's propionic acidemia, yet Sherise nevertheless stopped gaining weight for a period of several months. At the time, Dr. Silverman told Carolyn, "There's one good reason not to worry about her weight. Probably not a damn thing we can do about it. We know that she's getting enough calories, and decent nutrition, and [the failure to gain weight] is probably due to her condition." At the other end of the spectrum was Darren Holt, the young boy discussed in the last chapter who was diagnosed with citrullinemia, the same condition that Lupita Rodriguez had. Although Darren's parents did not follow the clinic's recommended dietary restrictions, Darren was quite fortunate not to have had a metabolic crisis. Dr. Silverman repeatedly assessed Darren as normal except for a minor speech delay, which he attributed to Darren's being a boy and growing up in a bilingual family, rather than to his metabolic disorder.

Inconsistencies such as these presented a real challenge to clinical authority since they mystified the stakes of the endgame of compliance. When the child of a "compliant" family develops unfavorable outcomes and a "noncompliant" family raises a perfectly healthy child, compliance loses some of its luster as the ultimate clinical goal. Thus, while the genetics staff often spoke of families' dietary noncompliance, they recognized its limits as an index of metabolic control. In many cases, then, noncompliance remained part of a diffuse rhetoric of suspicion rather than a problem to be solved through direct clinical intervention.

## Developmental Therapies

Ancillary developmental services such as speech, physical, and occupational therapies constituted another important component of care for symptomatic children. Nearly all of the symptomatic children experienced developmental delays, whether due to the direct effects of brain damage sustained during an early metabolic crisis or the secondary effects of nutritional deficiencies.[36] To limit the potential impact of developmental delay, the genetics staff tried to initiate therapeutic services through the family's local Regional Center as quickly as possible. As we described in the last chapter, Dr. Silverman often framed developmental therapies as preventive measures to normalize the use of therapeutic interventions during early development. For example, he told Carolyn Broderick and Gary Thompson at Sherise's five-month appointment that she was "perfectly normal" and getting physical therapy "just as a protection." Similarly, at

Diego Sanchez's four-month appointment, after inquiring whether Diego was receiving Regional Center services, Dr. Silverman said, "He doesn't have abnormalities at this time. It's just a precaution."

Over time, the symptomatic patients began to exhibit substantial delays that belied Dr. Silverman's initial reassurances. Dionna Walker's case is instructive. At nine months, Dr. Silverman described Dionna in the team meeting as "completely age-appropriate": she was babbling and sitting up on her own. When Dionna was a year old, Dr. Silverman said, "I would rate her as virtually normal. She's a little behind." Three months later, Dr. Silverman continued to assess her as "doing well," better than should be expected. She was not yet walking, but she was cruising on furniture, speaking 10 words, and her weight and height were good. At the two-year mark, however, his assessments evinced a decisive shift. In the team meeting, Dr. Silverman summarized her case as follows: "Dionna Walker is a patient with MMA picked up by newborn screening who did surprisingly well. Now she turned two and she is not doing well. She has only 25 to 30 words—single words and some two-word phrases. She is just beginning to walk, is quite hypotonic, and quite thin: 5 percent for weight and 50 percent for height. They give her a lot of table food. We are not doing much about it. It may not be bad. Too little protein is worse than too much. We may need a dietary intervention but we'll see after we have the test results back."

Most of the other symptomatic patients fared similarly poorly. By the time Diego Sanchez was eight months old, Dr. Silverman was describing him as "badly damaged" and a "disaster" in team meetings, noting several developmental problems: hypotonia (low muscle tone involving reduced strength), asymmetries between his right and left sides, and a large head.[37] At 15 months, Claribel Torres and Marisa Hidalgo could not sit up on their own; at 18 months, Reynaldo Gonzales was not walking; at two years old, Lupita Rodriguez spoke only five or six words; and at 31 months, Sherise Thompson was assessed by the Regional Center as a year and a half behind in cognitive development.

One of the most sobering consequences of our longitudinal ethnography was our ability to observe children return to the clinic every few months having made little developmental progress. In some cases, children regressed on previously attained developmental milestones after being hospitalized for a metabolic crisis. Such patients spent increasing amounts of time with developmental therapists who, in most cases, visited children in their homes, helping them to "catch up" on developmental goals. Some children received upward of eight hours of therapy a week from as many as four different therapists. Mothers were expected to participate actively in these sessions and to practice skills with children in their free time, extending their burden of care.[38] Inevitably, this added to the strain on families in caring for symptomatic children.

## Transplantation

Dietary management and developmental therapies are the only treatment that most children with metabolic disorders will ever get. However, for patients with MMA—the diagnosis shared by Dionna Walker, Marisa Hidalgo, Claribel Torres, and Julie Lee—liver or kidney transplant served as a final, last-resort option. In some respects, transplantation represents the ultimate preventive measure because the metabolic disorder is ostensibly eradicated when the transplanted liver begins to manufacture the previously deficient enzymes. In successful cases, protein restrictions have been mitigated and tube feeding has been eliminated.[39] However, even with transplantation, methylmalonic acid may still be produced in other organs, sustaining the neurological effects of the disorder. As with any organ transplant, there is a risk of mortality, and the efficacy of transplantation is not well known because MMA is so rare. While none of the patients in our study underwent transplantation, it became a topic of heated debate in the clinic when Julie Lee's family put pressure on Dr. Silverman to refer her for a transplant.

Julie Lee had long been a contentious case in the clinic due to the particular circumstances of her birth. Julie was born in Nevada, while her parents, who were not US citizens, were on a trip to attend a business conference. After Julie's diagnosis with MMA, the new family returned home to Taiwan, but Julie and her mother, Mimi, made periodic visits to California to visit the genetics clinic. The staff became suspicious of the couple's motives for giving birth in the United States when Mimi took steps to access a number of services provided by California that Julie was entitled to because she was born there. As one of the more complex cases in the clinic, Julie demanded significant time and attention, yet the staff members were never certain when she would be leaving California.

We first met Julie when she was three and a half years old. According to Dr. Silverman, by this point, Mimi had already been asking for a liver transplant for two years. At the first team meeting that we observed in which Julie's case was discussed, Dr. Silverman presented liver transplant as a poor option with a 20 percent risk for mortality. Julie did not return to the clinic for almost a year, when once again, Mimi asked for a transplant. This time, Dr. Silverman explained to Mimi that it would be premature to refer Julie for a transplant before they had attempted dietary control and emphasized that it was difficult for the clinic to monitor Julie from Taiwan. Lucy Chin, the dietitian, had gleaned from Mimi that Julie was taking "little bites" of everything, thereby exceeding her recommended protein intake. Dr. Silverman encouraged Mimi to remain in California so that they could work on Julie's diet together. In the team meeting, Dr. Silverman was firm: "I'm not gonna do a liver transplant."

Over the next few months, Mimi demonstrated that she had considered Dr. Silverman's advice seriously. She rented an apartment to establish a more permanent residence and worked closely with Lucy on Julie's diet. Monica remained skeptical: "She has an agenda. She wants a liver transplant." Over time, however, Lucy helped Mimi to improve Julie's dietary regulation. Still, Julie continued to do poorly and was hospitalized frequently. By the time that Julie was five years old, both Monica and Lucy pushed Dr. Silverman to approve the transplant. Dr. Silverman presented the case to the team: "Her methylmalonic acid levels are astronomical. She is constantly in the hospital. She is not manageable at home. Lucy is convinced that Mom is following the dietary rules. We assume that she is not managing medically. Julie's brain is well preserved [from the effects of the disease]. She is not retarded. The kidneys seem okay. We have no alternatives but a liver transplant. Everyone has treated her. The decision to transplant should be a collective one."

Multiple concerns were raised in the ensuing discussion. First, some of the team members had remained suspicious of Mimi Lee since she had traveled to the United States to give birth. While not much was known about Mimi's husband, the staff was under the general impression that he was a well-off businessman. Therefore, some questioned the Lees' use of state-funded healthcare services, finding them manipulative or disingenuous at best. Dr. Malvern noted that at Julie's last hospitalization, Mimi had only had enough formula left for two more feeds. Dr. Malvern found it incomprehensible that Mimi did not maintain a sufficient supply, implying that finances should not have been an issue. The geneticists ultimately agreed that these social factors did not bear on the medical necessity of the transplant.[40] But then there was the matter of the transplant itself. While it seemed that the transplant would decrease Julie's metabolic crises, she would not necessarily be spared the risk of brain damage, since methylmalonic acid could still be produced in the brain. Moreover, a liver transplant might complicate Julie's prospects for a kidney transplant further down the line—something everyone agreed was likely to become necessary.

Despite these concerns, the staff eventually agreed to endorse the transplant referral. However, at the time that our fieldwork was drawing to a close, Julie had not received a transplant because Mimi had not resolved which agency would pay for it. In the meantime, Mimi had gotten Julie on a waiting list for a transplant in Taiwan, but transplant regulations in Taiwan restricted a living donor transplant to a family member donor, and the Lees had not found a match in the family. (Cadaver donors were permitted but they were not as effective.) Thus, Julie could either wait for a cadaver donor in Taiwan, or the Lees could attempt to resolve the payment issues and have the transplant performed in California.[41]

Julie Lee's story illustrates that transplantation was a last-resort treatment for MMA mired by significant bureaucratic obstacles and medical uncertainties. Tragically, as Dr. Silverman observed, the genetics staff put off Mimi's requests for transplant for two years. As it is in other clinical settings, adherence to prescribed medical regimens was a prerequisite for transplantation, although geneticists may be somewhat unusual transplant gatekeepers. By the time Julie's quality of life had deteriorated enough that the clinic staff was prepared to seriously consider this option, transplant had become a desperate measure. Unfortunately, however, the infrastructural barriers to organ transplant were not easily resolved, Julie's life hung in a precarious balance, and the family continued to shuffle between California and Taiwan.[42]

## The Limits of Prevention

In team meetings over the course of our study, Dr. Flores repeatedly prefaced his discussions of Reynaldo Gonzales by introducing him as a "success story": a patient who was saved by newborn screening. Still, at three years old, Reynaldo had little verbal language abilities, noticeable cognitive delays, and persistent drooling problems. In the face of these problems, Dr. Flores's evaluative claims conveyed a subtle irony that the other geneticists grasped all too well. What does it mean to say that patients who face significant developmental delays, frequent hospitalizations, and serious risks of mortality have been "saved" by early intervention?

In contrast to the prolonged diagnostic odyssey for patients-in-waiting, for a small number of patients who experienced a metabolic crisis soon after birth, newborn screening helped to *reduce* the diagnostic odyssey by enabling physicians to identify the cause of their symptoms. In some of these cases appropriate treatment was already started, but the alleviation of diagnostic uncertainty, a major psychological burden for families, is a considerable achievement in its own right. Early diagnosis set in motion a wave of therapeutic interventions and bureaucratic oversight that aimed to keep children with symptomatic metabolic disorders under close medical surveillance and provide families with social and monetary resources to implement preventive measures. With this support in hand, families reorganized to meet the challenges of caring long-term for medically fragile children.

At the same time, we have also suggested that characterizations of success vis-à-vis newborn screening are ambiguous at best. In some cases, newborn screening results arrived too late, after a child had already sustained a devastating metabolic crisis and permanent brain damage. Once a diagnosis was in place, there were many infrastructural barriers to long-term management, and collaborative relationships between clinicians and families were challenged by the cultural tensions that proliferate in urban border zones. Even with perfect "compliance," a child could continue to lose weight and risk serious developmental consequences. The uncertain relationship between dietary regulation and health outcomes troubled families and clinicians alike, and complicated the authority of the clinic's message of prevention. Such lingering ambiguities highlight the recursive nature of biomedical uncertainty. Even if newborn screening reduces diagnostic uncertainty, prognostic uncertainty remains. Screening may settle a disease label, but it also creates pressing new questions about what the label will mean for a particular child.

This chapter has thus stressed that if newborn screening reduces the diagnostic odyssey for some families, the therapeutic odyssey is far from over. This second odyssey brings to light the various practices of care that help to sustain children with complex medical problems. In the genetics clinic, the nurse coordinator, dietitian, and social worker were crucial to the everyday management of children's metabolic disorders: they laid out essential daily routines and maintained open lines of communication, providing a foundation for trust and rapport. When problems arose, they were critical to finding solutions. Inevitably, resolving problems led to collisions between clinical and familial worldviews. But encounters are crucial to care, even when they yield uncomfortable frictions. Such frictions make clear that there is a darker side to care and its manifest value. As sociologist Renee Anspach has acknowledged, "Continuous contact has its shadow side, permitting emotions (including negative ones) to develop—emotions that may compromise the quality of an infant's care."[43] In a similar way, familiarity and sympathy may inhibit difficult clinical decisions because they may make it more difficult for clinicians to resist parental wishes.

In light of multiple ambiguities, the genetics staff acknowledged the difficulty of determining whether symptomatic patients fared better than they would have without newborn screening. As Monica put it: "And these kids . . . I can't really say. I—I think they're doing better than they would have done if we didn't know. But I don't—I *can't* know that." Reflecting on the gaps in scientific knowledge of newborn screening outcomes, Dr. Silverman offered a similar conclusion.

DR. SILVERMAN: So every one of these you might say, "Why are we doing [newborn screening for] propionic acidemia?" And the answer to that is—and methylmalonic—and the answer to that is because, firstly, when these sick patients have come in we've known immediately what the diagnosis is, as opposed to it being some child in the state of collapse, could it be sepsis, et cetera? Now, what we haven't shown is whether or not we affect the outcome.

STEFAN: It's just sort of a key rationale behind screening though, that you can affect the outcome.

DR. SILVERMAN: Yes.

STEFAN: Yes.

DR. SILVERMAN: And so we are vulnerable, if you will, on that basis.

In this candid exchange, Dr. Silverman acknowledged an important limitation of the newborn screening program: although it improved the timeline to diagnosis, it was not clear that it had improved the outcomes of metabolic disease for the most seriously affected children. Such comments point to gaps in the logic of prevention underlying expanded newborn screening, revealing one place where public health discourse rubs up against the realities of clinical practice and the limits of scientific knowledge. In light of such uncertainties, situations in which we "*can't* know," as Monica said, how do we define a public health success? In the next chapter, we begin to answer this question by directly addressing whether and how newborn screening saves lives.

## CHAPTER SIX

# Does Expanded Newborn Screening Save Lives?

During a staff meeting in November 2010, Dr. Dati asked the question that was on the minds of many working in newborn screening. He had seen a patient earlier that afternoon who had screened positive for glutaric acidemia type 1 (GA1), confirmed—but barely—by the patient's acylcarnitine levels, and with only one mutation implicated in the disease, not the two needed to feel confident about a diagnosis. During the clinic visit, Dr. Dati had taken a skin biopsy in another attempt to reach a more conclusive diagnosis. Both the boy and his mother had been crying. The stress of wondering, in Dr. Dati's words, "whether her son was going to die soon or whether he was fine" had taken its toll on the mother. Dr. Dati found it a deeply frustrating experience.

Later in the meeting, Dr. Flores reported on Marisa Hidalgo. Marisa had been diagnosed with methylmalonic acidemia (MMA) through newborn screening but at 26 months she was neither talking nor walking. All of the geneticists were familiar with Marisa because they had been on call during her recurring hospitalizations. On this particular day, she had just been discharged from yet another monthlong hospitalization. As Dr. Flores recounted these events, Dr. Dati interrupted and asked: "Are we actually doing any good with newborn screening? Do we have any data on whether we make a difference? Frankly, based on these meetings, I don't see that we are making a difference." After voicing this concern, he quickly backpedaled, adding, "You can never look at data this way." By this, Dr. Dati meant that you cannot draw any conclusions from anecdotal evidence: you have to look at the outcomes of newborn screening scientifically. He wondered whether after five years of expanded newborn screening there was any data that showed a positive health impact.

With these unsettling questions, Dr. Dati expressed a growing sense of unease with the outcomes of newborn screening. The staff saw many patients for whom newborn screening brought diagnostic ambiguity as well as symptomatic patients who did not seem to improve. And for the asymptomatic patients, there was always a lingering suspicion that perhaps these patients would have remained unaffected anyway. What was the public health impact of newborn screening? Are we, as the name of the parent advocacy group suggests, saving babies through screening? The ensuing discussion at the staff meeting offered a reflective diversion from the standardized case reports typically shared in staff meetings.

Dr. Silverman spoke first. He had the longest career in newborn screening. He explained that from the onset of the expansion, he had known that for the most severe disorders associated with the worst outcomes, such as MMA and propionic acidemia, newborn screening was unlikely to make a difference in outcomes. These conditions were, in his words, "guilty bystanders" of newborn screening. "You may treat these patients a little earlier," he explained, "but it will not change the outcome much." He added that with "milder" fatty acid oxidation disorders, such as MCADD, the outcomes seem to be better. But, he added, "the jury is still out" on whether some children diagnosed with disorders such as cobalamin C deficiency, 3-MCC, or carnitine deficiency truly benefit because with intervention at an early age, we never know if they would have developed symptoms.

While focusing on the diverse consequences of newborn screening for families and geneticists, we have remained agnostic about the official goal of newborn screening: to save babies through secondary prevention. Most of the immediate consequences of newborn screening do not directly pertain to lives saved. What stands out in clinic visits is the management of diagnostic uncertainty when newborn screening raises a red flag, or prognostic uncertainty in the care of symptomatic infants. Still, for public health officials and policymakers, newborn screening constitutes a health policy decision justified by the expectation of a reduction of morbidity and mortality. In this chapter, we turn to the lifesaving promise underlying newborn screening. Our starting point is the presumption that newborn screening does not save lives by itself. In the most fortunate of circumstances, newborn screening offers an opportunity for saving lives, but making a difference in health outcomes depends on a mixture of luck and hard work. Complicating causal narratives about newborn screening's lifesaving potential, we will argue that the window of opportunity to save lives may close prematurely due to remaining inequities in the US healthcare system.

To avoid misunderstandings, we would like to clarify up front that our study design does not allow us to evaluate the extent to which newborn screening has saved lives. Answering such epidemiological questions would require a different methodology. Because expanded newborn screening was implemented so recently, there is little data about long-term clinical outcomes. Data from pilot studies in the United States and elsewhere suggest that while infants diagnosed through newborn screening do experience better health outcomes than those diagnosed clinically, they may still experience significant morbidity and mortality.[1] In this chapter, we will focus on how the opportunity to save lives can be maximized, and point to some recurring barriers. Even then, our analysis is suggestive rather than definitive: we have not measured health outcomes but we can point to some social, cultural, and economic factors that likely impact lifesaving.

There are four logical possibilities that link newborn screening to health outcomes, as indicated in table 1. We use "doing well" and "doing poorly" as heuristics to indicate a stable or improving health course and a deteriorating health trajectory, respectively, recognizing that we are simplifying complex, multicausal processes. First, as Dr. Silverman's comments at the meeting and the situation of Marisa Hidalgo suggest, some children did poorly despite the advance knowledge provided by newborn screening.[2] In such cases, the main effect of newborn screening was to reduce the diagnostic odyssey once the children developed symptoms, and its inevitable counterpart, a period of "blissful ignorance"[3] during which parents could enjoy their as yet asymptomatic newborns unencumbered by the knowledge that their child had a life-threatening condition. As we discussed in the previous chapters, the goal of screening in such cases was to begin treatment promptly, address symptoms vigilantly, and keep the child out of the hospital for as long as possible. Newborn screening advocates hoped that earlier attention to metabolic diseases and a better understanding of their natural histories might lead to more effective therapies in the future. At this point, however, children might die in spite of early detection, as did three infants in our study, including Marisa, who passed away several

TABLE 1. **Four possible outcomes of expanded newborn screening**

|  | Positive outcome | Negative outcome |
| --- | --- | --- |
| Newborn screening makes a difference | Child doing well because of NBS | Child doing poorly because of NBS |
| Newborn screening is incidental | Child doing well regardless of NBS | Child doing poorly regardless of NBS |

months after the meeting we described in the beginning of the chapter. Researchers at Children's Hospital, Boston, also documented four sudden deaths in children with MCADD, despite identification via newborn screening. As the authors note, "While the frequency of sudden death in MCADD has probably been reduced by NBS it has not been eliminated."[4] Such cautionary tales demonstrate that even with early diagnosis, managing metabolic disorders is not a straightforward clinical task.[5]

Second, although it is impossible to know for sure without doing a randomized controlled trial, there is very likely a corollary at the other end of the lifesaving continuum: children who did well but whose good health might not be attributable to preventive measures. For these children, dietary regulation and other therapies were likely incidental to favorable outcomes. There is some evidence for this claim because the incidence rates of metabolic disorders have been significantly higher since the implementation of expanded newborn screening, which suggests that many patients with these disorders went undetected prior to population screening and went on to live healthy, symptom-free lives. As we discussed earlier, newborn screening has also lead to the diagnosis of metabolic disorders in asymptomatic mothers who had not been treated for their conditions but nevertheless had done fine.

One child in our study who fit into this category was Paul Wong, a boy diagnosed with GA1. Unlike Bailey Baio and Mike Honan, who had elevated metabolite levels with only one mutation, Paul's mutation analysis identified two mutations implicated in the disease and left no ambiguity that he indeed had the condition. Dr. Silverman explained his situation to a visiting medical student: "Paul was picked up on newborn screening as having glutaric acidemia type 1, and he definitely has it. His values, though, are not particularly high, the values of the telltale metabolites, but they were high enough for us to be fairly certain. And some patients, at least intermittently, are completely normal metabolically. We chose to sequence his glutaric-CoA dehydrogenase genes, and found two presumed pathological indications. . . . So he's got that. The Wongs sweated for two years. Two years is very important. After two years, damage does not frequently occur, at least acute damage, and after four years, virtually never." Paul had a fraternal twin brother who offered a ready comparison for his development. Based on language development, motor skills, and other developmental landmarks, Paul seemed ahead of his brother, which suggested that Paul was "normal."

The Wongs credited Dr. Silverman with saving their son's life. They even took a picture of Paul in Dr. Silverman's arms. Yet Dr. Silverman expressed reluctance to take credit for saving this child. He explained during a clinic visit, "We don't know if newborn screening is preventing anything in a kid like Paul. What we know is one thing: it scares the hell out of the parents." Paul's mother agreed: "Yeah, it sure did." Dr. Silverman continued: "I think now with the fact that he's doing this well and he's doing as well as his not-identical twin brother and that he hasn't had any episodes is very reassuring." Dr. Silverman then added that unlike for PKU, in which every untreated sibling had mental retardation, "from the earliest days of GA1, we had retarded kids who had normal siblings with the same mutations." Thus, some children diagnosed with GA1 did well without dietary treatment. Dr. Silverman could not be sure whether Paul was one of them or whether he did well because of the treatment. As Dr. Dati observed dryly in a meeting, "The kids with nondisease usually do fine."

A logical third group exists: those who undergo preventive measures that may harm them. We do not have evidence for such outcomes in our study, but the early history of PKU screening indicates that some patients were harmed because they had been unnecessarily deprived of essential nutrients. The full extent of iatrogenesis during the 1960–1970s is difficult to reconstruct because the medical literature is biased against publishing accounts of medical error.[6] Some case reports suggest failure to thrive, listlessness, and skin rashes in a few false positive PKU patients who were deprived of phenylalanine.[7] Similarly, past screening programs for histidinemia and the resulting low histidine diet may have caused psychological stress, unnecessary blood draws, and uncertainty about the future.[8] Monica mentioned that she occasionally had to talk pediatricians and parents out of implementing a restrictive diet as a preventive measure in cases where newborn screening results had not yet been confirmed. She also gave an example of potential iatrogenic harm in a child who screened positive for GA1. "You know, we actually were really scared that this was going to be a true positive, so we started the kid on diet, even though we didn't have a diagnosis," she recalled. "But we figured, 'Okay, it's just going to be a diet until we figure out, we'd just rather be safe than sorry, you know, just start this diet.' And then the kid started losing weight, because they started . . . I think we freaked them out about the protein and everything, and so the kid stopped breastfeeding and then they figured they would just give more formula. But the formula is not a complete formula . . . we figured out what was going on and we said, 'No, no, no. You know, go back, add formula, regular formula.' And I think at that time we'd figured out, the repeat test came back normal. So: 'Okay. Just go back. You know, go back to regular formula and everything.' "

The fourth possibility consists of the patients for whom there exists an opportunity for lifesaving preventive measures. This is the group of greatest interest to us, and we will devote the rest of this chapter to them. Since newborn screening is premised on the assumption that early intervention can save lives, geneticists and families had to take advantage of this early opportunity to intervene. Besides forming a working relationship with the genetics team, parents had to be vigilant every day. We offer the hypothesis that for some children with a positive newborn screen, the unrelenting work of parents and the genetics team could make a lifesaving difference. It is impossible to prove this conclusively because we do not know the counterfactual outcome of geneticists and parents not stepping up to the plate. We find some evidence in our data that acting on advance knowledge could tip the balance for fortunate children, presuming that the parents maintained an unwavering focus on keeping their child alive. Much of this mundane work to keep a child healthy is all-encompassing, infinite, and labor intensive. Clinicians delegate this work to parents but most of it remains invisible. Our goal here is to bring this critical yet often overlooked work into the open.

At the same time, parents' ability to keep the child alive was further circumscribed by certain features of the US healthcare system. In the context of the US healthcare economy, newborn screening is unusually democratic: every child is screened regardless of the family's ability to pay. Omnipresent inequities in the healthcare system, however, created structural barriers for some families that can offset the lifesaving benefits of screening. The problems related to accessing services, obtaining dietary interventions, follow-up testing, and transportation. Again, we do not have definitive evidence that healthcare barriers by themselves result in complications but our data indicate that such barriers may prematurely close the window of opportunity to make a difference in health outcomes. We suggest that an increasing complexity of problems and of coordinating care among multiple stakeholders combined with a lack of resources to circumvent barriers can have a negative impact on health outcomes.

## The Window of Opportunity

The geneticists' reference point for the potential success of newborn screening was their long experience with PKU. They had followed some patients with PKU for several decades and had observed how controlled phenylalanine levels could prevent mental retardation. The geneticists saw tremendous variety in cognitive outcomes in PKU patients: some patients exhibited age-appropriate intelligence, while others appeared to have serious cognitive deficits. The key point was that better cognitive outcomes correlated with lowered phenylalanine levels due to a phenylalanine-restricted diet at an early age. Although cognitive abilities could vary over the life course, an NIH consensus document argued that irreparable damage occurs if treatment is not started as early as 7 to 10 days after birth:

> Age at treatment initiation and level of metabolic control clearly influence outcomes. There is an inverse relationship between age at treatment initiation and IQ even in early treated PKU. Moreover, new evidence suggests that high plasma Phe levels during the first 2 weeks of life can affect the structural development of the visual system. Although the visual deficits are mild, this warrants efforts at earlier treatment initiation.[9]

There is thus a critical window of opportunity for starting lifelong health-preserving therapy.

Dr. Silverman noted the compelling logic of PKU prevention during a patient visit: "In PKU, 100 percent are retarded without treatment; 100 percent are normal with treatment." He then qualified that this correlation only worked for those children with classical PKU: "And of course, with PKU back in the late '60s and early '70s we discovered milder forms, partial effects, and if they had been included originally, well, it wouldn't have been 100 percent that we're talking." Further confidence for the correlation between diet and prevention came from a natural control group: the affected but undiagnosed older siblings. As Dr. Silverman explained, "Now, the other thing is when we looked at PKU families and there were other siblings who were not screened and not diagnosed, all of those affected had retardation. So we had an independent way of doing that." The take-home message was that newborn screening could lead to beneficial health outcomes if treatment was started early and sustained over the life course.

The question was, how many of the conditions added to the expanded newborn screening panel were similar to PKU? PKU is a condition detectable at birth in which effective treatment is available, and for which early intervention prevents morbidity and mortality. All of the screening targets on the expanded panel were detectable at birth, but they varied tremendously in terms of the availability and effectiveness of treatment and the benefits of early intervention. Even the ACMG report posited that only hypothyroidism, biotinidase deficiency, and MCADD were similar to PKU in the sense that "all" negative consequences could be prevented. For tyrosinemia type 1, carnitine transporter deficiency, VLCADD, and maple syrup urine disease, early interventions could avert the most negative consequences and clearly optimized individual outcomes. Early intervention in MMA, propionic acidemia, and classic galactosemia could prevent only some negative consequences. According to the report, developmental delay, seizures, and bone marrow suppression are common in propionic acidemia even with early intervention. Treatment for some forms of MMA had even more limited efficacy. For galactosemia, the literature review showed that poor growth and feeding, lethargy, jaundice, vomiting, and hypotonia could be prevented but that long-term complications involving the brain or ovaries still occurred in the majority of cases. For other conditions, less was known about the efficacy of early treatment. Early treatment for arginase deficiency could reduce some neurological dysfunction. Treating GA1 could help to avoid neurological degeneration, but early onset GA2 had not been successfully treated.[10]

If this anticipatory knowledge was correct, the window of opportunity to improve health varied across conditions and would be limited for some conditions targeted by newborn screening. Yet even in the most favorable situation, the key was to be able to act upon this window of opportunity. Next, we describe how one mother was able to capitalize upon the knowledge learned from newborn screening to keep her daughter healthy. Not surprisingly, this case concerns an MCADD diagnosis, for which treatment is straightforward and usually effective—although, as we mentioned, mortality has still occurred in spite of screening. We want to draw attention to the diligence required from this mother to advocate for her child and her ability to take responsibility when it really counted.[11]

## A Life Saved

Kari Buchanan was originally diagnosed with MCADD via newborn screening in New Zealand. In the eyes of the clinic staff, there was no ambiguity that Kari had MCADD. When she was a year old, her geneticists in New Zealand conducted a molecular analysis and found that Kari had one known MCADD mutation and one splice site mutation.[12] Kari also had consistently elevated levels of acylcarnitine, the biochemical marker for MCADD. At one early clinic visit after she moved to the United States,

Kari's C8-acylcarnitine levels measured 2.61 µmol/L, while in unaffected children the upper threshold of the normal range was 0.25 µmol/L. Kari's high levels indicated the accumulation of fatty acids in her blood. While still in New Zealand, Kari experienced two metabolic episodes following gastrointestinal illness, which required hospitalization for three and five days, respectively. Kari took carnitine supplements and cornstarch with milk before bedtime as a preventive measure.

Two years after Kari's family moved to the United States, Kari contracted the H1N1 virus (swine flu) and vomited repeatedly. This was an extraordinarily dangerous situation for a child with MCADD because she could not compensate for the lack of nutritional intake by breaking down her own fat reserves. With the emergency provisions in place, Kari was hospitalized for a week and came out of the episode relatively unscathed. Her mother, Samantha Buchanan, filled Dr. Silverman in during a clinic visit:

SAMANTHA: She had swine flu in October, and it was very awful. She was the sickest I've ever seen her. She had a 106 [degrees Fahrenheit] temperature, was puking everywhere. It was very bad, very, very bad. Very scary.

DR. SILVERMAN: You have to be hospitalized?

SAMANTHA: Oh yes, she was in the hospital for a week.

DR. SILVERMAN: But metabolically was she doing okay?

SAMANTHA: Yes. Oh, it was amazing. I don't even know how that was possible. She was so sick.

DR. SILVERMAN: Well, as soon as you get glucose you can protect them.

SAMANTHA: Well, just her onset, you know, it was really a rapid onset. And we had been to the doctor that day. And it was only 101 [degrees Fahrenheit], so we were just doing the temperature, you know. And she threw up the Zofran. And then she just went steadily downhill from there. Then, we had to go to the hospital at five in the afternoon. But it was great. They had people waiting out the wazoo, and you know, Dr. Martin [Kari's pediatrician] just rocks the house. He talked to the nurses, and got us in.

We don't know what would have happened if Kari had remained untreated during this episode, but based on a published record of MCADD patients with identical C8 values who underwent similar metabolic crises with fatal outcomes,[13] she seems to be the one patient in our study for whom newborn screening was most likely to be lifesaving. Kari was a precocious, active little girl, counting, recognizing the letters of the alphabet, and identifying colors by age three. Even this success story, however, was not predetermined by newborn screening. Knowing unquestionably that Kari had MCADD did not save her life. In fact, a diagnosis was simply the start of a years-long (and probably lifelong) commitment. Samantha engaged a singular focus on averting a metabolic crisis through prevention, including anticipating potential future problem situations. Because Kari did not have any symptoms or developmental delays, coordinating care with other specialties or securing medication was never an issue. Samantha also had reliable transportation, private health insurance for her daughter, a flexible work schedule that allowed her to visit the clinic, and the linguistic ability and cultural health capital to communicate clearly with the genetics staff. The number of issues that could go wrong in her situation was already limited. Even then, Samantha sometimes struggled to convince Dr. Silverman, Kari's father (whom she separated from two years after returning to the United States), and administrators at Kari's school about the seriousness of Kari's condition.

Samantha, who described herself as somewhat of a "hippie," emphasized during her clinic visits while Kari was busy making drawings or tracing letters that her former husband, Peter, was a great father. Still, Kari's MCADD became a hot-button issue in the separation. Peter saw Kari during the weekends while Samantha took care of her during the week. Samantha believed that Peter did not take MCADD as seriously as he should. There was the time that Kari came back from a weekend talking about the chocolate she had eaten, a no-no as far as Samantha was concerned. The point of major contention concerned Peter's desire to take Kari back to New Zealand, his birth country, for a holiday visit. Samantha refused to let Kari travel to New Zealand in case a metabolic crisis developed on the 15-hour flight. According to Samantha, the judge agreed with her that it was safer to wait until Kari was older.

Samantha and Dr. Silverman disagreed about the appropriateness of preventive measures for Kari's MCADD. Dr. Silverman considered MCADD to be a serious vulnerability that mattered mostly when a child was fasting due to illness. He aimed to convince Samantha to, as he put it in his early notes, "try to normalize [Kari's] life as much as possible." Samantha, in contrast, thought that Kari was continuously at risk for a metabolic crisis and required constant vigilance. Their discrepant views came to a head over the necessity of Kari's cornstarch routine. Since Kari had stopped breastfeeding, Samantha had fed her three tablespoons of cornstarch with six to eight ounces of soymilk before bedtime each night.

Cornstarch, a slow metabolizing carbohydrate, may counter hypoglycemia during the night by preventing the body from breaking down its own fats. The big glasses of milk led, according to Samantha, to a "zillion" nightly bathroom stops, and by age four and a half Kari was still not toilet-trained at night.

At the third clinic visit we attended, Samantha asked whether they could alter or decrease the amount of milk, suggesting that perhaps she could put the cornstarch in yogurt rather than milk or simply decrease the amount of liquid. To her surprise, Dr. Silverman replied that he did not "see any reason to take cornstarch at night." Samantha answered: "That's gonna make me nervous." She laughed. "It's gonna make me nervous now. Well, because she's always had something before she goes to bed." Sensing Samantha's resistance to his advice, Dr. Silverman suggested that she use a blood glucose monitor for the first couple of nights without cornstarch solution to see whether Kari's blood glucose levels were affected very much. But, he added, "an overnight fast in someone her age should be tolerated." Samantha understood the cornstarch solution as a necessary preventive measure to replace nighttime breastfeeding. When Dr. Silverman left, Samantha burst out, "Right now I'm not convinced that anybody really knows anything about MCADD." She contrasted Dr. Silverman's "let's wait and see what happens" attitude with the stakes of a metabolic crisis: "What's a little thing to them, is like life and death for her. If it's going to jeopardize her stability then this is not, you know, worth it. I'm happy to buy a pull-up until she's twelve." At the next visit, six months later, Kari was still drinking six ounces of soymilk with cornstarch before bedtime.

Samantha also struggled with overseeing Kari's mealtimes and food intake at preschool, and with the prospect of kindergarten. She told us months in advance that she had diligently interviewed teachers, principals, and school nurses to make sure that they understood MCADD. She was delighted with a magnet program in a public school that had experience with children with diabetes. Even this school, however, had regular cupcake parties. Samantha instructed her daughter that in such situations, she should cut the cupcake in half and scrape off the frosting. She recognized the danger of making her own cupcakes at home with applesauce, which could lead Kari to think that cupcakes were okay to eat at school: "Not all cupcakes are created equally. So we're trying to teach her about this stuff." Samantha's approach was to teach Kari how to deal with "social eating" situations in which there could be pressure not to eat too much or to eat the wrong kinds of food. She strategically fed Kari a diversity of foods "sufficient for survival" and taught her "about just being healthy and strong. Eating the right foods for our bodies and that, well, her body needs different things sometimes. We talked about listening to our body and, you know, when she needs to rest she rests, when she needs to, you know, eat she eats but it's still hard to know what's going on in her." Several times during preschool, Kari had come home with only a couple of bites taken out of her sandwich, which prompted Samantha to arrange meetings with Kari's teachers.

Some may dismiss these conflicts between Samantha and Peter, Dr. Silverman, and Kari's teachers as those of an overreacting or—worse—neurotic mother, suggesting a level of maternal irrationality. This tendency to psychologize mothers has deep roots in healthcare; see, for example, the convoluted history of mothers of children with autism and "schizophrenogenic" mothers over the course of the twentieth century.[14] Sociologically more interesting, however, is to ask how and under what circumstances Samantha's protectiveness makes sense. The conflicts developed in an environment where Samantha's role in keeping her daughter alive was critical yet unspecified. For every child diagnosed with a metabolic disorder, someone such as Samantha needed to take responsibility, but it was not specified how much care was sufficient. Samantha acted out of fear of losing Kari. She told us during the first visit that MCADD was "life-shadowing" and added that one of the major realizations for her was "learning that MCADD is not a death sentence." Samantha's actions suggested that MCADD did not have to be a cause of death, but it easily could become one if Kari strayed from her diet or stopped taking supplements. She had seen Kari "very, very, very sick." Therefore, Samantha not only always carried a bag with emergency food with her but also organized her entire life around the possibility of a metabolic crisis. She told us that she moved back to the United States in large part so that she would have a larger family support system to help with Kari.

The H1N1 flu episode was striking because it might have been interpreted as a validation of Samantha's perspective that her daughter remained in mortal danger. Dr. Silverman, however, saw the good outcome as an indication that Kari's MCADD was controllable and tried to dissuade Samantha from focusing her attention on the low-fat diet or food supplements. He repeated his basic message: "The most important thing is when they get sick, get them to a hospital, and make sure that they are eating. If they eat, they're protected. Although people talk about low-fat diets, talk about carnitine, the essential treatment is just not letting them become ill. With this condition, it's easy to treat, so that unless you live in the middle of nowhere—" Samantha interrupted him, her voice raised: "Or getting to the emergency room. Or have a doctor that will take you seriously. Or have a rapid onset disorder. You make it sound like it's so easy: like all you do is get them to the ER. So much happens before they get sick, and before you get to a [IV] drip." She added that during the H1N1 episode, the emergency department was full and it was only because of her strong relationship with Kari's pediatrician who called the hospital on her behalf that Kari was able to receive the intravenous glucose immediately.

In principle, it should be simple. Once you receive a diagnosis from newborn screening, you should be able to prevent the onset of disease, especially in a condition such as MCADD where the main objective is to keep the child from fasting. And once the child starts vomiting, intravenous glucose should save her. Yet diagnosis is not directly connected to prevention, nor vomiting to the drip. Making these connections requires the work of unspecified others to act on behalf of the child. Once a diagnosis was made, the work of keeping an infant alive was delegated to a primary caretaker, who had to take responsibility and inspire others to take equivalent responsibility. Social scientists have referred to the work that keeps things on track as *articulation work*.[15] This work is often invisible from an accounting or formal organizational perspective, but it is crucial to getting any job done. It is the work of countless administrative staff that allows an executive to multitask, or the work of taken-for-granted caregivers that allows the children of dual-income parents to attend soccer practice and a piano recital. And it is the work that in the current healthcare system increasingly has become the burden of parents of a sick or disabled child to manage the condition, regardless of available resources.[16]

Samantha's complaint, that Dr. Silverman "makes it sound like it's easy," was a cry for recognition of the work she had been doing to keep her child alive. Where Dr. Silverman focused on the effectiveness of emergency care, Samantha highlighted the erased work of recognizing Kari's signs of distress, communicating with her pediatrician,[17] rushing to the emergency department, not to mention spending a week with Kari in the hospital. Newborn screening makes saving some lives possible. Yet it is the chains of largely invisible and taken-for-granted work done by many people to mobilize and use resources—often coordinated by parents—that saves lives on a day-to-day basis. Dr. Silverman eventually recognized Samantha's role. In his notes from the last meeting, he wrote: "Really [Kari's] most important protection is her mother and her mother's diligence."

Kari's situation is the clearest case from our study that shows that newborn screening makes a difference. Most patients' health situations were more ambiguous to assess, or they were not doing as well. As Samantha's dedication showed, saving lives depended on connecting the promise of newborn screening with the available medical care. A collaborative effort by parents and healthcare providers may enable them to take advantage of the opportunity that newborn screening offers.

The downside of this portrayal, however, is that it might appear to suggest that saving lives can be reduced to the mother's desire to do the best for her child. Samantha was highly motivated to keep her daughter alive, but so were all of the mothers in the clinic, many with less fortunate outcomes. What mattered equally if not more than motivation was the parent's ability to tap into available medical services and social resources. This ability could be thwarted by mundane and frustrating bureaucratic issues at a critical crisis point. In the remainder of this chapter, we review the barriers that regularly emerged because of the way that expanded newborn screening fit in with the broader US healthcare system. Most of the time, these barriers were maddening inconveniences, but if they struck at the wrong time, they could undo the opportunity that newborn screening created.

## Old and New Forms of Citizenship

The screening program provides no direct benefit to untreated children. — (Botkin 2009, p. 167)

Universal newborn screening, with its public health rationale, sits uneasily in the for-profit landscape of US healthcare, and its success will be affected by the challenges to reach those least likely to have access to healthcare. The screening program has some structural advantages over other public health measures because it can dovetail with healthcare programs already available for newborns. But at some point, the inequities present in the healthcare system inevitably start to manifest themselves, squandering some of the public health benefits of universal screening. What good is it to screen a population and single out infants with rare diseases if follow-up care and preventive treatment is inaccessible?

Because screening for rare conditions has become a de facto birthright for those born on US soil, it raises the issue of citizenship, the process by which governments bestow rights and responsibilities to categories of people within a society. Citizenship reflects a series of civil, political, and social rights and obligations,[18] both a status and a set of practices. Citizenship has long been organized around biological characteristics, with beliefs about blood relationships organizing human beings, individuals, communities, and races. For example, people seeking a marriage license in Massachusetts are required to present a medical certificate that shows that the applicant is free of syphilis and was offered educational materials on AIDS. Physicians also need to offer women a voluntary rubella test.[19] Even genetics has offered a means of national and transnational governance for quite some time, most prominently with a morally mixed but largely dubious history of eugenics and racial hygiene.[20]

In the wake of rapid discoveries in biology, contemporary forms of "biological" citizenship have proliferated and scholars have noted significant differences from earlier racialized eugenic forms, which were aimed at population control by removing or enhancing purported inferiors.[21] A nation's "genetic stock" has scientific and commercial value, being mined for "biovalue" as in the many biobanks worldwide.[22] Anthropologist Adriana Petryna illustrated how damaged biology became a basis for state entitlement in the aftermath of the Chernobyl nuclear disaster when the young Ukrainian state offered financial and healthcare benefits to those exposed to radiation.[23] She highlighted that biological citizenship is a measure of last resort for the most marginal members of a society. Similarly, sociologist Steven Epstein explored how biopolitical citizenship captured the US government mandate to include racial minorities, women, and other underrepresented groups in federally funded research.[24] In each of these examples, biological differentiation is used to claim citizenship stakes and to classify, monitor, and regulate a population, often in deeply contested ways that pitch various stakeholders against each other. The moral stakes can still be high: hanging citizenship claims on the biology of gender or race institutionalizes a biological basis for race and gender in regulations, laws, and biomedical practices.[25]

Newborn screening constitutes a rare form of universal biological citizenship. In most instances, the presence of biologically distinguished characteristics stratifies a population and only specific groups qualify for state attention on biological grounds. Thus, the syphilis test is only required for Massachusetts couples seeking a marriage license, not for all residents. Only women planning to marry are offered the rubella test. And in most states, but not Massachusetts, a marriage license is available only to heterosexual couples. Newborn screening produces universal biological citizenship via state-funded public health when biology becomes an entry point in the prevention of population and individual disease at birth.

It bears repeating how unique the democratization of newborn screening is in the context of the US healthcare system. Americans are only guaranteed health insurance when they turn 65 and the entitlements of Medicare kick in,[26] yet virtually all US newborns are screened for rare conditions. One alternative to a public health model much more in line with the history of US healthcare would have been a commercial approach for newborn screening in which only the parents who were willing and able to pay would have their infants screened, forgoing the advantage of screening entire populations. Other alternatives would have been screening only high-risk groups (as was done for sickle cell disease screening in the 1970s) or making screening voluntary rather than mandatory. Newborn screening stands out because it is one of the few healthcare programs available to all in a country where healthcare access for most citizens is not a right but instead is dependent on one's ability to pay for it either directly out of pocket or through various public or private insurance plans.

Yet this novel form of distinguishing citizens based on their propensity for rare genetic diseases needs to be folded in with existing forms of citizenship, state actions, and professional power.[27] In newborn screening, public health quickly interfaces with privatized healthcare. And it is this transition we are interested in. Once the patient advocacy groups in partnership with commercial interests, professional groups, and regulators succeed in mandating screening, how does the infant-citizen newly identified with a rare metabolic disorder fare in a country where healthcare is not a citizenship right?

*Health Insurance*

Parents do not pay directly for newborn screening. The service is an item on the hospital or medical service birth bill and the screening test itself is funded by the state. In California during the time of our study, the cost for the specimen collection form was $1, the processing of the specimen cost $101.75, and service providers were allowed to charge $6 for collection of the specimen and handling. Public and private insurance companies covered these costs for their patients, and the state covered the costs for the uninsured.[28] Thus, no one failed to be screened due to an inability to pay.

State funding was more limited, however, in the domains of follow-up testing and treatment. The California Department of Public Health rolled out the newborn screening program in 2005. By 2008, the program had 30 percent more positive results, more submissions for biochemical and DNA follow-up tests, and more follow-up tests per infant than anticipated in 2005. As a cost-saving measure, the California Department of Public Health mandated: repeating newborn screening for positive NICU babies, rather than more expensive specialized follow-up testing; limiting follow-up tests to biochemical tests unless DNA analysis was done at the state-contracted laboratory; conducting qualitative rather than quantitative testing of organic acids for most disorders (i.e., providing information about whether results are abnormal rather than stating their specific values); and limiting testing of mothers to those with low carnitine levels.[29] The Department of Public Health thus envisioned screening as limited to diagnosis followed by a quick handover of the infant to the healthcare system.

One direct effect of screening is an increase in medical consumption. The 4,580 positive newborn screening patients referred to metabolic clinics in California between July 2005 and April 2009 made a combined 14,282 visits to specialty clinics during the same period.[30] This increase in medical consumption created additional costs for both public and private insurance companies, which occasionally affected families directly. One mother in our study, whose son screened positive for MCADD but was eventually dismissed as a false positive when he was six months old, told us that her insurance premiums were increased twice due to frequent emergency room visits during her son's first months of life.

Before visiting patients, we sat with the genetics team in a small office where they discussed the patients they were about to see. The staff taped a list of patients next to the door. The patient list included the patient's name, insurance, ID number, time of appointment, reason for consultation, and the patient's physician. There were five insurance categories: self-payment, two forms of private insurance—PPO (preferred provider organization) and HMO (health maintenance organization), and two public programs—Medi-Cal and California Children's Services (CCS). These categories set the bounds for what kind of care was available to a patient. We regularly observed that a physician or nurse would recommend a genetic test until someone—usually Monica, Lucy, or one of the genetic counselors—would double-check what kind of insurance the patient had. Upon learning the patient's insurance status, they often abruptly backed away from ordering the test saying: "Oh, then forget it. We'll never get authorization." Or: "We can't do an out-of-state DNA test." As other sociologists have observed, many decisions are consolidated before physicians even meet patients,[31] including whether testing is indicated, based on insurance status. There was thus considerable behind-the-scenes rationing of care based on patient insurance.

The five kinds of insurance influenced the follow-up care patients received. Self-paying patients were healthcare consumers in the most direct sense of the term: the genetics service "sells" services that the patients decide to "buy." This arrangement conforms to the old healthcare finance model of fee-for-service without insurance intermediaries. No patients in our study were self-paying, but it was more common in genetic testing for Huntington's disease, where confidentiality concerns were paramount. Next was private insurance. Some children received private health insurance through their parents' employer-based health insurance program. The PPO-insured patients received whatever services the physician deemed necessary. From a professional perspective, these were the easiest patients to treat because the staff did not have to take insurance into consideration, although there could still be hefty copayments. HMO patients were the most cumbersome: a clinic visit required a referral from a primary care physician and any intervention or test required prior authorization.

Next, a patchwork of public programs ensured that children received health insurance and healthcare access regardless of their parents' insurance status. US citizens are not automatically eligible for government health insurance programs such as Medicaid. They need to meet financial criteria and one other criterion such as pregnancy.[32] In California, low-income pregnant women are eligible for health insurance during pregnancy and 60 days after the child's birth through the state's Medicaid program, Medi-Cal. And for the most vulnerable group in terms of health insurance, the working poor who made too much money to qualify for Medi-Cal but did not receive health insurance through an employer, the state of California offered the Healthy Families program, a low-cost insurance program that offered health, vision, and dental care similar to Medi-Cal services. Some people with incomes higher than the Healthy Families program but without employer insurance could purchase reduced private or public rate insurance.

If a baby screened positive on newborn screening, the family was automatically referred to CCS, a state agency that provided care based on medical and financial needs and which, as a payer of last resort, reimbursed services for children from poor families under 21 years of age with covered health problems.[33] The state had a contract with a commercial laboratory service, which conducted the initial follow-up testing for diagnostic purposes. Once testing entered the domain of treatment, the care of publicly insured patients stayed with CCS but payment for the care of private patients was transferred to their individual insurers. Newborn screening patients from poor families could thus access health services relatively easily as long as the requested service conformed to the contract with the laboratory service and as long as they qualified for public insurance. When income levels rose or paperwork was lost, their services could be cut off. They were also at a disadvantage when they required specialized DNA mutation analysis from an out-of-state laboratory, which was not covered by CCS.

Despite these hurdles, patients with public insurance often had an easier time receiving healthcare services than patients with HMO insurance. Time was of the essence in follow-up testing but the required prior authorization could take weeks because it sometimes required a subsequent visit to a primary care physician. For HMO-insured families, the bureaucratic hurdles became yet another issue that they faced in addition to the unnerving news that their child might be affected by a metabolic disorder. Dr. Silverman explained to a mother with HMO insurance why he could not order a test for carnitine transporter deficiency for her newborn: "We can't do it today because what happens in the HMO world is they're just authorizing us to give an expert opinion. We're giving the opinion but we can't act on it. It's the primary care physician who can act on it." For one patient who required a skin biopsy, it took two weeks before the HMO authorized the procedure. In another case, the care of two siblings with carnitine deficiency had to be transferred to a different hospital when the HMO ended its contract with the academic hospital.

Private insurers could also institute expensive copayments for genetic mutation analysis, which, in turn, could affect whether a family decided to do the test. This was the case for genetic mutation analysis in MCADD patients until later in our study when it became part of the state's standard testing protocol for MCADD. In the following excerpt, Dr. Silverman informs a family that they will have an expensive copay for DNA analysis:

DR. SILVERMAN: So let's talk about the MCADD. What we're, what we're gonna recommend . . . it's just do DNA. I am looking on this chart and we may not do it today because of the fact that, uh, we may have to get insurance authorization. Do you have a PPO or?

MOTHER: HMO.

DR. SILVERMAN: HMO. We have to get then authorization and I don't know what your copay is but it's about nine hundred, thousand dollars.

This family decided to do the mutation analysis after Dr. Silverman floated the cost to them, but mutation analysis was held up for several months for Molly Martin while the staff and the family debated the pros and cons of the test. Kim and Dan Martin had a second child at the end of the study who was also diagnosed with MCADD, but by this point the genetic mutation analysis was done as part of routine follow-up testing.

Further insurance problems emerged when newborn screening identified mothers affected with metabolic disorders. As we showed earlier, the staff identified several mothers with metabolite levels outside of the normal range. In one case, the geneticists were stymied because the mother did not have health insurance. The contract with the commercial laboratory covered follow-up testing for mothers with carnitine deficiency because the possibility of maternal carnitine deficiency was known at the time of the contract renewal. But mothers with other conditions were not covered, and in those situations, financial concerns could make the difference in follow-up. Claudia Romero, a woman diagnosed with GA1 through her son's newborn screening,[34] had insurance for the first two months after the birth of her infant through emergency Medi-Cal. At a later visit, after her state insurance expired, Dr. Flores wanted to refer her for a cardiology consultation after she reported chest pain, but this was not possible because the cardiology group at the academic hospital did not take uninsured patients. The clinic staff "solved" the problem by referring her to a public county hospital. Monica reflected: "This is terrible because here we discovered something and then we can't help you. We're like: sorry."

The key point is that insurance status limited both the opportunity to conduct follow-up testing and the ease with which follow-up care could be delivered. Even within the medical center where our research took place, certain specialty clinics did not accept patients with public insurance or saw patients with some but not other forms of private insurance. Thus, Monica gave an example of a patient with private insurance that the genetics clinic accepted but the neurology clinic at the same institution did not. Because private insurance is tied to employment in the United States, insurance status—and with it access to healthcare—could change abruptly when people lost or changed jobs, decided to work part-time, divorced, or, most paradoxically, when people became sick and insurance rates went up. The remarkable universality of expanded newborn screening quickly encountered insurance barriers in matters of follow-up testing and care for chronic conditions.

## Medical Foods and Special Formulas

Similar private-public discrepancies plagued the provision of special formulas and medical foods. The FDA defines a medical food as "a food which is formulated to be consumed or administered enterally under the supervision of a physician and which is intended for the specific dietary management of a disease or condition for which distinctive nutritional requirements, based on recognized scientific principles, are established by medical evaluation."[35] While the definition of medical foods suggests a pharmaceutical status, the FDA considers medical foods to be more similar to food than to drugs or medical devices.[36] Many private health insurers and some state insurance programs do not cover medical foods, which may leave patients with annual out-of-pocket expenses of several thousands of dollars.[37] Medical formulas are nutritional supplements designed to correct metabolic imbalances in patients with particular disorders. Infants with galactosemia, for example, run the risk of liver disease, neurological damage, developmental delays, and other irreversible complications unless they drink a special lactose-free soy-based formula.

CCS and Medi-Cal insurance covered the cost of many medical foods and formulas. Even then, however, the process of obtaining them remained cumbersome. Lucy, the clinic's dietitian, provided free sample kits donated by various pharmaceutical companies to all families at the initial visit in which medical food treatment was recommended. She employed a policy of rotating the samples on a case-by-case basis to give every company the same access to patients. Then, the geneticist wrote a prescription. To fill the prescription, the pharmacy needed to obtain authorization from CCS and deliver the medical foods to the family "hopefully," Monica added, "before they run out of the sample kit." Monica recalled: "We had one case recently where they had CCS but you know, the mom called in frantically, you know, 'I'm out of formula. What do I do?' And I had sent the prescription I think like a week or two ago. And I figured it was taken care of, but I guess the paperwork got stuck somewhere. And then we had to fill out another form, I mean faxing it back and forth. And that took a lot of time to do all that."

Furthermore, publicly insured patients were at an advantage in accessing medical foods only insofar as the required foods were covered. At regular intervals, CCS reviewed the list of approved medical foods and substituted one food for another, leaving some families in the lurch.

For private insurers, the smoothness of the process depended on the specific disorder. California state law required the coverage of medical foods for patients with PKU.[38] Yet private insurers routinely denied authorization for formula and other medical foods for other conditions. In such cases, Monica and the geneticists wrote letters of medical necessity to the insurer and asked the families to become involved in the process of obtaining authorization by writing and calling in turn. Monica described the process as a "battle": "Everyone has to fight," she said. "Everyone has to go on the phone and, OK, press here, press here and go through to the whole 'you called the wrong number, you have to call this number' and blah blah blah.... You really have to be persistent. They almost always say no. You almost have to reach up to the level of the medical director and then you have to have Dr. Silverman on the phone with the medical director to make the case."

Understandably, some families did not fight. Paul Wong's family decided to pay for the formula out of pocket rather than fight their insurers. Others tried to receive reimbursement but remained unsuccessful:

MOTHER: Well we have to buy the food ourselves. Our insurance wouldn't cover it.
MONICA: Oh.
FATHER: Yeah we have [name of insurance] and they cover the medication too. But not the food. So.
MONICA: So try. You tried. They don't pay at all?
FATHER: Uh uh.
MONICA: No because—
FATHER: We tried for like a year.

Even if private insurers agreed to cover medical foods, the family had to pay a copayment, which was often quite hefty. Newborn screening policymakers have observed the barriers to accessing medical foods. Noting tremendous variation in reimbursement for medical foods and formulas across the states for some or all of the newborn screening metabolic conditions, they have suggested policy solutions to cover medical foods under health insurance.[39] At this point, however, coverage remains patchy.

### Therapeutic Service

The key determinant of access to therapeutic services was not insurance status but the age of the child: relatively generous services were publicly available until age three, after which they abruptly diminished. The provision of therapeutic services fell under the mandate of the state's Regional Centers for Developmental Services. The Regional Center has an Early Start program that offers therapeutic services to prevent or lessen developmental disabilities later in life to anyone who is at risk for developmental delays or mental retardation. After receiving a request from the clinic, the center sent out an early intervention specialist for a needs assessment. If a child was eligible for services, all services were free regardless of income, although the centers billed private and public insurance companies for medically indicated services. Newborn screening patients might qualify for respite nursing care, vision therapy, physical therapy, occupational therapy, and speech therapy.

Logistical hurdles routinely impeded timely therapeutic onset. To enroll children in Regional Center services, parents had to navigate complex bureaucracies through repeated phone calls and piles of paperwork and forms. Such tasks would be cumbersome for any parent caring for a young child at home, and were all the more onerous for those who also faced language barriers, such as Lena Sanchez, Carmen Rodriguez, Beatriz Hidalgo, and Clarice Muños. Families moved, changed phone numbers, or were overwhelmed with other caregiving responsibilities, and a connection was sometimes not made. Paperwork could linger on a desk at the Regional Center when therapists were not found. Such factors provided major obstacles. Denise Moskowitz, the social worker, described her job as a troubleshooter, coaxing families to services and ensuring that agencies followed through with services. While Denise was able to help some families navigate the vast minefield of social services, she was not always alerted about problems. Timeliness mattered because every month of delay of services meant one month less that the child would receive services and one month lost to make a difference.

The services covered by the Early Start program were considered "medically based." Once children turned three, however, they were no longer entitled to Early Start services and these same services no longer qualified as medical. Children requiring services might still qualify as Regional Center consumers but only if they had more severe physical disabilities.[40] The alternative was to contact the school district, but the school district only provided services that helped the child to access the classroom environment. Accessing any of those services past year three could require intervention from the geneticists and calls from the social worker. Such provisions were also subject to guidelines of progression: if the child did not progress, the services were cut.

## Transportation

The 15 metabolic clinics that served as newborn screening follow-up centers in California were centralized in major metropolitan areas. Geographic concentration implied that families might need to travel a long distance for clinic appointments. Many of the families living in rural areas were poor, and in such cases, transportation became an important barrier to care. One family traveled 64 miles on public transportation to get to the clinic by two in the afternoon:

MOTHER: We went to catch the Metro at eight forty-five this morning. We just got here like forty-five minutes, about an hour maybe.

STEFAN: From [name of city]?

MOTHER: Yeah, because we had to catch the Metro, then we had to get on a train, then we had to get on a bus.

Dr. Silverman was running behind schedule that afternoon and when we informed him that the family would have to leave by three to make the reverse trip home, he decided to forgo the blood draw he had planned for and asked the family to visit a local laboratory instead. This patient was eventually lost to follow-up, in part because his parents did not have a telephone in their home. Other families, including some with symptomatic children, had trouble making it to the clinic for transportation reasons.

There was some public funding available for transportation, but it was difficult to access. Indeed, there seemed to be a perception among service providers that transportation funding was ripe for abuse. The Westside Regional Center stated on its website: "Generally, parents or caregivers are responsible for transportation to social and recreational activities, as well as medical or therapy appointments." Marcella Torres had trouble getting her daughter Claribel to the genetics clinic because she did not drive, her husband worked, and the public transportation was too difficult to navigate. In desperation, she once took a taxi to the clinic but this was too expensive to be repeated. Claribel qualified for 40 hours per week nursing respite services from the Regional Center, in part because of her g-tube, but the g-tube did not entitle her to transportation assistance: the Regional Center case manager ruled that Claribel could take the bus with a g-tube.

Denise was occasionally able to obtain public transportation vouchers for patients from CCS or Regional Center, although each agency's first reaction was to delegate responsibility to the other. Basically, she had to put her authority on the line by vouching that the family absolutely needed help with transportation. "The advocacy has to come from me. Needs to have me calling and say, 'They need to come to the clinic. This is not a joke.' The squeaky wheel gets the oil." She also suggested families ask for help from their friends or churches. Once, she contacted a parish priest for help with transportation. The priest asked for help on a local radio program and secured rides for the family. Sometimes charity came through. A few patients who lived three hours away were able to secure a charity airlift from volunteer pilots. However, they did not have transportation from the airport to the clinic. In exceptional circumstances, the staff paid a patient's return bus ticket out of their own pockets. Transportation issues were most problematic for poor parents of children who required many appointments with various specialists. The unevenness of charity and public funding could lead to missed appointments or delay seeking care.

*Language*

Our study contained 16 monolingual Spanish-speaking families. The hospital had an interpreter service, which, on request, would send an interpreter to facilitate communication between the parents and the physician. However, this service was not always available at the time it was needed due to the high demand in the hospital. In such cases, family members translated, our research assistant Rocio filled in, or Dr. Silverman would try to get by with his rather elementary Spanish. We saw the weakness of these interpreting means when we observed Dr. Flores, a native Spanish speaker, communicate with Spanish-speaking families. Dr. Flores was sensitive to dialogue and pedagogy with all patients regardless of language. The ease and flow of his interaction with Spanish families, however, was striking. He typically set an agenda at the beginning of the meeting in which he told families that he wanted to ask them some questions first and then would explain the condition and answer their questions in turn. He was authoritative and to the point but also took the time to explain, carefully checking for understanding. Seeing Dr. Flores at work reminded us of the key message of the social model of disability: what many consider a disability is not inherently disadvantaging but rather depends on the social context. If everyone speaks sign language, deafness is not a liability.[41] Similarly, if your geneticist is fluent in Spanish, communicating in that language becomes less of an issue.

* * *

We have presented a number of factors that posed difficulties for capitalizing on the lifesaving opportunity that newborn screening provides. The universal inclusiveness of biological citizenship through newborn screening encounters well-known problems typical of any US healthcare interaction involving chronic diseases: different insurance systems with wide disparities between them, the coordination of care due to gaps in coverage, cumbersome and time-consuming bureaucratic rules, age-defined criteria of medical care, language gaps, and cost-shifting from one entity to another.[42] The result was substantial unevenness and a series of frustrating paradoxes: universal screening but highly fragmented follow-up and access to treatment, generous therapeutic services grinding to a halt by age three, and a superb genetic service but difficulty reaching it. The nurses, social worker, geneticists, and parents spent massive amounts of time and energy securing what should have been straightforward entitlements and fighting bureaucratic illogics. Universalism dissolved into stratification along resources.

We now provide an example of how such stratification might have featured in the death of Diego Sanchez, a patient with GA1. Again, we want to be careful. We do not make a causal argument between health service access and mortality: Diego was very sick and might not have survived with the best possible medical care. The clinicians that took care of him, however, wondered whether the interplay of various structural barriers might have contributed to an unfortunate outcome.

## A Life Lost

Diego Sanchez was the eighth child born to two Mexican immigrants. His father worked as a migrant farm laborer and the family lived three hours away from the clinic. One of his older siblings had passed away and a second one was diagnosed with cerebral palsy. After reviewing the family history, Dr. Silverman suspected that the deceased sibling and the sister with cerebral palsy were likely also affected with GA1. He wrote in Diego's patient file about the deceased sibling: "We believe that she probably suffered from glutaric acidemia as well. That remains to be determined." Dr. Silverman also suspected that his parents, Lena and Ricardo, were consanguineous. They grew up and met in a small Mexican village of about

200 people. Dr. Silverman inferred that in such a small community the probability for most people to be related to each other was high.

At the first visit, Dr. Silverman decided that he should test all of Diego's siblings to make sure that none of them were affected. Diego's levels of C5DC at newborn screening were 5.8 μmol/L with a normal upper limit of 0.35 μmol/L, and he received a "probable diagnosis of glutaric acidemia type 1." Dr. Silverman initiated a diet with a lysine-deficient formula. On repeat testing, Diego's levels were more than 30 times the normal level, confirming the diagnosis of GA1.

The genetics team saw Diego regularly. At two months, Diego seemed to be doing well. He ate constantly and was growing. Because his lysine levels were now low, the staff increased the amount of breastfeeding and decreased formula feeds from five times to twice daily. His head, however, was large—a possible symptom of GA1. Dr. Silverman noted in his report: "Hypotonia with head lag and there are excessive movements in the lower extremities, seemingly like pedaling, and he has fisting bilaterally with some spasticity in the extremities, but no clonus." Dr. Silverman again noted that he should test all of the siblings. At the third meeting, which we attended,[43] when Diego was four months old, Lena discussed her plans to go back to her factory job. She wondered about switching over from breast milk to formula and asked Dr. Silverman whether an unlicensed day care provider could provide the formula. Lena's understanding of GA1 was rather sketchy. She told us that Diego had a "high metabolism" for which he had to drink a special milk (a formula) with medications. Lena also remembered that the first four years of Diego's life were crucial. She ended up not returning to work.

Diego crashed right before he turned six months. His parents brought him to the local emergency department because he was "not acting himself." At that time, he had seizures that lasted 40 seconds to one minute. He was transferred to the academic hospital by helicopter and experienced more seizures during transportation. By the time he arrived, he had stopped seizing, but he was by then under the influence of heavy antiseizure medication.

At the next visit after this hospitalization, Dr. Silverman decided to admit Diego to the hospital again because he presented with a "spastic arching back," and was irritable, with limited food intake. At this point Diego was not only a genetics patient but was also followed by gastroenterology, neurology, and nephrology. The many specialties meant many different appointments, which created difficulties for the family. They did not have a car and depended on a friend for a ride or on public transportation.

Lena told us that she typically left at ten in the morning to make the three o'clock appointment in the genetics clinic and did not arrive back home until eight thirty at night. Diego's diagnosis was amended to "glutaric acidemia type 1 in a patient having sustained irreversible brain damage." He received a g-tube. Dr. Silverman requested one hour of physical therapy twice a week and noted that the parents had been instructed at discharge to "seek medical services emergently if they notice a change in behavior, cough, difficulty breathing, dizziness/fainting, signs of infection, unable to eat/drink or take medications, vomiting, or any other concerning symptoms." Dr. Silverman added that Diego's "prognosis remains guarded."

One month later, Diego was hospitalized again. Lena and Ricardo had taken him to the local hospital to replace the g-tube, and it was discovered after he was transferred to the academic center that the g-tube had been misplaced. Diego improved immediately after the g-tube was inserted correctly.

We interviewed Lena after this visit. Diego was lying on a blanket on the floor. She told us that she was torn about going back to work. Her husband's income was insufficient to pay the bills, and they desperately needed her income. She explained that the bills put her husband "in a bad mood and he almost did not sleep. He would come home from work angry." When she suggested that she could return to work and have her mother take care of Diego and his sister, her husband "told me to forget about work. Those kids are something else and my mom will not be able to take care of them. So he told me to stay at home and he would see how he could pull us through." During this period, the family also lost access to physical therapy services. The application was denied repeatedly because the submitted records lacked detail about the nature of Diego's disabilities.

The Sanchez family missed the next appointment because they could not find transportation. By the next visit, at 14 months, Dr. Silverman noted that Diego was neurologically severely compromised: "Severe episode of metabolic decompensation and is now neurologically impaired. For example, he does not sit without support, he does not stand, he has no language, but appears to understand language." Lena mentioned that now that Diego had turned one, she no longer received formula from the Women, Infants, and Children program. Dr. Silverman readjusted the diet to eliminate formula. At that meeting, Dr. Silverman also talked to Diego's 13-year-old brother and promised that they would check his levels. Monica arranged for Lena to bring all of the children to the laboratory to do at least a newborn screening test, but for unknown reasons, the tests were never done. The family came back when Diego was 17 months old and Dr. Silverman continued to tinker with his diet. During the staff meeting, Dr. Silverman explained that if a child suffers brain damage between age one and three, it does not bode well for the future. A visiting doctor agreed: "There was nothing to prevent this, the genetics are causative." Dr. Flores interrupted, saying, "You give genetics too much credit. You can prevent with early intervention."

Diego died three months later. His parents rushed him to the local emergency department following a metabolic crisis but he did not survive. In the e-mail message announcing Diego's death, Dr. Silverman wrote: "We will never know what his outcome would have been if he lived near a tertiary center and the parents responded rapidly. Given the circumstances there was little that we could have changed." Yet the question haunting the people who cared for Diego was whether the outcome would have been different if he had access to better medical services or if his parents were, in the words of Dr. Silverman, "more sophisticated," a euphemism signaling class and ethnic difference. If health service factors contributed to his outcome, there is not one critical factor that stands out but the cumulative effect of various barriers at critical moments. Beside the disease itself, the family's geographic distance from a hospital accustomed to caring for children with rare metabolic disorders, transportation problems, language barriers, difficulties securing therapeutic services, and additional effects of poverty may have contributed to the fatal outcome.

## Met and Unmet Opportunities

First aid lifesaving with resuscitation techniques is visually presented as "the chain of survival": early identification of an emergency and alerting of the emergency system connected to early CPR connected to early defibrillation connected to early advanced care offer the best chances for survival. The reality is that each one of these links requires not only a condition amenable to emergency care but also an infrastructure and public socialization to act appropriately in crisis situations.[44] Applying the metaphor of the chain of survival to expanded newborn screening, it is clear that newborn screening is only the first link in a chain of lifesaving events: it is equivalent to the warning system of first aid. To really save lives, the disease must be amenable to prevention, but many other links must also be made successfully. For some conditions, for some families, for some healthcare systems, and likely for some areas of the United States, this first link never connects to the next link required to save lives. Communication problems, barriers to follow-up treatment, insufficient funding for medical foods and services, insurance troubles, transportation issues, and other socioeconomic barriers mediate the opportunity to save lives. As in so many other US healthcare situations, expanded newborn screening holds out the promise of the best care possible but these promises quickly flounder for many stuck with the news that their infant is at risk for a metabolic crisis but who lack the resources to do something about it.

The barriers to follow-up care only make sense from a perverse bureaucratic and economic rationale guided by profit and cost-control motives rather than the principle of providing care to those who may benefit most. The logic of profit-making and expense reduction across the various insurance programs suggests that financial rewards lie with insuring those who least need care and by excluding those with highest risks. The patchwork of programs and exclusionary rules and cutoff points highlight that the fear that someone will take advantage of services trumps the provision of medical and therapeutic services. The spiraling US healthcare budget shows that such a competitive for-profit setup is not necessarily cheaper at the national level, although individual companies and providers may profit. Instead, everyone in the clinic, but especially Monica, Lucy, and Denise, spent much of his or her time determining whether they would be reimbursed for services and fighting for payment or services. For staff and patients, these barriers were illogical, random, frustrating, and consequential.

The universalism of newborn screening might have heralded a new US healthcare model centered on prevention in which follow-up treatment for screening required addressing the inequities of healthcare. There are some tentative steps in that direction, in the sense that we may eventually have federal legislation requiring funding for medical foods.[45] The actual practices of follow-up care, however, suggest a policy momentum in the other direction: the third-party payer system quickly eroded the still fragile collective responsibility and cost-sharing of population-based expanded newborn screening. A firm diagnosis became a problem for individuals who had to invest their own resources or fight for public or private insurance benefits. The California Department of Public Health substituted follow-up services with cheaper alternatives between 2005 and 2008. Such cost concerns could be telling of the likely future of newborn screening, in which cost-shifting and increasingly narrow reimbursement criteria might stifle the promise of screening.

# Conclusion

## *The Future of Newborn Screening*

We can find at least five contemporary omens that signal the possible futures of newborn screening. The first omen suggests a future in which screening for rare genetic disorders will become increasingly routinized and statistically monitored. In December 2010, a special issue of the journal *Genetics in Medicine* published the first available follow-up data from expanded newborn screening in California. Between July 7, 2005, and April 30, 2009, 2,105,119 newborns were screened. The program referred 4,580 newborns (or 0.22 percent) to a metabolic clinic for follow-up. Of those, 16 percent or 754 infants were diagnosed with a "resolved disorder," which we take to mean a true positive. Expanded newborn screening thus identified 36 infants with a metabolic disorder for every 100,000 live births, or, put differently, one true positive screen for every 2,778 births. Of the infants referred to a metabolic clinic, 3,334 were not confirmed to have a disorder. The false positive rate for newborn screening for patients referred to the clinic was thus 158 per 100,000 live births, or one false positive for every 633 births.[1] Of the remaining 492 infants referred to specialty follow-up clinics, 226 cases were still pending, 72 cases resulted in a maternal diagnosis, and 62 infants died prior to follow-up.[2] Several of the pending cases and false positives would probably fall under our category of patients-in-waiting. While this data does not prove that morbidity and mortality are prevented, it suggests that newborn screening succeeds in the basic goal of identifying rare conditions.

Another possible future became apparent in May 2010, when Kathleen Sebelius, US Secretary of Health and Human Services, added a 55th disorder, Severe Combined Immunodeficiency Disorder (SCID), to the recommended uniform screening panel. SCID is a genetic disorder that impairs the immune system, resulting in serious infections and, often, death within one year of birth. SCID is colloquially known as the "bubble boy" disease because its most famous afflicted patient, David Vetter, spent most of his 12 years in a sterile bubble-like structure at Texas Children's Hospital, until his death in 1984. Unlike most of the conditions discussed in this book, SCID may be cured by successful hematopoietic stem cell transplantation within three months of life, although survival rates vary.[3] The addition of SCID to the recommended uniform screening panel implied a future in which newborn screening programs cast an even wider net in the prevention of rare genetic conditions.

The third omen signals a more cautionary stance toward newborn screening program expansion, suggesting that program retrenchment and cost-cutting measures could stifle its continued growth. In May 2011, a crowd of leading experts in US newborn screening gathered in Washington, DC, for the 24th meeting of the Secretary's Advisory Committee on Heritable Disorders in Newborns and Children.[4] On the agenda for the meeting was a discussion of the report to Secretary Sebelius regarding the status of newborn screening for SCID. At the time of the meeting, California, Louisiana, and Massachusetts had implemented pilot programs in which newborn screening for SCID was universally offered but not yet required. In Michigan and Texas, screening was required by law but had not yet been implemented. Only New York and Wisconsin had implemented mandatory screening programs.[5] At the meeting, Fred Lorey, acting director of the Genetic Disease Laboratory at the California Department of Public Health and one of the directors of the pilot SCID screening program, spoke about California's experience in an unscheduled commentary.[6] According to Lorey, the pilot program had been very successful, but due to rising budget constraints in California and elsewhere, they faced considerable hurdles in securing legislative approval to implement the program permanently. Lorey cited data from a state congressional budget committee, which suggested that the program would cost $7 million, while the savings would only be $1 million per year.[7] Lorey indicated that he doubted the accuracy of these statistics: "We're having to deal with people who make monetary decisions who don't really care about what we have to say about the disorders."

A fourth sign of the future of newborn screening should be familiar to readers of this book. In May 2011, just weeks after the Secretary's Advisory Committee meeting, the headline of an msnbc.com article proclaimed: BABIES' BLOOD TESTS CAN END IN FALSE-POSITIVE SCREENING SCARES. "When they're correct, such tests are invaluable," health correspondent JoNel Aleccia wrote about newborn screening. "But," she added, "when they're not—and they're not a lot—parents and kids can endure months of repeated tests, special sleeping schedules and stringent diets, plus lingering uncertainty and anxiety, health experts say."[8] The false positives Aleccia described are an inevitable consequence of any screening program needing to strike a balance between specificity and sensitivity, and research has documented that false positives may cause anxiety and other adverse effects.[9]

Although the article is not remarkable (except for some dubious statistics), the reactions in the comment section stand out as emblematic of the pro-screening narrative circulating within the newborn screening advocacy community. Very soon after the article appeared, newborn screening activists mobilized to skewer with scathing commentary Aleccia, the families quoted in the article, and any blogger who endorsed the article's message. Many of the hundreds of reactions followed a similar script. Respondents identified themselves both as organizers in the newborn screening community and as parents, mostly mothers, of a child with a genetic condition for whom they would have loved to have received a false positive result. The commentators argued that Aleccia's article does a disservice to newborn screening because newborn screening programs save lives every day and ultimately, any negative consequences of false positive results pale in comparison to the harmful effects of devastating disorders. Such narratives both disregard the need for evidence of newborn screening's lifesaving capacity and effectively shut out of the conversation any newborn screening stakeholder who does not have a child diagnosed with a life-changing genetic disorder. Two days after the article's publication, the American College of Medical Genetics (ACMG) weighed in on the comment section with a statement that the organization was working hard to reduce false positives and that newborn screening was "one of the most significant, effective and well-run public health program [sic] of the past 50+ years."[10]

A final omen signals a different sort of challenge for the future of newborn screening. One important consequence of expanded newborn screening that has captured widespread public attention is the retention, by state governments, of dried blood samples from nearly every US newborn. Newborn screening programs collect more dried bloodspots than are necessary to perform the screening tests, and the residual samples have been used for program evaluation and quality control measures. For many scientists, however, these biobanks constitute a treasure trove for population research and technological innovation: they have been used to detect seropositivity rates, to determine toxicity levels in the blood, and to test for environmental exposures.[11] Yet because newborn screening blood samples are collected, in most cases, without parental informed consent, making them available to researchers without specific authorization may exceed the legal mandate of state newborn screening programs. Parents in several states have filed lawsuits against state governments for storing blood samples indefinitely and making them available without parental permission. A widely publicized Texas lawsuit revealed that the state had already given 800 blood samples to the US Armed Forces Pathology laboratory for use in a forensics database.[12] A review of the legal statutes regarding retention and use of newborn screening blood samples showed limited parental control over the ownership, period of retention, and future use of dried blood samples:

> In most states, there is no requirement that parents be informed that their child's dried blood sample may be retained for future use. Eight states require that parents be provided information regarding the retention of dried-blood samples.... Parents retain control over the disposition of their infants' dried-blood sample in only a few states.[13]

The study authors concluded that the boundaries of what was considered research were not always clear, and that efforts to protect privacy and confidentiality varied widely.

While some ethicists have argued for obtaining parental consent for the retention and use of newborn screening blood samples, policymakers have feared that introducing an informed consent model might open the door for parents to opt out of newborn screening altogether.[14] Others have argued that parents should be offered the opportunity to opt out of long-term storage and retention, but only after the samples have been collected, so as not to jeopardize the public health aims of newborn screening.[15] At a workshop hosted by the Institute of Medicine to discuss the challenges of using residual newborn screening blood samples in translational research, attendees acknowledged that newborn screening cannot be successful without public trust.[16] This fifth sign, then, heralds the possibility of growing public dissatisfaction with newborn screening based on proprietary concerns about government control of personal information.

## "Success" as a Contested Category

How to read these mixed signals? Expanded newborn screening is a technology in the process of settling both in the clinic and in the broader healthcare landscape. The follow-up data from California underscore the exceptional status of mandatory screening for rare conditions in US healthcare. Newborn screening is quasi-universal in a country where preciously few health services are universally available. With few exceptions, the program bypasses informed consent, a cornerstone of the autonomy principle in bioethics. Still, this government program goes to great expense to identify rare diseases. As physician historian Jeffrey Brosco has noted:

> Organized medicine and the general public have historically resisted attempts of government bodies to provide direct medical services, and organized governmental programs have focused on specific populations such as military veterans or persons living in poverty. The initiation of universal [newborn screening] programs, in contrast, required that state governments invest in detection and treatment of specific medical conditions with relatively low incidence and no threat of contagion.[17]

We should add that government is involved in spite of lingering questions about efficacy. In the previous chapter, we showed that while newborn screening may prevent the onset of disease in fortunate circumstances, screening is insufficient to save all children from the devastation of metabolic disorders. In light of ongoing morbidity and mortality, the health payoff of screening is likely to be lower than the number of true positives might otherwise imply.

The varied omens suggest that judgments of "success" remain contested but critical to the future of newborn screening. The concept of "success" performs important cultural work in highlighting desirable biomedical outcomes. For example, it is well known in the field of resuscitation that first aid lifesaving techniques have a wide range of effects: they may restore life in rare circumstances but they may also be ineffective, or worse, cause harm. Resuscitation techniques are typically evaluated solely in terms of "survival rates" because this is the intended outcome. The concept of "survival rate" not only defines success narrowly by ignoring quality-of-life issues but also overlooks morbidity due to resuscitation attempts.[18] How should we evaluate newborn screening? What counts as a "success"? In this book, we have eschewed the notion that every outcome of newborn screening is beneficial, or that only the beneficial outcomes of screening should be considered. We have examined the *consequences* of screening, leaving open the question of whether such consequences are beneficial. Indeed, rendering these consequences "beneficial" or public health "successes" requires interpretive practices, which, as the five omens show, remain debated.

Fred Lorey's impromptu testimony at the 24th Secretary's Advisory Committee meeting regarding the legislative hurdles to newborn screening for SCID raises important questions about how policymakers should evaluate a newborn screening program as a public health "success." Is the program successful if it identifies asymptomatic infants with rare disorders, results in favorable health outcomes, demonstrates cost-effectiveness, or fulfills another criterion? According to Lorey and a report from the Secretary's Advisory Committee, the pilot screening program for SCID had been very successful.[19] Yet out of the 385,000 infants screened in the first nine months of the California pilot screening program, only 11 screened positive for SCID.[20] While this incidence rate was much higher than previously anticipated—estimates had put the incidence at 1/100,000 live births[21]—there was nevertheless no doubt that SCID was a very rare disorder. In Louisiana, not a single case had been identified. How can a public health program that yields so few identifiable cases, let alone lives saved, be considered a success? Where were the secondary targets and false positives in Lorey's discussion, and how do they figure into a calculus of net success? The low identification rate for SCID captures a key paradox of population screening for rare conditions: while a negative result may be good for the patient, some positive results are necessary in order to justify screening.[22] The logic of public health intervention suggests that success be defined at the population, rather than the individual, level.

Other committee members present at the meeting mentioned different indicators of success. Jeffrey Botkin, an early critic of the ACMG report, questioned the lack of outcome data from SCID screening and suggested that the interim report on SCID would benefit from more information about cost. Indeed, the California data showed that newborn screening between 2005 and 2009 cost about $231 million.[23] This means that the average cost of identifying a child with a true positive disorder is more than $300,000. This figure only indicates the actual screening cost and does not include the cost of additional laboratory testing, treatment, or other opportunity costs. At the same time, it also does not account for the possible savings in healthcare costs incurred by early identification and preventive treatment. While Lorey scoffed at the legislators' doubts about costs, bioethicists have argued persuasively that cost is a critical ethical issue because the collective resources used for screening might always have been spent on other worthy causes and lifesaving aims.[24]

Success may also be hampered by beneficiaries themselves. In her review of preventive medicine policies in the 1960–1980s, political scientist Deborah Stone noted the striking discrepancy that "enthusiasm for large-scale adoption of public health techniques ran into resistance by the very people prevention was supposed to help."[25] Stone's work has shown that beneficiaries are not a stable category. The strong negative reactions of newborn screening advocates to a predictable effect of screening programs—anxiety due to false positives—contrast with wider public concern about the residual use of dried bloodspots following newborn screening. In the comment section to Aleccia's article, we find people who were convinced that they would have benefited from screening if a program had been in place when their child was born. Members of this small but vocal minority not only present themselves as the true beneficiaries of expanded newborn screening but also have been officially recognized as spokespeople through their involvement at various policy levels. However, concerns about governmental research abuse and the commercial use of newborn screening bloodspots mobilize a much larger constituency. Every parent whose child was tested and every future generation of US citizens now become stakeholders. Their attitudes may be informed by suspicion of government overreach and highly publicized stories of researcher's misappropriation of organs and tissues.[26] Advocacy cuts both ways.

The future of newborn screening will hinge upon what stakeholders consider the program's most relevant outcomes in light of the invested resources. Considering the countervailing forces, it is too early to predict the program's historical momentum. Because much of newborn screening's potential is realized in the encounters between clinicians and families, it is likely that the clinic will play a major role in defining the program's long-term viability. Here, we highlight some salient ways in which newborn screening's outcomes are conceptualized in the clinic, how they contrast with views of newborn screening in the policy world, and how both worlds influence each other.

## Newborn Screening in the Clinic

*Favorable Impressions and Collateral Damage*

In his study of breast cancer, Robert Aronowitz noted the counterintuitive finding that most women who received false positives from breast cancer screening tests nevertheless supported the screening paradigm. These women were deeply alarmed to learn that they might have breast cancer and engaged in difficult diagnostic procedures, which they later learned were unnecessary. Yet they still viewed the screening program positively.[27] Similarly, in spite of having a difficult time with newborn screening, nearly all of the families in our study regarded the screening program favorably. For families, newborn screening presented an opportunity for anticipatory action in a healthcare context in which the value of prevention is often overlooked. As one parent put it, "Western medicine, the way it's practiced, it tends to be very reactive. And this is—this presents a situation that can actually be proactive." Thus, while many parents expressed their desire for various programmatic improvements—such as quicker testing and delivery of results, better education about screening, and a reduction in the rate of false positives—they were willing to endure these shortcomings because the perceived benefits outweighed the cost.[28] For example, when we asked Renee Baio about how she reconciled her difficult experience with Bailey's false positive with her pro-screening agenda, she responded: "Well, that's Washington's gripe. They said, 'Why put these families and these first-time parents through hell that they don't need, it's unnecessary.' And we welcome it. We would rather go through 10 weeks of the hell we went through than a lifetime of having a special needs child without having the opportunity to know from day one or day five."

Many parents shared Renee's views. Aronowitz surmised that for women undergoing cancer screening, "being given a cancer diagnosis and then having it taken away is experienced as a victory over cancer, leading to a greater sense of control over cancer and fears of cancer."[29] Similarly, parents of patients-in-waiting were initially shocked to learn that their child screened positive, but the sequence of clinic visits aimed to reassure them that the situation was not as bad as originally thought. Most of the time, clinicians brought good news after initial bad news. And for symptomatic patients, the daily struggle of dealing with numerous health problems confirmed the need for screening because it offered the promise of early interventions. For their parents, criticisms of the program focused on a desire to receive results even sooner.

The outlier in our study was Gemma Jacek-Love, whose son Ian was diagnosed with SCADD via newborn screening and remained completely asymptomatic. When Ian was two, Gemma became pregnant again and decided with her husband to undergo prenatal testing test for SCADD. The results came back positive, and the couple made plans to visit the genetics clinic with their baby soon after the birth. Interestingly, however, despite having the genetic mutation associated with SCADD, the couple's second son, whom they named Marshall, did not have high enough C4 levels to trigger a follow-up on newborn screening. It appeared that Marshall was abnormal at the genotypic level, yet was phenotypically normal. If Marshall's older brother had not already been diagnosed with SCADD, the family would never have discovered his genetic status. When reflecting on her attitudes about newborn screening in an interview several months after Marshall's birth, Gemma said, "With this there's a part of me that feels, gee, if they didn't have this newborn screening, we probably would have gone through all our lives without ever having to think about this. But then there's a small part of me that says, well, what if in the future there's a reason that I need to know this? Like, let's say, God forbid, one of them is—I mean, now I do take slightly more precautions probably than another person or parent would. So let's just say if one of them was really sick for months I'd think now, do they need an IV? So there is a slight accommodation for the 'what if' kind of thing now. I would never wake them up at night to feed them or something like that. So I don't know. I have to say I struggle with it and I'm not sure. There's a big part of me that wishes that they both had been like Marshall's. Their C4 is just a little higher so there would have been a chance that Ian's had never registered."

Gemma's ambivalence toward newborn screening more closely reflects the attitudes of the clinicians we studied, who expressed a sense of shared uncertainty about the benefits of newborn screening. Admittedly, there were few moments of reflexivity, as when Dr. Dati asked, as we cited earlier, "Are we actually doing any good with newborn screening?" Yet we gathered through the side commentary and joking behind closed doors that no staff members would characterize expanded newborn screening as an unmitigated success. Whenever Dr. Flores would describe a patient as a newborn screening "success story," a colleague would invariably diminish his optimistic assessment with a follow-up question about the child's metabolic levels, as in the following example from our fieldnotes:

> Dr. Flores described Reynaldo Gonzales as a "success story" and Dr. Silverman knocked on wood before asking what his leucine levels were like. Dr. Flores replied, "Don't ask me that. Now you're gonna poop my party." After some laughter, Dr. Flores said that the levels were 600. Dr. Silverman said, "That's a little high." Dr. Flores responded, "See, I told you so!"

Even typically sanguine Dr. Flores had his more cynical moments, as when he reported, when introducing a patient in a team meeting, "Unfortunately, Dr. Malvern saved her life." When pressed to explain why this lifesaving had been unfortunate, Dr. Flores explained that the child was doing quite poorly and had extensive developmental delays and impairments; it was thus unclear what her quality of life would be like.

The geneticists' doubts about the benefits of newborn screening were not limited to their most symptomatic patients. As we have hinted throughout the book, they also expressed substantial concerns about the consequences of newborn screening for the families of asymptomatic patients. These families, as Dr. Silverman once explained, were the "collateral damage" of newborn screening: they were not the primary intended beneficiaries, and screening arguably did them as much harm as good. Thus, after finding Clara and Sybil Miner on his case docket and realizing that Sybil might have a metabolic disorder rather than her daughter, Dr. Dati asked, "See how newborn screening screws up people's lives?" Concerns about unbridled medicalization made the geneticists sensitive to the possible dangers of medical interventions that were designed to help a small segment of society by acting on the whole. By employing the language of medicalization, the geneticists revealed themselves to be sophisticated social commentators, deliberately borrowing social scientific disciplinary lingo to illustrate how medical intervention can disrupt the status quo in ways that clinicians might otherwise overlook. The geneticists were unmistakably aware of working within a powerful double bind: they knew that newborn screening produced many unanticipated and sometimes harmful consequences, but they were ethically and legally bound to follow up on the results.

Collateral damage or beneficent innovation? Social scientists Sarah Franklin and Celia Roberts, writing about preimplantation genetic diagnosis (PGD), note that such diverging opinions may coexist uneasily:

> It is perfectly possible to feel deeply ambivalent about PGD, while ultimately feeling it is right to offer it as carefully as possible to as many people as possible, and indeed to ever more groups of people for an ever-widening range of conditions. This cannot be described as a dilemma produced by the technology "itself," much as it often appears to have "a life of its own," which, in a sense, it now does. PGD came into being out of the same complex matrix of emotional desires— of wanting to help, wanting to relieve suffering, wanting to be able to know and do more, and never knowing "how far to go"—that characterize it today.[30]

Wanting to know but not knowing how far to go characterizes the lingering sense of ambivalence among the frontline workers of expanded newborn screening. While even the most skeptical parents could not put the "what if" scenario out of their minds, clinicians wondered if the long periods of uncertainty might have been avoided. Therefore, they tailored their care to the patient situation at hand. They harnessed clinical judgment to avoid collateral damage as much as possible, realizing that available resources and a contractual obligation to follow up on newborn screening circumscribed their possible actions. Clinicians dealing with patients on a day-to-day basis thus enacted their own nuanced understanding of "public health success," in which saving lives is qualified with various unintended consequences.

## Biomedical Uncertainty and Knocking on Wood

I am not superstitious (knock on wood). — Shel Silverstein, *Superstitious*

Often, when the geneticists—especially Dr. Silverman and Dr. Flores but also other staff—announced that a baby was doing well during a clinic visit or staff meeting, they knocked on wood. Sometimes, they added the expression "knock on wood" midsentence. Other times, they rapped their knuckles almost reflexively on a piece of wood while they described how healthy an infant was. In still other instances, they simply conjured the expression by searching the examination room for a piece of wood to knock on. Considering the stature of the genetics team as scientific experts, we found this well-ingrained superstitious practice striking.

"Knocking on wood" generally signals that simply acknowledging someone's well-being might initiate a turn for the worse. The series of knocks served as a protective physical and social antidote to a verbal statement that might be "tempting fate." In his study of prognosis at the end of life, sociologist Nicholas Christakis noted that some physicians fear stating a prognostic message because they are afraid of hexing the process.[31] In the genetics clinic, the practice more likely reflected an attempt to safeguard a situation lacking control and understanding. The act of knocking on wood momentarily interrupted the flow of conversation to insert a specific future orientation. With this subtle gesture, geneticists conveyed that health could be precarious, but that they hoped that the child would continue to do well.

Geneticists' knocking on wood did not originate from incompetence but rather from the desire for a favorable outcome in spite of inevitable unknowns. The geneticists in our study knew as well as their colleagues the possibilities and limitations of newborn screening technologies. Although they had significant experience with newborn screening and metabolic conditions as researchers, clinicians, and some as policymakers, they realized that their knowledge—anyone's knowledge about newborn screening—was pushing its limits. Many newborn screening patients were first-of-a-kind. In fact, the clinicians did not know exactly what kind they were. Newborn screening cases often posed clinical puzzles with respect to disease knowledge and patient care. Knocking on wood provided a bit of extra insurance, faith against fate, when the geneticist was not really certain whether a good outcome could be attributed to therapeutic action or to other contingencies.

As social scientists have foreseen, using technological means to reduce uncertainty generates new forms of uncertainty. In our study, the recursive and iterative nature of biomedical uncertainty manifested itself along a large number of practical, moral, economic, and scientific dimensions, affecting both families and clinicians. Regardless of whether the screening results were deemed to be true or false positives, or whether the baby became symptomatic, uncertainty came down to the existential question of the kind of life a baby would lead. "Newborn screening," as Dr. Silverman put it, "upset the applecart." For asymptomatic patients, the question was whether the child would be normal and for symptomatic patients, the question was how normal the child would be. How normality was assessed and how these assessments were marshaled to foreshadow the child's possible future remained flexible across patient visits. Our concept of *normalizing subjunctivity*, a type of normalization that describes things as we wish they might be, highlights the ways in which uncertainty can serve as a valuable resource to preserve hope for an unknown future. Thus, parents and clinicians collectively redrew the boundaries of normality while adjusting to changing disease parameters.

The traditional response to biomedical uncertainty is to search for more conclusive information. For many of the uncertainties facing the genetics staff, however, definitive knowledge remained elusive. Instead, the staff aimed to establish trusting relationships that would facilitate families' cooperation with tests with unknown clinical payoff, intrusive dietary and lifestyle changes, and repeated clinic visits that kept the child's health status in limbo. While newborn screening upset the applecart, the clinicians were also ready to help pick up fallen and bruised apples, and worked to avoid bumps in the road for the remainder of the journey. The clinical staff conveyed that they would take care of families, treat each one according to its needs, and aim to resolve the situation in the best way possible. This caring relationship was apparent in small gestures such as handing the parents a business card at the first encounter and encouraging families to call if they had questions, stating explicitly that the parents would have as much time as they needed for questions to be answered, explaining genetics concepts with helpful metaphors and drawings, and conveying a desire for a favorable outcome by knocking on wood.

Another manifestation of care was acknowledging uncertainty to families. Many of the geneticists' statements contained metacommentary reflecting on the state of newborn screening, disease knowledge, and the many unknowns. The clinical staff laid bare its vulnerabilities and offered a plan to deal with it. The plan was tentative and flexible but the intent was patient-centered, in the sense of finding common ground in the management not only of the condition but also of the information conveyed.[32] Still, there was a downside to focusing clinical care strongly on intimacy with families: such close personal relationships made tough decisions even more difficult. One such difficult decision that emerged several times in the genetics clinic, but only once with the newborn screening patients, was a debate over whether to call Child Protective Services (CPS) when parents did not follow the recommended dietary regulations. The staff members were reluctant to engage CPS because they were afraid that this would turn the family away from the clinic, or worse, rupture the family. As a result, they focused their efforts on persuading families based on their personal relationships.

Biomedical uncertainty also gave way to the rapid proliferation of disease-related knowledge. Over a three-year period, we observed that the MCADD patient of the past was diagnosed, treated, and managed differently from the MCADD patients of the present. We examined the emergence of a new knowledge ecology linking clinics and laboratories and building upon the experiences of clinicians and researchers across the country. Although the clinic we studied was part of an effort toward long-term follow-up and collection of outcome data in California,[33] the geneticists thought that more in-depth prospective follow-up studies for specific conditions should be implemented.

Newborn screening brings the relationship between knowledge, uncertainty, and ignorance into sharp relief. Social scientists have noted that knowledge and uncertainty are often presented as opposites in the sense that additional knowledge resolves uncertainty. Yet the counterfactual to knowledge is not uncertainty but ignorance, a state where one does not even know that there was something to be known. Our study demonstrates that uncertainty is also a form of knowledge, but one where the content remains unsettled.

Uncertainty presumes doubt about the correct action and a search for guidance about how to act, but it does not involve an inability to act, or an inability to know. We saw over and over again clinicians and parents facing various uncertainties engaged in trial and error processes to see what worked for the practical issue at hand. In biomedicine, then, uncertainty and knowledge are recursively linked: bits of biomedical knowledge continually raise additional questions about how findings apply to the situation at hand, what should be done, and what is implied for the future.

Once a baby is screened, the knowledge-uncertainty interface can no longer be undone to return to a state of ignorance, but rather has a momentum of its own that embeds itself in people's lives. This momentum is institutionally supported because the state requires follow-up for positive screens. Newborn screening challenges parents to specify what they are willing and able to do to save their babies. The uncertainty surrounding what to do and which child will respond to preventive measures further adds to their moral quandary. Parents do not meet such challenges equally or similarly: we saw how some families drew different moral lines around the possibility of disability, had widely disparate resources, and had more biologically favorable windows of opportunity. The salient experience of newborn screening in the clinic is not only facing the practical dilemma of acting under uncertainty but also an irrevocable loss of ignorance.

The staff's acknowledgment of biomedical uncertainty by knocking on wood and their active knowledge production contributed to a gradually evolving consensus of what newborn screening had to offer to patients and families. Increasingly, this consensus was at odds with the understanding of newborn screening benefits that circulated in policy circles, where the program was held up as a means to save babies' lives. Instead, the interactions in the clinic addressed uncertainty with care, repertoires of reassurance, and new scientific knowledge.

## Emotional Expression Outside and Inside the Clinic

Parent advocacy played a critical role in the expansion of newborn screening in the United States. The March of Dimes and other advocacy organizations carefully orchestrated a persuasive case for screening by showcasing the tragic stories of parents who had lost a child due to a metabolic disorder that might have been detected by screening, followed by those of families whose children had been doing fine following screening and early intervention. The implied causal narrative suggested that newborn screening was sufficient to save babies' lives, and sent the message to legislators that they could help parents to avoid the unspeakable pain of losing a newborn by giving the green light to expanded newborn screening. We characterized this situation as an *affective economy* because health advocates enacted and elicited emotional responses for social and political ends, such that affect came to serve as its own currency and yielded its own profits and costs.[34] Marshaling emotion for political gain has long been a common strategy in health advocacy, as studies of HIV/AIDS,[35] breast cancer,[36] and abortion[37] activism have made clear. However, the affective scripts imposed by the March of Dimes and other advocacy organizations truncate the full range of emotions experienced by families whose newborn screening trajectories did not fit the mold of saving babies through screening.

For some parents, the raw emotions experienced in the clinic set the stage for later political engagement. One father testified to the California legislature and another couple launched its own advocacy organization. One mother wrote a children's book about her daughter's metabolic disorder to raise awareness about the condition and funds for its treatment. Another planned to write a book about her experience after her son turned six. The genetics staff explicitly enlisted families to participate in such advocacy efforts. As Dr. Flores told one family: "It's up to the medical community and parents to come together and say, is it really helping or not. We think it is. And if you do, please advocate for the program, and talk to other parents who are part of the—there's a very active newborn screening community. If you guys want to participate then go out there and say, 'Yes, this is something that's worthwhile, it changed our lives.' And that will help other people change their lives, too."

Interestingly, however, there was a noticeable gap between emotional expression in the policy arena and that which we observed in the clinic. In the public forums where some of the families in our study advocated for the expansion of newborn screening programs, emotional expression focused on the capacity of newborn screening technologies to prevent tragedies and save lives. Yet in the clinic, we witnessed a wider range of emotions that called into question the view put forth in advocacy narratives that newborn screening saved lives and had only positive effects. The most striking emotion we observed in the clinic was anxiety, but parents also expressed shame, anger, and sadness. Parents cried, cradled their infants, paced nervously, held on to each other, cooed at their babies, and articulated their worries. A few outliers expressed mild outrage at being part of an "experiment" or reluctance to label their children at birth. Still others presented a remarkably calm façade in the face of persistent medical challenges that cast the lifesaving promise of newborn screening into doubt.

Emotions experienced in the clinic are part of the everyday politics of US healthcare, in which patients and their families clamor not only for medical treatment but also for answers to existential questions about suffering. For parents of newborn screening patients, the distress provoked by screening results emerged from threatened biographical flows: a positive newborn screening result raised the possibility of a baby who might die prematurely or live with long-term disabilities. Listening carefully to the metaphors parents used to describe the unexpected news of positive newborn screening results, we found recurring images of rupture and shock.

With physicians, nurses, social workers, and ethnographers acting as witnesses, affective displays became interactive cues that clinicians used to guide actions and structure support for families. Explicitly acknowledging emotions offered an interactional opening to explore the reasons for parents' anxiety and address it, when appropriate, with subtle repertoires of reassurance. With little probing, parents revealed complicated family medical histories, fertility problems, and fears of sudden death and disability, all of which helped to contextualize their emotional responses. Yet despite such helpful clues, clinical emotional expression also came with its costs. Not all affect was considered appropriate, and impassivity, anger toward the staff, or the perception of melodramatic reactions could send misleading signals and divert interactions. Occasionally, then, managing parents' emotions became the sole purpose of clinical consultations, displacing other important care.[38]

Although affective displays in the clinic are not as scripted and purposeful as testifying before a legislative committee, clinical emotional expression also constitutes a public display. Yet we found little continuity between the affective displays in the clinic and those in the policy arena. By emphasizing only successes and lifesaving benefits, the narratives that circulated within policy forums eclipsed the complex array of distressing emotions implicated in screening.

## Abduction in the Clinic

In the clinic, newborn screening does not make sense as a straightforward lifesaving technology. Too many ambiguous results, too many unex-

pected reactions, too many contradictions, and too much variation in consequences render screening results a work in progress. The diverse signals
of distressing emotions, appeals to fate, and "collateral damage" signify
the need for a creative refitting of what newborn screening is in the clinic.
In these instances, we can observe abductive reasoning at work. Faced
with surprising situations in which expectations did not meet the available signs or circumstances, clinicians conjectured new hypotheses requiring further trial and error to resolve interpretive ambiguities. Abductive
insights emerge from the failure of analogy. Parents and clinicians search
for models of what the situation at hand resembles. When no immediate
referents come to mind, they try to fit the situation into a new interpretive
frame. Abduction rests on deciphering the critical elements of the misfit.
In the process of defining possible solutions, particular problematic elements gain saliency. Thus, when Dr. Silverman encountered a surprisingly
rapidly recovering infant, the situation did not register as anomalous until
he spoke with a colleague at a conference and pondered the possibility of
maternal disease. The "aha" moment simultaneously defines problem and
solution, although the steps for reaching those solutions can remain unspecified, and other outcomes might be possible.[39]

Abductive reasoning thrives in medical settings, where it is guided by
a decision-making process centered on differential diagnosis, multiple
rounds of testing, and interdisciplinary consultations.[40] Thus, abduction
flourishes in newborn screening clinics. The far-reaching search for biomarkers only loosely tied to disease categories is bound to reveal anomalous findings.[41] Consistent with Renee Fox's writings on uncertainty in
medical education,[42] abduction may occur when individual clinicians lack
familiarity with medical signs or when the biomedical knowledge base is
insufficient. In medical settings, the ability to engage abductive insights
is limited by the institutional impetus to process patients in standardized
ways and the fear—fueled by liability concerns—of discharging a patient
with ambiguous symptoms that could develop into complications.

The ad hoc generation of conjectural registers to deal with surprises
indicates the general mechanism by which the reality of newborn screening diverged from the hopes and aspirations expressed at the policy level.
The end result of abductively tinkering in newborn screening clinics was
a gradual redefinition of the accomplishable goals of newborn screening, appropriate patient populations, knowledge base of diseases, and the
successes of screening. Emotions salient in the clinic were filtered out in
legislative venues. Disease-based knowledge acquired in the clinic no lon-

ger corresponded to the evidence summarized in the ACMG report that opened the door for expanded screening. The effect of newborn screening was not only a saved life but also the realization that screening is insufficient to impede disability and death. In response to local practical concerns, newborn screening in the clinic drifted from the way screening was framed in policy circles.

## Newborn Screening in the Policy Arena

### Public Health Genomics

In December 2010, the National Institute of Child Health and Human Development, the National Human Genome Research Institute, and the NIH Office of Rare Diseases Research sponsored a workshop in Rockville, Maryland, to set a research agenda for the future of newborn screening.[43] This imaginary future, as articulated by the academic and industry experts and federal agency officials who attended the meeting, went far beyond the omens we presented at the beginning of this chapter. They imagined the implementation of comprehensive genetic sequencing technologies at birth to identify a wide spectrum of adult onset diseases and additional medically relevant information, such as behavioral traits, drug response, and carrier status. In this paradigm, parents might be informed that their infant would experience an alcohol flush reaction, had a warfarin (Coumadin) sensitivity, or carried a mutation on the BRCA1 gene associated with an increased risk of breast cancer. Such screening would take place soon after birth alongside screening for an expansive number of traditional newborn screening targets. Screening of newborns would depend on a variety of emergent genomic technologies such as targeted array, whole exome, or whole genome sequencing, and could be integrated into electronic health records to provide a set of personalized health guidelines. Although the workshop participants agreed that the technology for such screening was still too slow, imprecise, and costly, they discussed preliminary pilot studies that could test the feasibility of their visions.

This workshop highlights that the understanding of newborn screening in policy circles did not remain stable, either: the push to use newborn screening as the platform for comprehensive public health genomics at birth expands the program's promise to detect rare disorders to encompass every aspect of health management. We need to be cautious not to be swept away by visions of the radical transformation of newborn screening.

The history of genetics is littered with unfulfilled prophecies of high-risk/ high-reward innovations. Still, contemporary newborn screening offers an important example of a close interface between population screening and genetic technologies. Here, we examine how newborn screening with its links to genetics has become the harbinger of public health genomics in the policy world. We note that newborn screening, as either a method for identifying rare genetic conditions or a pathway to personalized medicine, sits somewhat uneasily in the broader field of public health, which is traditionally focused on population-based outcomes.

Sociologist David Armstrong has linked the preventive logic of public health to the imperatives of screening with his conceptualization of surveillance medicine, a new form of medicine based on monitoring healthy populations rather than care for the sick that emerged in the early twentieth century.[44] Armstrong observed that surveillance medicine alters the temporality of illness by transforming the possibility of disease—rather than disease itself—into the grounds for therapeutic action, creating a new optics of "hidden" disease. From this perspective, population screening becomes the practical means of realizing the preventive gaze of surveillance medicine. Screening programs not only serve the beneficent aims of promoting and maintaining health but also control and regulate patients' bodies, habits, and activities in much broader—and sometimes troubling—ways. In this way, population screening is both a medical and a social intervention, in which patients' bodies become the grounds for a larger set of moral and political debates about state control and responsibility for illness.[45]

The current face of surveillance medicine appears remarkably different. Newborn screening has ushered in a new age of "public health genetics,"[46] in which surveillance is practiced at the molecular level. This field addresses problems of a different scale and scope than the major health problems that public health has traditionally targeted. Historically, public health efforts focused on the deleterious consequences of infectious disease, through interventions targeting sanitation issues, infant mortality, and more recently, HIV/AIDS. Following the epidemiological transition and the decreasing prevalence of infectious diseases, public health experts began to target chronic diseases such as cancer and heart disease, which have become the major foci for contemporary screening programs in the West. In contrast to these conditions, single gene genetic disorders affect a much smaller segment of the population, and force us to reexamine the relationship between individual and societal level concerns in light of public health objectives.

What public health values are reflected in a societal emphasis on genetic technologies aimed at detecting rare disorders or providing a platform for personalized medicine? Renee Anspach, in her pivotal ethnography of neonatal intensive care, highlights the seductive power of healthcare technologies for societal advancement in the global marketplace.[47] In a similar way, investing in high-tech genetic technologies reveals a cultural logic of hidden priorities and values that reaches far beyond the execution of seemingly benevolent public health aims. If any society has access to a finite amount of resources, then investing in one program instead of another necessarily asserts a claim about the moral worthiness of that particular cause. From this perspective, public health serves as a moral gatekeeper on both medicine and social life.[48]

We noted in the introduction that a key remaining question following the routinization of genetics was whether the influx of genetic information reinforced old ways of stratifying the world or produced new classification systems. Public health genetics raises concerns about the emergence of a so-called genetic underclass due to the possibility for insurance and employment discrimination following genetic testing.[49] Theoretically, such a group would be socially, economically, and politically marginalized due to disadvantages and inequalities resulting from putative biological inferiority. Many of the early fears of this possibility have not been borne out, and the passing of the 2010 Affordable Care Act in the United States has substantially decreased the likelihood of medical insurance companies discriminating against individuals with genetic disorders, due to the prohibition of excluding subscribers from coverage on the basis of "preexisting conditions." But as sociologist Susan Kelly has persuasively argued, public health genetics may lead to other forms of genetic stratification beyond overt discrimination.[50] For example, single mothers of children with genetic disorders may remain unmarried long-term so as not to be disqualified from state-funded services that could be rescinded as a result of combined incomes. Summarizing her study of outreach programs for genetic services in rural Kentucky, Kelly concludes:

> In these cases neither the genetic condition nor initial poverty alone appear to explain the patterns of cumulative social and economic disadvantage and marginalization experienced. Rather, the analysis points to interactive processes among genetics (the experience of a genetic condition and availability of genetic services and expertise) and social and structural forces including policy and social services, rural economic disadvantage, and social exclusion. The data collected to date suggest that a genetic underclass might be constituted through

cumulative stresses on the lives of families resulting from poorly coordinated, underfunded and punitive health and social service structures, stresses that encourage marital dissolution, unemployment, and reliance on state-provided health insurance, that ultimately reproduce social biases.[51]

For Kelly, then, public health genetics may inadvertently collude in the further entrenchment of social inequalities through policies and services that poorly serve families already struggling with poverty.

Our research on newborn screening lends further support to these claims. For state governments to provide funding for diagnostic testing but to stop short of ensuring access to clinical services for geographically isolated families and the provision of medical foods and formulas to families who cannot afford to pay appears to be a myopic take on what is meant by "public health genetics." Public health has long been concerned with inequalities of many kinds and origins and has accumulated extensive evidence that resources matter greatly to health outcomes. We demonstrated in the previous chapters that the network of technologies, actors, and practices that constitute newborn screening provide a window of opportunity during which healthcare providers and families may act on behalf of infants. Yet many other conditions must be in place for the lifesaving potential to be realized. For newborn screening to be effective, the infant must also have access to healthcare, insurance to pay for it, adequate medication and dietary supplements, and family caregivers able to administer treatment on a day-to-day basis. Our claim is that these factors form the conditions of possibility for newborn screening to "work," and thus impose necessary constraints on its public health success.

Another matter of debate from the perspective of public health is when in the life course it is appropriate to screen for genetic disorders. At the Rockville workshop, Arthur Beaudet of the Baylor College of Medicine argued that many of the screens now performed at birth could be performed in utero, or earlier, through carrier screening. Carrier and prenatal screening have not been routinely employed for the conditions on the uniform newborn screening panel due to their rarity and the expense of testing. However, the technologies currently available may already identify genetic mutations that cause over 100 Mendelian disorders as well as more than 440 severe recessive disorders.[52] Carrier screening programs for thalassemia in Cyprus and Tay-Sachs disease among Ashkenazi Jews have been extremely effective at reducing morbidity and mortality.[53] Sequencing of fetal DNA in maternal plasma also has diagnostic implications. Yet prenatal genetic screening raises the contested flashpoints of abortion and fetal surgery, and both carrier and prenatal screening technologies have tremendous social, ethical, and public health implications. Indeed, abortion is the great elephant in the room of newborn screening policy: why screen postnatally if the same tests can be used prenatally? The uncertainty we observed in the clinic will be nothing compared to the challenges facing parents told that a fetus will have 3-MCC, glutaric acidemia, or, buying into the visions of the workshop, have a greater risk for Alzheimer's disease, male-pattern baldness, or a low caffeine tolerance. How to weigh such information?

Our discussion of public health and newborn screening would be remiss if we did not point out the big picture issue: the United States ranks 30th worldwide in infant mortality, with rates that have remained stable for several years, even as it stands at the vanguard of innovation in newborn screening technology.[54] In the broader landscape of US healthcare, policymakers have struggled to weigh individual cases against overall public welfare and measure opportunity costs.[55] Newborn screening may make a world of difference in individual families, but no available data has shown that newborn screening is associated with a reduction of infant mortality at the population level. In contrast, other "lifesaving" technologies, particularly surfactant therapy in neonatal intensive care units, have been directly correlated with a reduction of infant mortality.[56] Moreover, the history of newborn screening suggests that epidemiological outcomes may fall short of lifesaving expectations. Although PKU screening was initially presented as a means to prevent mental retardation, and has undoubtedly changed the lives of many families, it has not altered mental retardation rates because PKU accounts for a relatively small proportion of mental retardation.[57]

Sociologist Paul Starr has shown that over the course of the twentieth century, professional opposition succeeded in defeating many large-scale preventive public health interventions.[58] Professional medical organizations advocated for a limited role of government in healthcare. The history of PKU screening showed that such opposition may be surmounted with determined patient advocacy. The irony of expanded newborn screening is that the United States instituted a public health program aimed at prevention for very rare conditions. When combined with widespread inequities in healthcare access, the rarity of the conditions will make it difficult to demonstrate the health payoff of newborn screening and to use universal newborn screening as a model for similar programs in the future.

Newborn screening makes the most sense as a mandatory public health program if all of the conditions screened require interventions in the first days of life to prevent devastating harm. This was the case for PKU, congenital hypothyroidism, and congenital adrenal hyperplasia. But urgency is not an issue for all of the conditions on the recommended universal screening panel, and treatment efficacy remains variable. Offering a comprehensive genetic screen at birth to set the stage for personalized medicine without clearly established pathways from diagnostic information to disease outcomes will inevitably have rapidly diminishing population health returns. Some observers have questioned whether the investment in expanded newborn screening has already come at the expense of other children's health programs.[59] The key question for public health is whether its future includes becoming the standard bearer for personalized medicine on a genomic platform.

## Newborn Screening in Policy and in the Clinic

While clinic-based research depicts newborn screening as a technology with stark limitations, unintended consequences, and opportunity costs, policymakers still dream of seizing the newborn screening infrastructure for comprehensive genome sequencing at birth, further imbuing screening with lifesaving potential. The clinic and the policy world move in opposite directions. In this last section, we explain why this is so and what these divergent movements hold for the future of screening.

Newborn screening can be considered a biomedical platform that involves at least two arenas where screening is made and enacted: the regulatory policy-advocacy realm and that of the clinic.[60] In a biomedical platform, arenas are work sites where people work on similar tasks. They have a distinct character but remain interdependent. The policy world presumes to speak for the clinic, and in turn, the clinical world operates within the parameters set by policymakers. Although spatially distinct, the two arenas are interdependent with loose connections. The connections are loose because each realm reacts to different pressures. Policy actors have redefined the aims of newborn screening in reaction to funding challenges, public opinion, scientific evidence, and technological advancement, while clinicians face the exigency of doing the best for an infant with a positive screen. Each of these worlds has its own practical concerns, resources, and regulations that need to be reconciled in order for newborn screening to work. Consequently, these arenas may drift apart in their understanding of newborn screening, and conflicts may emerge that require a more explicit reframing of what the program is.

What are the links between the clinic and the policy arena? Or more precisely, how can we trace back the effects of the encounter between a genetics fellow and alarmed parents to something that a legislative committee in Washington, DC, decided some years ago? The extent to which the policy world influences the clinic matters for our understanding of the effects of screening, the persistence of health inequities, and the barriers that will need to be overcome to improve the current situation. We can understand the strength of the connections between the clinic and the policy world by examining how policy issues become salient in the clinic and vice versa.

Interactional clues about the relevance of broader policy processes abounded throughout our research. Clinicians, among themselves and in conversations with families, discussed the logic for including certain conditions rather than others in the screening panel, the state of knowledge about the burden of disease, the availability of therapies, tricks to formulate insurance requests, best practices for rationing formula samples, or work-arounds for the lengthy wait at the phlebotomy laboratory. In many cases, they circumvented perceived limitations by writing letters, telephoning pharmacies, and plotting to bypass barriers to care. At other times, they became more proactive, lobbying for changes in the state newborn screening program by communicating directly with program officials. Dr. Silverman, in particular, was multiply implicated in both the policy and clinic arena as a leading clinical expert on metabolic conditions, an investigator of a pilot screening study that preceded the expansion, and an active participant in the legislative process.

The key point is that clinicians and parents experienced friction when acting on newborn screening findings that they directly and indirectly related to off-site policy decisions. Regardless of whether their understanding of policy workings was correct, clinicians and parents responded to emergent interpretations of what policymakers do. This situated problemsolving within a local culture of managing newborn screening results in light of policy constraints. In backroom and end-of-day conversations, clinicians triaged and rationalized what they could do based on their understandings of what was possible in the broader context in which they were operating. The staff thus developed a contextual understanding of what newborn screening was. The resulting ecology of connections between the clinic and policy arenas offered a picture of what policy looks like from the perspective of the clinic, where practical dilemmas were framed as policy issues with their own logic and mechanisms of action.

Our notion of *bridging work* captures the work of anticipating and fixing policy logics from within the clinic. Bridging work refers to the work of aligning the promise of medical technologies as formulated in the policy arena with the realities of their implementation in the clinic. The introduction of new technologies affects a workplace at multiple levels, including the incorporation of technology into available health services, the divisions of labor between medical subspecialties and, importantly, the lives of beneficiaries and others affected directly and indirectly by the technology. Consequently, bridging work has multiple dimensions: making the technology work in terms of finances, information systems, organizations, and epistemologies in the clinic. Earlier we examined how clinicians created new knowledge about newborn screening targets. This kind of bridging work was necessary, we argued, because the designers of newborn screening had an inadequate understanding of disease properties and the screened conditions differed from what biomedical researchers thought they knew.

The clinicians in our study adopted a view of newborn screening success that diverged from the official accounts of policymakers and parent advocates. This discontinuity rarely came into the spotlight because the clinical staff buffered the sharp edges and unintended consequences of newborn screening. An unintended effect of the road maps clinicians offered families to navigate the detours and switchbacks of US and state health policy is that much of the frictions of newborn screening policy never entered public awareness. The same medical object may coexist in very different forms, precisely because it is spatially distributed and entails different prevailing concerns.[61] Such differences may be exposed as conflicts when they seem to lead to contradictions. The experience of a false positive that journalist Aleccia reported or the experience of a patient-in-waiting that we described may bring into the open the discrepancy between what policymakers claim newborn screening does and what the clinical reality is.[62]

Actors in the policy-advocacy arena adopted two primary responses to research findings demonstrating that newborn screening has unexpected consequences for families. The first was to offer the possibility of a technological fix: they suggested that improving the precision of newborn screening technologies could help to avoid false positives and negatives. An extraordinary international data sharing collaboration has helped to improve the designation of clinical parameters. The collaboration was formed in reaction to the proprietary nature of older newborn screening data: only commercial companies who had been offering newborn screening prior to universal screening had sufficient data to help define cutoff values, but these companies were unwilling to share their data. Initially, individual states introduced their own cutoff values and tinkered with them in an ad hoc fashion when too many false positives or a false negative occurred. This was not an advisable strategy considering the rarity of conditions. To address this problem, one of the Regional Genetics and Newborn Screening Collaboratives funded by the Health Resources and Service Administration of the Maternal and Child Health Bureau created a web-based data reporting and collection system to pool newborn screening data. By March 2011, the project had gathered data from 47 US states and Puerto Rico and an additional 80 newborn screening programs in 45 countries. This enabled researchers to compare data from approximately 25–30 million screen negative newborns with 10,742 true positive cases.[63] With this data, the researchers were able to define screening cutoffs point for various biomarkers.[64] This collaborative was thus aimed at avoiding needlessly alarming parents by reducing false positives, and avoiding potentially preventable morbidity and mortality by reducing false negatives. However, although improving the analytical sensitivity and clinical utility of newborn screening will affect the number of babies picked up by the screen, it is unlikely to change how parents are informed of results or to provide them with clearer guidance.

As is apparent from the unsubstantiated assertion that newborn screening is "one of the most significant, effective and well-run public health programs of the past 50+ years," the second strategy of how policy advocates dealt with gaps between intended effects and actual consequences was to ignore the experiences of certain families, deny any negative consequences of screening, and assert authoritatively that everyone who receives a positive screen benefits. The authoritarian nature of newborn screening is exemplified by the lack of parental consent to screening procedures with largely pro forma religious or other exemptions. The lack of parental informed consent prior to screening has been a topic of debate in the bioethics literature since the 1970s and has become relevant again in light of the scientific "gold mine" of research opportunities for dried bloodspots.[65] Although support is high among the public for newborn screening in general, research has shown that for conditions for which there is less urgency, such as adult-onset conditions, some parents would prefer not to have their children tested.[66] Policy stakeholders realized that "newborn screening programs are a multifaceted system of education, screening, diagnosis and referral, treatment and care management, and ongoing evaluation of the effectiveness of all components," in which "communication with the family is key."[67] Yet their efforts and resources have not been matched in the realm of health communication, health psychology, and the social sciences. In spite of a well-documented history that every screening program has unexpected consequences, they embraced a strategy of simply asserting that families benefit.

A fundamental structural and power asymmetry exists in the relationship between the clinic and the policy arena: clinicians work actively to manage the contradictory incentives and bureaucratic hurdles originating from a broadly conceived policy world. For policymakers, however, frontline work in clinics may have little saliency for the budgetary and political issues that they face. The difference is clear in each group's attitude toward false positives. Policymakers consider research attention to false positives and patients-in-waiting as doing a "disservice" to expanded newborn screening, although they also aim to reduce such instances.[68] For clinicians, however, false positives that take a long time to resolve result in difficult interactions with deeply worried parents and extensive bridging work to resolve interpretive ambiguities.

Regardless of what the future holds, the exceptional character of US newborn screening and the fragile relationship between the clinic and policy arenas call for greater responsibility for what parents experience *now*. Parents dealing with the first positive newborn screens are moral pioneers:[69] they are the first to go through the program and work out the dilemmas of care and treatment in light of the possibilities of sudden death and disability. One of our goals in writing this book has been to bring a wider range of clinician and family experiences into the open. All of the parents in our study appreciated that their baby had been screened, but, like the Baios, many also wished that they did not have to go through the experience the way it played out. Considering the changes we witnessed over a three-year period, it is clear that neither the length nor the intensity of these experiences is inevitable. With different protocols, communication scripts, more uniform insurance provisions, and faster and more targeted follow-up care, the sharp edges of newborn screening can be blunted, although every intervention will likely produce new unintended consequences. Currently, much of this moderating occurs in an ad hoc fashion, depending on the sensitivities of an already overburdened clinic staff rather than on a systematic learning process in which a science of informing and communicating with parents is developed. Policymakers, in particular, have ignored the many ways newborn screening affects families and clinicians, focusing instead on fixes to the screening technologies. Similarly, most of the policy barriers are tackled on a case-by-case basis rather than systematically. Much energy is wasted on addressing similar issues in family after family.

We don't know how the drift between the clinic and policy arenas will affect the future of newborn screening. It is unclear whether the ongoing controversies reviewed here represent minor or potentially fatal challenges for the future of newborn screening. The history of medical technologies and health professions has shown that moneyed, networked advocates should never be underestimated. The American College of Medical Genetics has reinvented itself with its leadership on newborn screening and has received considerable NIH funding to advance newborn screening. At the Maryland workshop, PerkinElmer, Luminex, and Advanced Liquid Logic made presentations about their technologies. PerkinElmer is already a global leader in newborn screening, but Luminex issued a press release to mark its intent to seek a piece of the newborn screening market, which the CEO estimated at a $100-plus million opportunity.[70] The discrepancy between intended and actual consequences and the lack of clear measures of public health outcomes may still be made moot by new technological innovations that expand newborn screening even further or a mandate to secure informed consent from parents, which would shift the entire discussion from how to interpret findings to how to entice parents to participate in screening programs. The field may also shift from neonatal to prenatal screening, again upending the current terms of debate with more complex ethical questions. Or, we may enter the world of personalized medicine with whole genome sequencing at birth. If any of these changes come to pass, they may once again transform the work in clinics, creating new claims about benefits and success, with unintended consequences.

# Notes

## Introduction

1. See http://www.baileybaioangelfoundation.com/ for more information.

2. (Watson et al. 2006).

3. (McCabe and McCabe 2008).

4. Except when indicated, all names of research participants in our study are pseudonyms. The Baios consented to using their real names.

5. See, for example, their interview in *People* magazine: http://celebritybabies.people.com/2008/06/16/scott-and-ren-1/, accessed December 9, 2011.

6. http://www.cdph.ca.gov/programs/nbs/Pages/NBSProgrOVforProviders.aspx, accessed December 16, 2010.

7. See, for example, Lloyd-Puryear and Brower (2010); Weaver et al. (2010).

8. See President's Council on Bioethics (2008). Massachusetts had a period of informed consent during a pilot study.

9. (Toiv et al. 2003, pp. 22–23).

10. http://www.childrensmercy.org/content/cmbc/VIEW.ASPX?ID=11768, accessed June 3, 2011.

11. Newborn screening also detects cystic fibrosis and hematological and endocrine disorders, but these fell outside the scope of our study.

12. (Watson et al. 2006, p. 15S).

13. Scott's reluctance to bond with Bailey bears a striking resemblance to Barbara Katz Rothman's (1993) discussion of how women suspend a commitment to pregnancy while waiting for the delivery of amniocentesis results.

14. (Reichertz 2007).

15. (Sewell 1992).

16. (Groopman 2007; Montgomery 2005).

17. (James 1981 [1907], p. 44).

18. Sociologists such as Anthony Giddens and Ulrich Beck have also singled out uncertainty as an epochal characteristic of modern life.

19. (Fox 1957, 1980, 2000).

20. (Timmermans and Angell 2001).

21. (Armstrong 2002).

22. (Armstrong and Ogden 2006). See also Prosser and Walley (2006).

23. (Mykhalovskiy and Weir 2004).

24. (Timmermans and Angell 2001).

25. The remainder of this paragraph draws from Han, Klein, and Arora's (2011) conceptual taxonomy of uncertainty.

26. (McGowan, Fishman, and Lambrix 2010).

27. (Raspberry and Skinner 2011).

28. (Sulik 2009).

29. (Babrow and Kline 2000).

30. (Konrad 2003).

31. (McCoyd 2010; Rapp 2000b).

32. (Glaser and Strauss 1965; Groopman 2004; Whitmarsh et al. 2007).

33. See, for example, Sulik (2009).

34. Further complicating the issue, the time of an isolated dyadic relationship between patient and physician is largely gone. Medical care is now provided by teams of medical specialists and allied semiprofessionals, which, in virtue of their added complexity, will require coordination and ironing out of conflicting priorities. These clinical teams are further constrained by various third parties, such as insurance companies, government regulators, and pharmaceutical interests. Each of these third parties may create opportunities and roadblocks that further fuel distrust. Furthermore, many people now have access to medical information online. Within this rapidly changing ecology of competing interests, the management of biomedical uncertainty forms a decisive test of what it means to be a medical professional and a patient in technology-driven fields.

35. (Barker 2005; Brown and Zavestoski 2004; Conrad and Stults 2010; Dumit 2006; Haug and Lavin 1983; Hibbard and Weeks 1987; Nettleton 2006; Stockl 2007).

36. (Brown 2009).

37. (Mollering 2006).

38. (Atkinson 1984).

39. (Locke, Golden-Biddle, and Feldman 2008).

40. Tandem mass spectrometry existed long before it was applied to newborn screening. This has been a common pattern in medical innovations: countless biologics and medical instruments have created medical needs de novo, rather than responding to such needs. This pattern of diffusion likely represents the wave of the future in genetic medicine; as whole exome and genome sequencing become more affordable and faster, they are technologies in search of clinical applications.

41. (Berg 1997; de Laet and Mol 2000; Suchman 2007).

42. (Oudshoorn and Pinch 2003; Suchman 2007; Woolgar 1991).

43. (Woolgar 1991).

44. (Timmermans and Berg 1997).

45. See especially Berg (1997).

46. (Stinchcombe 2001).

47. (Akrich 1992).

48. (de Laet and Mol 2000).

49. (Bijker, Hughes, and Pinch 1989).

50. (Suchman 2007).

51. (Keating and Cambrosio 2003).

52. (Lakoff 2005, 2007; Petryna 2009).

53. On invisible work, see Star (1991b).

54. (Timmermans and Berg 2003b).

55. (Wailoo et al. 2010).

56. (Sachs 1995).

57. (Greene 2007).

58. (Armstrong 1995).

59. (Aronowitz 2009).

60. (Ibid.).

61. (Brownlee and Lenzer 2011).

62. (Browner et al. 2003; Ehrich and Williams 2010; Franklin and Roberts 2006; Parthasarathy 2005).

63. (Breen and Meissner 2005; Stone 1986).

64. (Aronowitz 2007; Breen and Meissner 2005; Kolata 2011).

65. (Howson 1999).

66. (Atkin and Ahmad 1998).

67. (Good 1994, p. 133).

68. (Sachs 1995).

69. (Kerr and Cunningham-Burley 2000; Rose 2010).

70. (Paul and Brosco, forthcoming, chapter 5).

71. (Collins 2010).

72. (Lippman 1991).

73. (Conrad 1997; Duster 1990; Nelkin and Andrews 1999; Nelkin and Tancredi 1989). For a review, see Freese and Shostak (2009).

74. (Boyer 2010, p. 62).

75. (Novas and Rose 2000, p. 487).

76. (Hacking 2004, p. 287).

77. (Bearman 2008, p. i).

78. (Atkinson, Parsons, and Featherstone 2001; Bharadwaj 2002; Bourret and Rabeharisoa 2008; Browner and Preloran 2010; Callon and Rabeharisoa 2004; Conrad and Gabe 1999; Finkler 2000, 2005; Latimer et al. 2006; Palladino 2002; Rabeharisoa 2006; Rabeharisoa and Bourret 2009; Raz and Vizner 2008; Sarangi and Clarke 2002; Wood, Prior, and Gray 2003).

79. (Browner and Preloran 2010).

80. (Barker 2005; Dumit 2006).

81. (McLaughlin 2008; Whitmarsh et al. 2007).

82. (Scott et al. 2005).

83. (Saukko et al. 2006).

84. (Bogardus, Holmboe, and Jekel 1999).

85. (Latimer et al. 2006).

86. (Hedgecoe 2003; Keating and Cambrosio 2000; Miller et al. 2005; Vailly 2008).

87. (Rabeharisoa and Bourret 2009, p. 699). See also Sarangi et al. (2003).

88. Besides genetics, Rabinow (1996) also singled out advances in immunology and environmental sciences.

89. (Rabinow 1996, p. 103).

90. (Callon and Rabeharisoa 2008).

91. (Epstein 1995; Klawiter 2009; Kolker 2004).

92. (Duster 1990).

93. (Duster 1990; Fujimura, Duster, and Rajagopalan 2008; Fullwiley 2007, 2008; Nelson 2008; Reardon 2005).

94. (Shim 2002).

95. (Franklin, Lury, and Stacey 2000).

96. (Featherstone et al. 2006).

97. (Buchbinder and Timmermans 2011; Finkler 2005).

98. (Strathern 1992). This may counter the movement of reproductive technologies to expand the notion of families beyond the normative model of father and mother (Franklin and Edwards 1999).

99. (Franklin 2003, p. 71).

100. (Chilibeck, Lock, and Sehdev 2011, p. 1774). See also Scott et al. (2005).

101. (Cox and McKellin 1999).

102. (Konrad 2003).

103. (Hacking 1986, 1991, 2007).

104. (Morgan 2009).

105. The few collections housed in natural history museums provide one notable exception.

106. (Taylor 2008).

107. (Bowker and Star 1999).

108. (Hughes 1971 [1945]).

109. Besides Mara and Stefan, the research team in the clinic included John Heritage and Rocio Rosales. We observed 28 families once and 25 families twice. We saw 6 families 3 times, 7 families 4 times, 1 family 5 times, 3 families 6 times, and 2 families 7 times. We saw 1 family 9 times, another 11 times, and a third family 12 times. Sixteen families spoke only Spanish; the remaining families were all English-speaking.

110. Two families were ineligible for our study because they spoke neither Spanish nor English. Five families refused participation, mostly because they objected to audiotaping. The first refusal was from a family of Eastern European immigrants. When the father saw our recorder, he said, "no taping" before we had a chance to explain the study. The mother of the second child told us that she was not interested in the study. The third child was believed to be a false positive for an ultra-rare condition. In the fourth family, the mother and grandmother would have been happy to participate but the father nixed it based on the legal language of the HIPAA form. We did not get to speak to the fifth family. The parents were very anxious because they had been led to believe, prior to their visit, that they would simply be having a conversation rather than a formal medical consultation. They also objected to the nurse recording their child's height and weight.

111. (Timmermans and Tavory 2007).

112. (Marcus 1998; Nader 1972; Ortner 2010).

113. (Bosk 1992).

## Chapter One

1. The other country is Canada.

2. Watson et al. (2006) was published in 2006 but was available for public comments in 2005.

3. Urine-based screening programs existed in some parts of the country in the 1950s, prior to Guthrie's developments.

4. http://www.thearc.org/NetCommunity/Page.aspx?pid=183&srcid=403, accessed August 13, 2008. The organization was founded in 1950 as the National Association of Parents and Friends of Mentally Retarded Children.

5. (Bickel, Gerrard, and Hickmans 1953; Woolf and Vulliamy 1951).

6. Chromatography and the McCaman-Robins fluorometric method were added to the Guthrie inhibition assay in the early years of PKU screening (McCaman and Robins 1962).

7. (Paul 1997). In addition, the United States did not have home visiting nurses to do well-baby visits, as the United Kingdom did (Lindee 2005).

8. (California State Department of Public Health 1963).

9. (Ibid.).

10. (Guthrie 1992, p. 12).

11. (Starr 1982).

12. (American Academy of Pediatrics 1967).

13. (Koch 1997).

14. (National Academy of Sciences 1975).

15. (Ibid., pp. 288–293).

16. (Ibid., p. 50).

17. (McCabe and McCabe 2002).

18. (Pass et al. 2000).

19. In the latter discussion, universal screening for PKU was held up as an example that genetics is not necessarily destiny: dietary interventions at an early age can offset mental retardation due to a genetic mutation (Paul 1997). See also Scriver (2007).

20. (Berman et al. 1969).

21. (Frankenburg et al. 1968).

22. (Lenke and Levy 1980, p. 390).

23. (Brosco et al. 2008; Brosco, Seider, and Dunn 2006; Fost 1992).

24. (Abram 1983; Holtzman, Meek, and Mellits 1974).

25. (McCabe and McCabe 2008, p. 166).

26. (AAP Newborn Screening Task Force 2000).

27. (National Academy of Sciences 1975).

28. (Ibid., p. 93).

29. (Ibid., p. 91).

30. (Andrews et al. 1994, p. 66).

31. (Paul 1997, p. 149).

32. (Andermann et al. 2008).

33. (Wilson and Jungner 1968, p. 27).

34. (Andrews et al. 1994, p. 67).

35. (Abram 1983, p. 6).

36. (Ibid., p. 47).

37. (Andrews et al. 1994, p. 6, italics in original; National Academy of Sciences 1975, p. 91).

38. (Holtzman and Watson 1998, p. xiii).

39. (Halpern 2004).

40. (Wilson and Jungner 1968, pp. 26–27).

41. (AAP Newborn Screening Task Force 2000, pp. 394–395). On the concept of medical home, see Sia et al. (2004).

42. (Star 1991a).

43. Many of these organizations have joined forces in the "Genetic Alliance," an umbrella advocacy organization committed to improving health through genetics.

44. (Howse, Weiss, and Green 2006).

45. http://www.hrsa.gov/heritabledisorderscommittee/presentations/04june .htm, accessed August 25, 2008.

46. (Ahmed 2004).

47. (Ibid., p. 119, emphasis in original).

48. On the notion of "will" to live and to tackle disease, see Biehl (2009).

49. (Howell 2006b, p. 1800).

50. (Howell 2006b; Howse, Weiss, and Green 2006).

51. (Howse, Weiss, and Green 2006).

52. http://www.hrsa.gov/heritabledisorderscommittee/presentations/04june
.htm accessed August 25, 2008.

53. (AAP Newborn Screening Task Force 2000, p. 394).

54. (Howse and Katz 2000).

55. (Howse, Weiss, and Green 2006).

56. (Atkinson et al. 2001).

57. (HGSA-RACP 2004; Pandor et al. 2004; Pollitt 2006).

58. (King 2000, p. 333).

59. (Watson et al. 2006, p. 17S).

60. (Bailey, Skinner, and Warren 2005).

61. (Ibid., p. 1889).

62. (Watson et al. 2006, p. 30S). See also Bailey et al. (2006).

63. (Bailey et al. 2006).

64. See, for example, Abram (1983).

65. (Howell 2006b, p. 1803).

66. (Baily and Murray 2008; Botkin et al. 2006; Kerruish and Robertson 2005;
Moyer et al. 2008; Natowicz 2005; President's Council on Bioethics 2008; Tarini
2007).

67. (Baily and Murray 2008, p. 28).

68. (Baily and Murray 2008, p. 29). See also Moyer et al. (2008, p. 34) and Tarini
(2007).

69. (Moyer et al. 2008).

70. (Ibid., p. 35).

71. (Kerruish and Robertson 2005, p. 397).

72. (Watson et al. 2006, p. 36S).

73. (Ibid., p. 19S).

74. (Ibid., p. 17S).

75. (Greene 2007).

76. In some states, high-performance liquid chromatography is used to test for
sickle cell disease (Eastman et al. 1996).

77. (Millington et al. 1990).

78. (Garg and Dasouki 2006).

79. (GAO 2003).

80. (Holtzman 2003).

81. (Therrell 2001).

82. The term "throughput" refers to the productivity of a machine or other
technology.

83. (Watson et al. 2006, p. 41S).

84. (Baily and Murray 2008; Botkin et al. 2006; Harrell 2009; Holtzman 2003;
Moyer et al. 2008).

85. (Moreira 2005; Timmermans and Berg 2003a).

86. (Bluhm 2005).

87. The ACMG committee used a variant of this hierarchy of evidence but then added expert opinion to it and used the evaluations to obtain evidence for an ad hoc scoring system. At the end of the process, the scoring system was further tweaked to account for exceptions. The strong impression is that this was a system based on expert opinion, which is exactly the kind of evidence that evidence-based medicine tries to supplant.

88. (Moyer et al. 2008, p. 37).

89. (Ibid., p . 38).

90. (Botkin et al. 2006; Kerruish and Robertson 2005; Moyer et al. 2008; Natowicz 2005; Tarini 2007).

91. (Pandor et al. 2004).

92. (Grosse 2009).

93. (Watson et al. 2006, p. 40S).

94. (Vaughan 1996).

95. For more detail, see Vaughan (1996, 2004).

96. (Hogle 2009; Timmermans 2002).

97. (Weimer 2007). In addition, a black market exists for purchasing kidneys from living donors despite prohibitory laws. See, for example, Scheper-Hughes (2004).

98. See statistics at http://www2.uthscsa.edu/nnsis/, accessed August, 21 2008.

99. (Howse, Weiss, and Green 2006).

100. (Burke and Rosenbaum 2005).

101. (Burke and Rosenbaum 2005; Kraszewski, Burke, and Rosenbaum 2006).

102. (Botkin et al. 2006, p. 1797).

103. (Howell 2006b, p. 1802).

104. (Lloyd-Puryear and Brower 2010; Weaver et al. 2010).

105. (Campbell and Ross 2003; Detmar et al. 2007).

106. (GAO 2003). The lack of informed consent in newborn screening has generated an extensive and nuanced bioethics literature. See, for example, Ross (2011).

107. (Grob 2011; Gurian et al. 2006; Harrell 2009; Waisbren et al. 2003).

108. But see Scriver (2007).

109. (Schweitzer-Krantz 2003).

110. (Marsden, Larson, and Levy 2006; Yusopov et al. 2010).

111. (Watson 2006; Watson et al. 2006).

112. (Watson et al. 2006, p. 35S).

113. (Scriver 2007).

114. (Watson et al. 2006, p. 36S).

115. (Marsden, Larson, and Levy 2006).

116. (Teach, Lillis, and Grossi 1998).

117. (Timmermans and Buchbinder 2012).

118. (Berg 1997).

**Chapter Two**

1. (Watson et al. 2006, p. 29S).
2. (Landsman 1998; Rothshild 2005).
3. (Star and Gerson 1986; Timmermans 2011).
4. (Hughes 1971 [1945]).
5. (Dewey 2005 [1910], p. 10).
6. See Parsons (1951) on the sharing of the patient role between parents and children.
7. On the concept of trajectory, see Strauss et al. (1985) and Timmermans (1999a).
8. Sociologist Rachel Grob (2011) documented similar reactions to the delivery of cystic fibrosis newborn screening results among the parents in her study.
9. See also Schaffer, Kuczynski, and Skinner (2008).
10. The equilibrium related to PKU was upset, however, with the 2007 introduction of sapropterin dihydrochloride (brand name Kuvan), an expensive drug that enabled some patients with PKU to relax the traditional restrictive diet. (http://www.ncbi.nlm.nih.gov/pubmedhealth/PMH0000447, accessed October 19, 2010). During our study, the genetics team was in the process of testing who responded to Kuvan, appropriate dosage, and follow-up testing. They also debated whether Kuvan was indicated for young children.
11. Hyperprolinemia was not part of the recommended uniform screening panel, but it was still part of the California panel.
12. For an early and likely outdated ethnographic account of this modus operandi, see Bosk (1992). Bosk describes a time when geneticists did not have a clear clinical domain of practice. The geneticists in his study self-describe as providing "mop-up" services for biological quirks and organizational problems. The geneticists in our study had a more defined area of expertise that was recognized by colleagues. See also Bourret and Rabeharisoa (2008), Browner and Preloran (2010), Featherstone et al. (2005), Latimer et al. (2006), Rabeharisoa and Bourret (2009), and Taussig (2009).
13. (Latimer et al. 2006).
14. (Star 1994).
15. (Rosenberg 2007).
16. (Becker 1960, p. 35).
17. (Latimer et al. 2006).
18. The C14 level was 13.
19. Dr. Silverman misspoke here—Sylvia underwent a chorionic villus sampling test (CVS) rather than amniocentesis.
20. (Armstrong 1995).
21. (Cederbaum et al. 2001).
22. (Grineski 2009).

23. (Feuchtbaum, Dowray, and Lorey 2010, p. S244).

24. (Ibid., p. S249).

25. (Hughes 1971 [1945]).

26. (Rosenberg 2007).

27. (Gillespie 2009).

## Chapter Three

1. (Mol 2002).

2. (Aronowitz 2008; Rosenberg 2007).

3. (Kirk and Kutchins 1992; Shostak, Conrad, and Horwitz 2008).

4. (Epstein 1996).

5. (Greene 2007; Kerr 2005).

6. (Rosenberg 2007).

7. (Greene 2007; Lakoff 2005).

8. (Bowker and Star 1999).

9. (Kerr 2005).

10. (Armstrong 1979).

11. (Paul 1997).

12. (Wailoo and Pemberton 2006).

13. (Kleven, McCudden, and Willis 2008).

14. (Howson 2001).

15. (McBride et al. 2010).

16. (Keating and Cambrosio 2003).

17. (Latimer et al. 2006).

18. (Rabeharisoa and Bourret 2009, p. 699).

19. (Hedgecoe 2004).

20. (Yang, Latntz, and Ibdah 2007).

21. (Iafolla, Thompson, and Roe 1994).

22. (Gregersen et al. 1993).

23. (Andresen et al. 2001, p. 1408).

24. C8 is a measure of fatty acids in the blood and is considered to be the principal biochemical indicator of MCADD.

25. (Smith et al. 2010, p. 241).

26. (Ibid., p. 245).

27. (Ibid., p. 245). Note, however, that the classification did not extrapolate to physical symptoms but to biochemical changes. The correlation is between genetic mutations and biochemical changes. Severity thus refers to severity of biochemical changes.

28. C2 and C10 measure different fatty acids, and hexanoylglycine is an indicator of MCADD in urine.

29. (Maier et al. 2005; Waddell et al. 2006).

30. (Maier et al. 2005).

31. Dr. Flores cited Smith et al. (2010, p. 247).

32. (Fujimura, Duster, and Rajagopalan 2008).

33. In fact, the most salient element of Osiel's case was the consanguinity of his parents because consanguinity leads to higher risk for genetic disorders. Geneticists routinely asked about consanguinity when taking a family pedigree during the first clinic visit. In some Latino families who migrated from small "pueblitas," geneticists asked a follow-up question about how many people lived in the village. Their assumption was that in small villages, everyone was likely related to everyone else. But they asked the consanguinity question indiscriminately to US-born and foreign-born patients. Dr. Nazif, an Egyptian born genetics fellow, encouraged us to study the prevalence of consanguinity in her home country.

34. (Wilcken 2010, pp. 501, 504).

35. (Yusopov et al. 2010).

36. Fred Lorey, California Department of Public Health, personal communication.

37. http://ghr.nlm.nih.gov/condition/hyperprolinemia, accessed March 12, 2009.

38. (Stanley 2004).

39. (Karpati et al. 1975).

40. (Shoji et al. 1998; Tamai et al. 1998; Wu et al. 1998).

41. (Stanley 2004). This article also distinguished a second form of carnitine deficiency due to chronic administration of pivalate-conjugated antibiotics. Such antibiotic treatment did not come up in our study.

42. Two articles were published around the same time: Schimmenti et al. (2007) and Vijay et al. (2006).

43. (Schimmenti et al. 2007, p. 443).

44. (Crombez et al. 2008).

45. (Hinton et al. 2010).

46. (Lin et al. 2009).

47. (Koeberl et al. 2003).

48. (Leydiker et al. 2011).

49. (Schimmenti et al. 2007, p. 444).

50. (El-Hattab et al. 2010, p. 22).

51. The practice of testing mothers but not fathers reflects a gendered logic of screening follow-up that stems from a long history of medical surveillance of pregnant women (Armstrong 2003; Levy 1982).

52. (Rosenberg 1979; Star 1995).

53. (Becker 1993).

54. (Feuchtbaum, Dowray, and Lorey 2010). Similar studies exist in different states. See Berry, Lloyd-Puryear, and Watson (2010).

55. (Kuhn 1962).

## Chapter Four

1. (Parker, Zuckerman, and Augustyn 2004).

2. (Ablon 1990; Landsman 2003; Mattingly and Lawlor 2003).

3. Of course, the geneticists' instructions to treat the newborn screening patients "as" or "like" normal babies highlight the sense of mutual pretense necessary to accomplish this goal. This language implies that they were not completely normal, since parents should act *as if* they were. Deborah Kent, a congenitally blind woman, illustrates the importance of this distinction in a published account: "As I was growing up people called my parents 'wonderful.' They were praised for raising me 'like a normal child.' As far as I could tell, my parents were like most of the others in my neighborhood—sometimes wonderful and sometimes annoying. And from my point of view, I wasn't *like* a normal child—I *was* normal" (Kent 2000, p. 57). With instructions to treat their babies *as* normal children, the geneticists attempted to reconcile the seeming incommensurability of being normal with having a genetic disorder.

4. This definition of normalization is informed by Hacking's (1990) account of the origins of statistical thinking in the late nineteenth century. Population screening is itself predicated upon such normalization, since a positive newborn screen indicates a biochemical value lying outside a preestablished normal (i.e., statistical average) range.

5. (Daston and Galison 2007; Porter 1995).

6. We are indebted to Wong (1994) for this chapter heading, and much of the discussion that follows.

7. (Davis 1995; Landsman 2009; Lauritzen 1997; Leiter 2007; Press et al. 1998).

8. (Ariès 1965; Mintz 2006; Zelizer 1994).

9. (Hacking 1990, 2007).

10. (Armstrong 1986; Meckel 1998).

11. (Armstrong 1994; Meckel 1998; Weaver et al. 2010).

12. (Rose 1999).

13. (Armstrong 1995).

14. (Canguilhem 1991[1978]).

15. (Rose 1999, p. 144).

16. (Burman 1994).

17. (Kelle 2010).

18. See, for example, Burman (1994) and James (2004).

19. (Kelle 2010).

20. According to Lampl and Thompson (2007), growth charts are designed to characterize the size of an individual relative to a group of peers. In practice, however, they have become tools for monitoring individual progress. This use of growth charts is misleading because location on a lower centile curve is not neces-

sarily an indicator of a clinical condition or poor health status, although it may be interpreted as such. Furthermore, there is significant evidence to suggest that the biology of human growth involves episodic bursts that are not well represented through growth curves.

21. (Heritage and Lindstrom 1998; Lauritzen 1997).

22. (Hacking 1990). See also Hogle (2005), Lock (2000), and Vailly (2008).

23. (Rose 2009).

24. (Ibid., p. 74).

25. See Grob (2011), Raspberry and Skinner (2007), and Whitmarsh et al. (2007).

26. (Ehrich and Williams 2010; Press et al. 1998; Remenick 2006).

27. See Mattingly (2010) and Strathmann and Hay (2009) for related analyses of the clinic waiting room and hospital lobby as liminal spaces.

28. A study of Mexican-origin women's uptake of amniocentesis in California similarly found that reassurance from genetic counseling about the likelihood of false positive screening results could lead to misunderstandings about the importance of further testing (Browner et al. 2003).

29. (Porter 1995, p. 3). Daston and Galison (2007) suggest that what we now think of as objectivity actually consists of a diverse, sociohistorical layering of several different types of objectivity, including empirical reliability, procedural correctness, impersonality, and emotional detachment.

30. (Boyd and Heritage 2005).

31. (Adolph and Berger 2005).

32. When the case was discussed at the team meeting later that day, Dr. Silverman expressed his reluctance to prescribe speech therapy for a child that "is that normal and looks that normal" because it would "medicalize the baby." One genetic counselor disagreed, however, arguing instead that the child was in a critical period of development where he could benefit significantly from speech therapy, and would qualify because of his diagnosis. Ultimately, he did receive speech therapy, though not until several months later, after returning from a two-month vacation out of the country, when his delay became more pronounced. See Gill and Maynard (1995) for a discussion of how clinicians minimize the social implications of developmental disability diagnoses.

33. (Latimer 2007, p. 113).

34. (Daston and Galison 2007; Porter 1995).

35. Ben-Joseph, Dowshen, and Izenberg (2009) suggest that parental understanding of growth charts is lacking, despite their widespread use. In an Internet survey of 1,000 US parents, they found that only 65 percent of respondents believed that they understood the information conveyed by a sample growth chart, and charts with plotted points proved difficult for respondents to interpret. Interestingly, 40 percent of respondents indicated a desire to see a growth chart as a visual verification of the clinician's verbal assessments, which corroborates the significance of mechanical objectivity.

36. Lampl and Thompson (2007) provide a useful overview of the design of growth charts.

37. Of course, absent from this explanation is any discussion of *which* children her age—typically children of European descent—have been used to establish the norms.

38. (Foucault 1976).

39. (Porter 1995).

40. (Daston and Galison 2007, p. 48). See also Goodwin's (1994) incisive account of how members of a professional community shape objects of knowledge through socially situated perceptual practices.

41. (Porter 1995, pp. 213–214). Similarly, Latimer et al. (2006) and Rabeharisoa and Bourret (2009) have demonstrated that mechanical objectivity has not completely subsumed clinical judgment in the genomic era.

42. As we mentioned earlier, Kyle Stardust was not ultimately diagnosed with glutaric acidemia type 1 and was eventually dismissed from the clinic.

43. *Positional plagiocephaly*, or flattened head, has become more common in infants since the practice of supine sleeping has been widely adopted to prevent sudden infant death syndrome. There is some evidence to suggest that it is associated with developmental delays over time (Hutchinson, Stewart, and Mitchell 2009; Miller and Clarren 2000; Steinbok et al. 2007).

44. (Ben-Joseph, Dowshen, and Izenberg 2009; Laraway et al. 2010).

45. (Rapp 2000a, p. 197).

46. (Good and Good 1994, p. 837).

47. (Bruner 1986, p. 26) cited in Good and Good (1994, p. 838).

48. (McLaughlin 2008; Whitmarsh et al. 2007).

49. (Raspberry and Skinner 2007, p. 366).

50. (Burman 1994; James 2004).

## Chapter Five

1. (Mattingly 2006, 2010).

2. Even if such a correlation were statistically valid, it would not provide evidence for a causal relationship between social and biogenetic variables, since causality could plausibly work in either direction. Recent work in epigenetics has moved past claims about the biological basis of certain racial health disparities to elucidate a biocultural framework for understanding how social inequalities "get under the skin" to influence biological outcomes (Kuzawa and Sweet 2009). Another possible explanation for higher rates of metabolic disorders in certain immigrant populations would be higher rates of consanguinity in isolated populations.

3. (Mattingly 2010, p. 495).

4. Layne (1996) tracks the use of the roller coaster metaphor to describe how parents experience a child's hospitalization in a neonatal intensive care unit. She

notes that while the up-and-down nature of the roller coaster does "seem to capture the alternating moments of hope and despair" as well as the cyclical sense of "getting nowhere making no progress," (p. 633) the NICU experience embodies a real, rather than imagined, danger.

5. See Heimer and Staffen (1998), Landsman (2009), Leiter (2007), Mattingly (2010), Mattingly and Lawlor (2003), and Rapp (2000b), among others.

6. See Anspach (1993) and Mesman (2005) for a discussion of prognostic uncertainty in NICU settings.

7. (Davidson 2001; Elderkin-Thompson, Cohen Silver, and Waitzkin 2001; Hsieh 2007; Simon et al. 2006).

8. (Feuchtbaum et al. 2006).

9. Although prenatal screening is contentious and ethically fraught (Duster 1990; Raz 2009; Shakespeare 2005; Taussig, Rapp, and Heath 2003), the fact that newborn screening in some cases does not come early enough raises the question of whether (or perhaps, when) prenatal screening might be pursued as an alternative course of action that might potentially afford better outcomes, albeit with a new set of social and ethical challenges (Bombard et al. 2010). Cowan (2008) offers a relevant discussion of the implementation of a multitiered genetic screening program for thalassemia in Cyprus.

10. Skinner and Weisner (2007) provide a useful review of sociocultural approaches to understanding how family ecologies adapt to children's disabilities.

11. (Baker et al. 2010; Leiter 2004; Lewis, Kagan, and Heaton 2000; McKeever and Miller 2004; Skinner, Lachicotte, and Burton 2007; Skinner and Weisner 2007; Timmermans and Freidin 2007).

12. (Acs and Loprest 1999; Powers 1999).

13. (Bernheimer, Weisner, and Lowe 2003; Skinner, Lachicotte, and Burton 2007).

14. With Denise's assistance, Lena eventually procured state-funded health insurance for her children.

15. Carolyn Broderick also reported insurance difficulties. Prior to Sherise's birth, Carolyn and Gary received insurance for their family through Carolyn's employer. Because Gary worked as a freelance writer and could not receive employer-based health insurance, they purchased private insurance in preparation for Carolyn to leave her job. However, their new insurance company refused to cover Sherise when Carolyn tried to enroll her because they deemed her propionic acidemia a preexisting condition. Sherise was eventually covered by the state insurance plan, but Carolyn had to switch to a different pediatrician.

16. Anthropologists have referred to this phenomenon as "stratified reproduction" (Ginsburg and Rapp 1991).

17. Rapp (2000a) and Weiss (1994) have noted that having a child that appears physically different raises a different set of concerns than invisible illness, insofar as it threatens the foundation of kinship and relatedness.

18. Mol (2008) argues that chronic illness management should be guided by a

logic of *care*, which she views as a collective endeavor, in contrast to the logic of patient *choice*, which seeks above all to preserve patient autonomy and has come to dominate Western biomedical thinking.

19. (Heimer and Staffen 1998).

20. An important point of contrast between the families of symptomatic and asymptomatic patients is that in most cases, the families of symptomatic patients accepted the gaps in medical knowledge with equanimity, while the families of asymptomatic patients were more visibly frustrated. While it is likely that differences in class positioning contribute to this distinction, it is also possible that higher stakes and grimmer prognoses mitigated the anxiety of the families of symptomatic patients.

21. This example illustrates how caring has its limits: emotional concern for a family's welfare may lead physicians to overlook important factors. For similar reasons, Groopman (2007) argues that patients are not necessarily best served by physicians who accommodate patients' preferences.

22. For example, Conrad (1985).

23. (Hunt and Arar 2001).

24. (Weaver et al. 2010). The US Food and Drug Administration defines special dietary use of foods as those used to supply specific dietary needs that exist in virtue of physiological disorders (American Academy of Pediatrics 2003).

25. See Craig and Scambler (2006).

26. Mattingly (2010) observes that clinicians may speak of individual differences because it is not acceptable to speak of social difference. She explains, "Direct racial talk is silenced among clinicians in part because strong moral codes in healthcare make it difficult for clinicians to consider the possibility that they are drawing upon racial classifications in their dealings with patients. While they may find it perfectly reasonable to recognize differences at an *individual* level, it is highly problematic to speak of difference among *social categories*" (p. 93).

27. (Shim 2010).

28.(Ibid., p. 3).

29. For example, Dr. Silverman often prefaced his clinical explanations with judgments of parents as "sophisticated" or "educated." These implicit (sophisticated) and explicit (educated) markers of class lay bare the social logic by which Dr. Silverman evaluated whether parents were capable of understanding complex medical information. See also Anspach (1993, pp. 104–110) and Heimer and Staffen (1998, pp. 178–225).

30. (Mattingly 2006, p. 496).

31. Similarly to infant growth charts, diet diaries serve as surveillance technologies that extend the medical gaze beyond the confines of the office visit (Armstrong 1995).

32. For related investigations of how clinicians confront similar dilemmas of care in their everyday practice, see Brodwin (2008), Chambliss (1996), Fitzgerald (2008), Kaufman (2005), Mattingly (1998), and Robins (2001).

33. Sadly, Marisa died due to complications with the dietary management of her MMA shortly after we concluded our study.

34. (Fadiman 1997).

35. See, for example, Ferzacca (2000), Kaljee and Beardsley (1992), Rouse (2010), Trostle (1988), and Whitmarsh (2009).

36. Julie Lee, who was deemed at five years old to have normal speech and physical development despite astronomically high levels of methylmalonic acid, was an important exception to this rule.

37. Diego ultimately died as a result of his metabolic disorder.

38. See Leiter (2004) and Mattingly and Lawlor (2003).

39. (Morioka et al. 2007).

40. White (2002) offers a relevant analysis of clinical team meetings in pediatric settings as a site of moral deliberation over parental behavior. Of course, medical necessity and psychosocial criteria have historically been conflated in decisions about which patients should receive a transplant (Fox and Swazey 1974, pp. 240–279; Gordon 2000).

41. There is tremendous international variation in the regulation of organ transplantation. See Lock and Nguyen (2010) for an overview. In some ways, the Lees' efforts to procure a transplant for Julie in the United States can be seen as a form of what Scheper-Hughes (2003) has called "transplant tourism." While space constraints preclude us from offering a comprehensive review of the transplantation literature here, it is worth noting that live donor transplantation has been hotly contested.

42. Koenig and Hogle (1995) have observed that despite a rich scholarly literature on organ transplantation, relatively less work has examined the broader socioeconomic forces shaping local organ transplantation practices. They note, "There is almost no mention of the enormously high cost of transplantation, nor its potential to create public policy chaos if the current high demand for transplant procedures is no longer kept in check by the supply-side constraint of organ availability" (p. 396).

43. (Anspach 1993, p. 78).

### Chapter Six

1. (Berry et al. 2010; Berry, Lloyd-Puryear, and Watson 2010; Feuchtbaum, Dowray, and Lorey 2010; Kennedy et al. 2010; Powell et al. 2010; Widhalm and Virmani 1994; Wilcken 2008, 2010).

2. Another possibility of a child doing poorly in spite of newborn screening was the emergence of false negatives: infants with a negative screen who were actually affected by the metabolic conditions. In such situations, screening results may give false assurance. We did not observe any false negatives during our study, but we learned that the clinicians treated one false negative after our study ended.

3. (Botkin 2009, p. 175). In our study, the period of blissful ignorance was rather short for many of the symptomatic patients, because they developed symptoms soon after birth. See also Grob (2011).

4. Yusupov et al. (2010, p. 34).

5. The issue of death despite screening and early diagnosis provoked some controversy on the newborn screening Listserv in November 2011, when Jill Levy-Fisch, president of the Save Babies Through Screening Foundation, wrote in to share the story of a Colorado infant who had died due to complications of MCADD following a delay in the processing of his newborn screening bloodspot. http://www.thedenverchannel.com/news/29759209/detail.html?taf=den, accessed December 16, 2011. Interestingly, while Levy-Fisch had written to suggest that regular shipping (versus a courier service) had contributed to this delay, her e-mail prompted a mixed response. Fred Lorey, acting director of the Genetic Disease Laboratory at the California Department of Public Health, wrote in to say: "This is an unfortunate occurrence that several states have experienced since beginning ms/ms testing, but there is sadly more going on in addition to the transport method. . . . A 3 and 4 day test result is pretty hard to beat when everything goes right. Although there are many cases that can clearly be blamed on delayed collection, transport, loss, inadequacy etc and everything should be done to improve these, I'm afraid these early death MCADD cases will continue to occur, though rarely." Additional respondents wrote that screening is only one part of preventing the serious consequences of genetic disorders.

6. (Brosco et al. 2008; Brosco, Seider, and Dunn 2006).

7. (Rouse 1966). See also Brosco et al. (2008).

8. (Brosco et al. 2010; Widhalm and Virmani 1994).

9. (Phenylketonuria: Screening and Management 2000). http://consensus.nih.gov/2000/2000Phenylketonuria113html.htm, accessed June 23, 2011.

10. (Watson et al. 2006). For page numbers in the report: hypothyroidism (p. 80S), classic galactosemia (p. 85S), biotinidase deficiency (p. 103S), PKU (p. 150S), MCAD (p. 173S), MSUD (p. 146S), tyrosinemia (p. 152S), carnitine uptake deficiency (p. 165S), VLCADD (p. 183S), MMA (p. 210S), propionic acidemia (p. 214S), arginase deficiency (p. 128S), glutaric acidemia type I (p. 198S), and glutaric acidemia type 2 (p. 169S). See also Bailey et al. (2006). The Yusupov article shows that not all negative consequences may be prevented for MCADD (Yusupov et al. 2010).

11. (Heimer and Staffen 1998).

12. A splice site mutation refers to a genetic mutation that modifies or deletes a number of nucleotides. The splice site indicates the place where the splicing of an intron takes place.

13. (Kennedy et al. 2010).

14. (Fromm-Reichmann 1948; Silverman 2012).

15. (Star 1991a; Star 1991b; Strauss et al. 1985).

16. (England 2005; Garro et al. 2005; Glazer 1993; Glendinning 1983; Guillemin and Holstrom 1986; Harrington Meyer 2000; MacDonald 2002; Morris 2001; Tardy 2000; Timmermans and Freidin 2007; Traustadottir 1991).

17. It is interesting that Samantha called the pediatrician rather than Dr. Silverman during the H1N1 episode. She had told us that she had a much better relationship with the pediatrician and the original team of geneticists in New Zealand than with Dr. Silverman. By not calling the California geneticist and not transferring Kari to the academic hospital, she also prevented Dr. Silverman and his team from seeing Kari in a metabolic crisis.

18. (Marshall 1950). Marshall's classification has been criticized for being evolutionary and Anglo-centric (Mann 1987).

19. See http://www.natickma.gov/public_documents/NatickMA_Clerk/marquest .pdf, accessed April 26, 2010.

20. Reviewing the policies instituted in the name of eugenics, Cowan (2008, chapter 1) notes that some countries developed involuntary sterilization programs and racist immigration policies, but other countries produced proactive family benefits.

21. (Rose 2007).

22. (Tutton 2010; Waldby 2000).

23. (Petryna 2002).

24. (Epstein 2007).

25. (Ibid.).

26. We write this while the fate of the Obama healthcare reform is still uncertain. Even if these reforms are implemented as planned, the Congressional Budget Office estimates that 23 million Americans will still remain uninsured by 2019, http://www.cbo.gov/ftpdocs/113xx/doc11355/hr4872.pdf, accessed May 15, 2011.

27. (Kerr 2003).

28. http://www.cdph.ca.gov/programs/nbs/Pages/NBSSpecimenCollection Procedures.aspx, accessed December 16, 2010.

29. Letter from Kathleen Velazquez Chief of the California Department of Public Health Newborn Screening Branch of June 12, 2008, to metabolic centers.

30. (Feuchtbaum, Dowray, and Lorey 2010, p. S244).

31. (Anspach 1993).

32. Medicaid is a collaboration between individual states and the federal government. For the other criteria in California, see http://www.dhcs.ca.gov/services/ medi-cal/Pages/Medi-CalFAQs.aspx#whocangetmedi-cal, accessed June 9, 2011.

33. For eligibility criteria, see http://www.dhcs.ca.gov/services/ccs/Pages/qualify .aspx, accessed January 24, 2011.

34. Glutaric acidemia type 1 causes secondary carnitine deficiency.

35. Section 5(b) of the Orphan Drug Act (21 U.S.C. 360ee [b] [3]).

36. http://www.fda.gov/Food/GuidanceComplianceRegulatoryInformation/ GuidanceDocuments/MedicalFoods/UCM054048#q2, accessed January 25, 2011.

37. (Weaver et al. 2010).

38. (Ibid.). This requirement is different in other states.

39. (Ibid.). They suggested developing model state Medicaid coverage policy, amending existing Medicaid legislation, enacting federal legislation to require third-party payer health insurance coverage of medical foods, or changing the FDA's classification of medical food from food to pharmaceuticals.

40. http://www.dhcs.ca.gov/services/ccs/Pages/medicaleligibility.aspx, accessed February 29, 2012.

41. (Groce 1985).

42. (Lutfey and Freese 2005).

43. Diego was born during our project. We did not enroll him in our study until his third clinic visit because we did not yet have IRB approval to recruit Spanish-speaking families.

44. (Timmermans 1999b).

45. The legislation is still pending: http://www.opencongress.org/bill/112-h1311/show, accessed June 24, 2011.


## Conclusion

1. The actual false positive rate would be higher than this number, since many false positives are eliminated before they are referred to the specialty follow-up center.

2. The remaining cases were accounted for as follows: in 25 cases the screening program was unable to obtain a response from the parents; in 27 cases the parents refused follow-up; in 31 cases the infant was lost to follow-up; the infant was diagnosed with a nonscreened disorder in 19 cases; and 30 cases were assigned to an "other" category (Feuchtbaum, Dowray, and Lorey 2010).

3. (Baker et al. 2010; Bell et al. 2011; Brown et al. 2011; McGhee, Stiehm, and McCabe 2005).

4. Hereafter, we refer to this committee as the Secretary's Advisory Committee.

5. Information updated as of May 9, 2011, accessed via http://genesrus.uthscsa.edu/nbsdisorders.htm. Arizona and New Mexico pursued targeted screening among Navajo Indians, a group that is considered to be at high risk for SCID due to its higher incidence rates. See Baker et al. (2010) for a report on the implementation of SCID screening in Wisconsin.

6. The Secretary's Advisory Committee meetings are open to the public and Mara had the opportunity to attend the 24th meeting.

7. In general, there is very little cost-effectiveness data on newborn screening for SCID. The evidence review committee that provided the impetus for the Secretary's Advisory Committee to recommend universal screening noted "limited evidence regarding the costs or cost-effectiveness of screening for SCID" (Lipstein

et al. 2010:e1230) in an article published in *Pediatrics*. The committee found only one study that addressed the cost-effectiveness of newborn screening for SCID, which found an 86 percent likelihood of screening being cost-effective at a threshold of $100,000 per quality-adjusted life-year. However, the authors noted significant uncertainty in the model due to limited data on SCID screening (McGhee, Stiehm, and McCabe 2005).

8. http://today.msnbc.msn.com/id/42829175/ns/today-today_health/t/babies -blood-tests-can-end-false-positive-screening-scares/, accessed May 30, 2011.

9. (Gurian et al. 2006; Morrison and Clayton 2011).

10. Similar language was employed in a critical response to one of the early articles that we published from this study (Watson, Howell, and Rinaldo 2011). Michael Watson, the lead author, is the executive director of the ACMG.

11. (Olson and Berger 2010).

12. http://www.texastribune.org/texas-state-agencies/department-of-state -health-services/dshs-turned-over-hundreds-of-dna-samples-to-feds/, accessed June 13, 2011. The lawsuit was settled, and the Texas newborn screening laws were changed to authorize the retention of blood samples, but Texas agreed to destroy five million samples that were retained prior to the new legislation taking effect.

13. (Lewis et al. 2011, p. 706).

14. (Ross 2011; Rothwell, Anderson, and Botkin 2010; Rothwell et al. 2011).

15. (Olson and Berger 2010).

16. (Ibid.).

17. (Brosco 2011, p. 591).

18. (Timmermans 1999b).

19. http://www.hrsa.gov/heritabledisorderscommittee/reports/, accessed July 5, 2011.

20. These statistics were cited in a press release from the Save Babies Through Screening Foundation distributed to the newborn screening Listserv on October 6, 2011. T lymphocyte disorders are secondary targets of SCID screening.

21. (Lipstein et al. 2010).

22. (Lee 2010).

23. http://www.cdph.ca.gov/programs/nbs/Pages/NBSSpecimenCollection Procedures.aspx, accessed November 28, 2011. The $109.75 cost per screened infant is split up as follows: "The Specimen Collection Form or Test request Form (TRF) for Newborn Screening is provided to every perinatal licensed health facility by the Genetic Disease Screening Program (GDSP) at a cost of $1.00 per form. GDSP also bills the facility a program fee of $101.75 for each completed specimen received. The facilities in turn can charge $1.00 plus the program fee per newborn for the total screening process. (This includes the initial test and any necessary repeat or recall testing until the newborn screen is resolved.) In addition, each facility may charge up to $6.00 for specimen collection and handling. Medi-Cal covers the complete screening process, including the specimen collection fee.

Private insurance generally covers both the newborn screening and the specimen collection fee."

We multiplied the cost of screening with the number of patients screened in California as reported in (Feuchtbaum, Dowray, and Lorey 2010), thus 2,105,119 x $109.75 = $231,036,810.

24. (Baily and Murray 2008).

25. (Stone 1986, p. 689).

26. See, for example, Landecker (2007) and Scheper-Hughes (2004).

27. (Aronowitz 2007). See also Forss et al. (2004) and Scott et al. (2005).

28. It is important to note that when parents are surveyed about their attitudes regarding newborn screening, they are typically asked whether screening is a good idea, without considerations of the opportunity cost. Baily (2009) has argued that the wording of such questions should make the opportunity cost clear by including examples of the hypothetical benefits of devoting these same resources to other causes.

29. (Aronowitz 2009, p. 425).

30. (Franklin and Roberts 2006, p. 227).

31. (Christakis 1999, chapter 6). Christakis focuses on physicians' reluctance to make a poor prognosis at the end of life out of fear of initiating a bad outcome. At the beginning of life, when children are doing well, the fear centers on hexing a favorable process.

32. (Stewart et al. 1995).

33. (Feuchtbaum, Dowray, and Lorey 2010).

34. We develop this idea in more detail in Buchbinder and Timmermans (n.d.).

35. (Epstein 1996).

36. (Klawiter 2009).

37. (Luker 1985).

38. Physicians usually kept their own emotions to themselves, but one genetics fellow wrote up a narrative to cope with the death of a patient she had cared for.

39. (Helmreich 2009, pp. 172–173).

40. (Saunders 2008).

41. (Epstein 1997).

42. (Fox 1957, 1980, 2000).

43. http://www.genome.gov/Pages/PolicyEthics/StaffArticles/Newborn_Screening_Meeting_Summary.pdf, accessed June 2, 2011.

44. (Armstrong 1995).

45. For example, Patricia Kaufert (2000) describes how the Pap smear and the mammogram have rendered women's bodies public spaces for which formerly intimate decisions are now a matter of hotly debated public policy.

46. In the past few years, a scholarly journal, Centers for Disease Control office, and several academic institutes have sprung up bearing this moniker or the related term public health genomics, and there is at least one PhD-granting pro-

gram. (See, for example, the Institute for Public Health Genetics at the University of Washington.)

47. (Anspach 1993). See also Good (2007).

48. (Lupton 1995).

49. (Lee 1993; Nelkin and Tancredi 1989; Novas and Rose 2000).

50. (Kelly 2002).

51. (Ibid., p. 181).

52. (Bell et al. 2011; Lo et al. 2010).

53. (Cowan 2008; Wailoo and Pemberton 2006).

54. (MacDorman and Mathews 2009).

55. (McKie and Richardson 2003) .

56. (Frisbie et al. 2004; Malloy and Freeman 2000).

57. (Paul 1997).

58. (Starr 1982).

59. (Baily and Murray 2008).

60. (Keating and Cambrosio 2003). There is at least a third level, the laboratory, which we bracket here. Other arenas might have been possible if we had approached newborn screening from a different perspective. For example, if we had examined how newborn screening became a billable category in insurance reimbursement, we might have had to disassemble the policy arena into different sites in which various stakeholders negotiated with public and private insurers.

61. (Mol 2002).

62. This discrepancy, and the frictions implied, was brought home to us when our research was met with a critical response from several key policy stakeholders. When we published an early version of chapter 2 in the *Journal of Health and Social Behavior* (Timmermans and Buchbinder 2010), Michael Watson, Rodney Howell, and Piero Rinaldo wrote a critical letter to the editor objecting to our research and conclusions (Watson, Howell, and Rinaldo 2011). Watson is the executive director of the ACMG; Howell chairs the Secretary's Advisory Committee; and Rinaldo, a pathologist and geneticist at the Mayo Clinic, has been credited with essential scientific work underlying the expansion of newborn screening. All three authors were key players in the 2006 ACMG report that launched expanded newborn screening and continue to shepherd national policy on newborn screening; none were seeing newborn screening patients clinically at the time of their writing. The respondents made several criticisms of our research that reflected the imposition of biomedical criteria onto a social science project, which we pointed out in our reply (Timmermans and Buchbinder 2011). Their negative reaction seemed to originate from a growing insecurity about the fate of expanded newborn screening. The letter ended with the unsubstantiated assertion that newborn screening is "the most significant public health program of the past 50+ years" (p. 278). Given that the public health achievements of the last half century include establishing the causal link between cigarette smoking and lung cancer, the trans-

formation of HIV from an acute to a chronic condition, and a 60 percent reduction in US cardiac mortality, this statement does not stand up to scrutiny. Without supporting evidence, these claims only make sense as wishful political statements by stakeholders feeling threatened. At the same time, they confirm a growing disconnect between the worlds of policy and the clinic.

63. Not all individual data is entered for screen negative cases. The different sites provide data about the 1 percent, 10 percent, 50 percent, 90 percent and 99 percent of all markers in the population at large. The authors note "the current percentile values of the Minnesota program alone are derived from 517,283 newborns screened by MS/MS between July 1, 2004, and August 31, 2010" (McHugh et al. 2011, p. 235).

64. The high target range is defined as the interval between the cumulative 99th percentile of the normal population and the lowest 5th percentile of the disorder range. The low target range is defined as the interval between the highest 99th percentile of disorder ranges and the 1st percentile of the normal population (Ibid., p. 237).

65. (Couzin-Frankel 2009; Ross 2011).

66. (Davis et al. 2006; Hasegawa et al. 2010; Skinner et al. 2011).

67. (Lloyd-Puryear and Brower 2010, p. S256). Michele Lloyd-Puryear is affiliated with the Genetic Services Branch of the Maternal and Child Health Bureau, Health Resources and Services Administration.

68. (Watson, Howell, and Rinaldo 2011).

69. (Rapp 2000b).

70. http://laboratory-manager.advanceweb.com/News/Daily-News-Watch/Luminex-Will-Enter-Newborn-Screening-Market.aspx, accessed June 8, 2011. Here, then, is another new face for public health: its capacity to generate medical consumption markets for private companies.

# References

AAP Newborn Screening Task Force. 2000. Newborn Screening: A Blueprint for the Future. *Pediatrics* 106 (2): 389–427.

Ablon, Joan. 1990. Ambiguity and Difference: Families with Dwarf Children. *Social Science and Medicine* 30 (8): 879–887.

Abram, Morris. 1983. Screening and Counseling for Genetic Conditions. Washington, DC: President's Commission for the Study of Ethical Problems in Medicine and Biomedical and Behavioral Research.

Acs, Gregory, and Pamela Loprest. 1999. The Effects of Disabilities on Exits from AFDC. *Journal of Policy Analysis and Management* 18 (1): 28–49.

Adolph, Karen, and Sarah Berger. 2005. Physical and Motor Development. In *Developmental Science: An Advanced Textbook*, edited by Marc Bornstein and Michael Lamb. Mahwah, NJ: Lawrence Erlbaum.

Ahmed, Sara. 2004. Affective Economies. *Social Text* 22 (2): 117–139.

Akrich, Madeleine. 1992. The De-Scription of Technical Objects. In *Shaping Technology/Building Society: Studies in Sociotechnical Change*, edited by W. Bijker and J. Law. Cambridge, MA: MIT Press.

American Academy of Pediatrics. 1967. Statement on Compulsory Testing of Newborn Infants for Hereditary Metabolic Diseases. *Pediatrics* 39: 623–624.

American Academy of Pediatrics, Committee on Nutrition. 2003. Reimbursement for Foods for Special Dietary Use. *Pediatrics* 111 (5): 1117–1119.

Andermann, Anne, Ingeborg Blancquaert, Sylvie Beauchamp, and Veronique Dery. 2008. Revisiting Wilson and Jungner in the Genomic Era: A Review of Screening Criteria over the past 40 Years. *Bulletin of the World Health Organization* 86 (4): 317–319.

Andresen, Brage S., Steve F. Dobrowolski, Linda O'Reilly, Joseph Muenzer, Shawn E. McCandless, Dianne M. Frazier, Szabolcs Udvari, et al. 2001. Medium-chain acyl-CoA Dehydrogenase (MCAD) Mutations Identified by MS/MS-based Prospective Screening of Newborns Differ from Those Observed in Patients with Clinical Symptoms: Identification and Characterization of a New,

Prevalent Mutation That Results in Mild MCAD Deficiency. *American Journal of Human Genetics* 68 (6): 1408–1418.

Andrews, Lori B., Jane E. Fullarton, Neil A. Holtzman, and Arno G. Motulsky. 1994. *Assessing Genetic Risks: Implications for Health and Social Policy.* Washington, DC: National Academy Press.

Anspach, Renee. 1993. *Deciding Who Lives: Fateful Choices in the Intensive Care Nursery.* Berkeley: University of California Press.

Ariès, Philippe. 1965. *Centuries of Childhood: A Social History of Family Life.* Translated by R. Baldick. New York: Vintage Books.

Armstrong, David. 1979. Child Development and Medical Ontology. *Social Science and Medicine* 13 (1): 9–12.

———. 1986. The Invention of Infant Mortality. *Sociology of Health and Illness* 8 (3): 211–232.

———. 1994. Medical Surveillance of Normal Populations. In *Technologies of Modern Medicine,* edited by G. Lawrence. London: Science Museum.

———. 1995. The Rise of Surveillance Medicine. *Sociology of Health and Illness* 17 (3): 393–404.

———. 2002. Clinical Autonomy, Individual and Collective: The Problem of Changing Doctors' Behaviour. *Social Science and Medicine* 55 (10): 1771–1777.

Armstrong, David, and Jane Ogden. 2006. The Role of Etiquette and Experimentation in Explaining How Doctors Change Behavior: A Qualitative Study. *Sociology of Health and Illness* 28 (7): 951–968.

Armstrong, Elisabeth M. 2003. *Conceiving Risk, Bearing Responsibility.* Baltimore: Johns Hopkins University Press.

Aronowitz, Robert A. 2007. *Unnatural History: Breast Cancer and American Society.* Cambridge: Cambridge University Press.

———. 2008. Framing Disease: An Underappreciated Mechanism for the Social Patterning of Health. *Social Science and Medicine* 67 (1): 1–9.

———. 2009. The Converged Experience of Risk and Disease. *Milbank Quarterly* 87 (2): 417–442.

Atkin, Karl, and Waqar I. U. Ahmad. 1998. Genetic Screening and Haemoglobinopathies: Ethics, Politics, and Practice. *Social Science and Medicine* 46 (3): 445–458.

Atkinson, Kathleen, Barry Zuckerman, Joshua M. Sharfstein, Donna Levin, Robin J. R. Blatt, and Howard K. Koh. 2001. A Public Health Response to Emerging Technology: Expansion of the Massachusetts Newborn Screening Program. *Public Health Reports* 116 (2): 122–131.

Atkinson, Paul. 1984. Training for Certainty. *Social Science and Medicine* 19 (9): 949–956.

Atkinson, Paul, Evelyn Parsons, and Katie Featherstone. 2001. Professional Constructions of Family and Kinship in Medical Genetics. *New Genetics and Society* 20 (1): 5–24.

Babrow, Austin S., and Kimberly N. Kline. 2000. From "Reducing" to "Coping with" Uncertainty: Reconceptualizing the Central Challenge in Breast Self Exams. *Social Science and Medicine* 51 (12): 1805–1816.

Bailey, Donald B., Laura M. Beskow, Arlene M. Davis, and Debra Skinner. 2006. Changing Perspectives on the Benefits of Newborn Screening. *Mental Retardation and Developmental Disabilities Research Reviews* 12 (4): 270–279.

Bailey, Donald B., Debra Skinner, and Steven F. Warren. 2005. Newborn Screening for Developmental Disabilities: Reframing Resumptive Benefit. *American Journal of Public Health* 95 (11): 1889–1893.

Baily, Mary Ann. 2009. Fair Distribution of Newborn Screening Costs and Benefits. In *Ethics and Newborn Genetic Screening: New Technologies, New Challenges*, edited by M. A. Baily and T. Murray. Baltimore: Johns Hopkins University Press.

Baily, Mary Ann, and Thomas H. Murray. 2008. Ethics, Evidence, and Cost in Newborn Screening. *Hastings Center Report* 38 (3): 23–31.

Baker, Mei Wang, Ronald H. Laessig, Murray L. Katcher, John M. Routes, William J. Grossman, James Verbsky, Daniel F. Kurtycz, and Charles D. Brokopp. 2010. Implementing Routine Testing for Severe Combined Immunodeficiency Within Wisconsin's Newborn Screening Program. *Public Health Reports* 125 (Suppl 2): 88–95.

Barker, Kristin Kay. 2005. *The Fibromyalgia Story: Medical Authority and Women's Worlds of Pain*. Philadelphia: Temple University Press.

Bearman, Peter. 2008. Exploring Genetics and Social Structure. *American Journal of Sociology* 114 (Suppl): v–x.

Becker, Howard S. 1960. Notes on the Concept of Commitment. *American Journal of Sociology* 66 (1): 32–40.

———. 1993. How I Learned What a Crock Was. *Journal of Contemporary Ethnography* 22 (1): 28–35.

Bell, Callum J., Darrell L. Dinwiddie, Neil A. Miller, Shannon L. Hateley, Elena E. Ganusova, Joann Mudge, Ray J. Langley, et al. 2011. Carrier Testing for Severe Childhood Recessive Diseases by Next-Generation Sequencing. *Science Translational Medicine* 65 (3): 65ra4.

Ben-Joseph, Elana, Steven Dowshen, and Neil Izenberg. 2009. Do Parents Understand Growth Charts? A National, Internet-Based Survey. *Pediatrics* 124 (4): 1100–1109.

Berg, Marc. 1997. *Rationalizing Medical Work: Decision Support Techniques and Medical Practices*. Cambridge, MA: MIT Press.

Berman, Julian L., George C. Cunningham, Robert W. Day, Robin Ford, and David Y. Hsia. 1969. Causes for High Phenylalanine with Normal Tyrosine in Newborn Screening Programs. *American Journal of Diseases of Children* 117 (1): 54–65.

Bernheimer, Lucinda, Thomas Weisner, and Edward Lowe. 2003. Impacts of Children with Troubles on Working Poor Families: Mixed-Methods and Experimental Evidence. *Mental Retardation* 41 (6): 403–419.

Berry, Susan A., Anne M. Jurek, Carolyn Anderson, and Kristi Bentler. 2010. The Inborn Errors of Metabolism Information System: A Project of the Region 4 Genetics Collaborative Priority 2 Workgroup. *Genetics in Medicine* 12 (Suppl 12): S215–S219.

Berry, Susan A., Michele A. Lloyd-Puryear, and Michael S. Watson. 2010. Long-Term Follow-Up of Newborn Screening Patients. *Genetics in Medicine* 12 (Suppl 12): S267–S268.

Bharadwaj, Aditya. 2002. Uncertain Risk: Genetic Screening for Susceptibility to Haemochromatosis. *Health, Risk and Society* 4 (3): 227–240.

Bickel, Horst, John Gerrard, and Evelyn M. Hickmans. 1953. The Influence of Phenylalanine Intake on the Chemistry and Behaviour of a Phenylketonuric Child. *Acta Paediatrica Scandinavia* 43 (1): 64–88.

Biehl, João. 2009. *The Will to Live: AIDS Therapies and the Politics of Survival*. Princeton, NJ: Princeton University Press.

Bijker, Wiebe E., Thomas P. Hughes, and Trevor Pinch. 1989. *The Social Construction of Technological Systems*. Cambridge, MA: MIT Press.

Bluhm, Robyn. 2005. From Hierarchy to Network: A Richer View of Evidence for Evidence-Based Medicine. *Perspectives in Biology and Medicine* 48 (4): 535–548.

Bogardus, Sidney T., Eric Holmboe, and James F. Jekel. 1999. Perils, Pitfalls, and Possibilities in Talking about Medical Risk. *JAMA* 281 (11): 1037–1047.

Bombard, Yvonne, Fiona Miller, Robin Hayeems, Denise Avard, and Bartha Knoppers. 2010. Reconsidering Reproductive Benefit through Newborn Screening: A Systematic Review of Guidelines on Preconception, Prenatal, and Newborn Screening. *European Journal of Human Genetics* 18: 751–760.

Bosk, Charles L. 1992. *All God's Mistakes: Genetic Counseling in a Pediatric Hospital*. Chicago: Chicago University Press.

Botkin, Jeffrey R. 2009. Assessing the New Criteria for Newborn Screening. *Health Matrix Cleveland* 19 (1): 163–186.

Botkin, Jeffrey R., Ellen Wright Clayton, Norma C. Fost, Wylie Burke, Thomas H. Murray, Mary Ann Baily, Benjamin Wilfond, Alfred Berg, and Lainie Friedman Ross. 2006. Newborn Screening Technology: Proceed With Caution. *Pediatrics* 117 (5): 1793–1799.

Bourret, Pascale, and Vololona Rabeharisoa. 2008. Medical Judgment and Medical Decision-Making in a High-Uncertainty Situation: When Clinical Practices Meet Genetics. *Sciences Sociales et Sante* 26 (1): 33–66.

Bowker, Geoffrey, and S. Leigh Star. 1999. *Sorting Things Out*. Cambridge, MA: MIT Press.

Boyd, Elizabeth, and John Heritage. 2005. Taking the History: Questioning during Comprehensive History-Taking. In *Communication in Medical Care: Inter-*

*action Between Primary Care Physicians and Patients*, edited by J. Heritage and D. Maynard. Cambridge: Cambridge University Press.

Boyer, Peter J. 2010. The Covenant: Francis Collins, a Fervent Christian, Thought He Had Resolved the Stem-Cell Debate. A Judge Disagreed. *New Yorker*, September 6.

Breen, Nancy, and Helen I. Meissner. 2005. Toward a System of Cancer Screening in the United States: Trends and Opportunities. *Annual Review of Public Health* 26: 561–582.

Brodwin, Paul. 2008. The Coproduction of Moral Discourse in US Community Psychiatry. *Medical Anthropology Quarterly* 22 (2): 127–147.

Brosco, Jeffrey P. 2011. Hidden in the Sixties: Newborn Screening Programs and State Authority. *Archives of Pediatrics and Adolescent Medicine* 165 (7): 589–591.

Brosco, Jeffrey P., Lee M. Sanders, Robin Dharia, Ghislaine Guez, and Chris Feudtner. 2010. The Lure of Treatment: Expanded Newborn Screening and the Curious Case of Histidinemia. *Pediatrics* 125 (3): 417–419.

Brosco, Jeffrey P., Lee M. Sanders, Michael I. Seider, and Angela C. Dunn. 2008. Adverse Medical Outcomes of Early Newborn Screening Programs for Phenylketonuria. *Pediatrics* 122 (1): 192–197.

Brosco, Jeffrey P., Michael I. Seider, and Angela C. Dunn. 2006. Universal Newborn Screening and Adverse Medical Outcomes: A Historical Note. *Mental Retardation and Developmental Disabilities Research Reviews* 12 (4): 262–269.

Brown, Lucinda, Jinhua Xu-Bayford, Zoe Allwood, Mary Slatter, Andrew Cant, E. Graham Davies, Paul Veys, Andrew R. Gennery, and H. Bobby Gaspar. 2011. Neonatal Diagnosis of Severe Combined Immunodeficiency Leads to Significantly Improved Survival Outcome: The Case for Newborn Screening. *Blood* 117 (11): 3243–3246.

Brown, Patrick R. 2009. The Phenomenology of Trust: A Schutzian Analysis of the Social Construction of Knowledge by Gynae-Oncology Patients. *Health, Risk and Society* 11 (5): 391–407.

Brown, Phil, and Stephen Zavestoski. 2004. Social Movements in Health: An Introduction. *Sociology of Health and Illness* 26 (6): 679–694.

Browner, Carole H., and H. Mabel Preloran. 2010. *Neurogenetic Diagnoses: The Power of Hope and the Limits of Today's Medicine*. New York: Routledge.

Browner, Carole H., H. Mabel Preloran, Maria Christina Casado, Harold N. Bass, and Ann P. Walker. 2003. Genetic Counseling Gone Awry: Miscommunication between Prenatal Genetic Service Providers and Mexican-Origin Clients. *Social Science and Medicine* 56 (9): 1933–1946.

Brownlee, Shannon, and Jeanne Lenzer. 2011. Can Cancer Ever Be Ignored? *New York Times*, October 5.

Bruner, Jerome. 1986. *Actual Minds, Possible Worlds*. Cambridge, MA: Harvard University Press.

Buchbinder, Mara, and Stefan Timmermans. 2011. Newborn Screening and Maternal Diagnosis: Rethinking Family Benefit. *Social Science and Medicine* 73 (7):
1014–1018.
———. n.d. Affective Economies and the Politics of Saving Babies' Lives. Unpub-
lished manuscript.
Burke, Taylor, and Sara Rosenbaum. 2005. Molloy v Meier and the Expanding
Standard of Medical Care: Implications for Public Health Policy and Practice.
*Public Health Reports* 120 (2): 209–210.
Burman, Erica. 1994. *Deconstructing Developmental Psychology*. London: Rout-
ledge.
California State Department of Public Health. 1963. Phenylketonuria, and Guthrie
Inhibition Assay Screening Procedure. *Pediatrics* 32 (3): 344–346.
Callon, Michel, and Vololona Rabeharisoa. 2004. Gino's Lesson on Humanity:
Genetics, Mutual Entanglements and the Sociologist's Role. *Economy and
Society* 33 (1): 1–27.
———. 2008. The Growing Engagement of Emergent Concerned Groups in
Political and Economic Life: Lessons from the French Association of Neu-
romuscular Disease Patients. *Science, Technology, and Human Values* 33 (2):
230–261.
Campbell, Elizabeth, and Lanie Friedman Ross. 2003. Parental Attitudes Regard-
ing Newborn Screening of PKU and DMD. *American Journal of Medical
Genetics A* 120A (2): 209–214.
Canguilhem, Georges. 1991 [1978]. *The Normal and the Pathological*. Translated by
C. Fawcett. New York: Zone Books.
Cederbaum, Julie A., Cynthia LeMons, Mindy Rosen, Mary Ahrens, Sharon
Vonachen, and Stephen D. Cederbaum. 2001. Psychosocial Issues and Coping
Strategies in Families Affected by Urea Cycle Disorders. *Journal of Pediatrics*
138 (1): S72–S80.
Chambliss, Daniel F. 1996. *Beyond Caring: Hospitals, Nurses, and the Social Orga-
nization of Ethics*. Chicago: University of Chicago Press.
Chilibeck, Gillian, Margaret Lock, and Megha Sehdev. 2011. Postgenomics, Uncer-
tain Futures, and the Familiarization of Susceptibility Genes. *Social Science and
Medicine* 72 (11): 1768–1775.
Christakis, Nicholas A. 1999. *Death Foretold: Prophecy and Prognosis in Medical
Care*. Chicago: University of Chicago Press.
Collins, Francis C. 2010. *The Language of Life*. New York: HarperCollins.
Conrad, Peter. 1985. The Meanings of Medication: Another Look at Compliance.
*Social Science and Medicine* 20 (1): 29–37.
———. 1997. Public Eyes and Private Genes: Historical Frames, New Construc-
tions, and Social Problems. *Social Problems* 44 (2): 139–154.
Conrad, Peter, and Jonathan Gabe, eds. 1999. *Sociological Perspectives on the New
Genetics*. Oxford, UK: Blackwell.

Conrad, Peter, and Cheryl Stults. 2010. The Internet and the Experience of Illness. In *Handbook of Medical Sociology*, edited by C. E. Bird, P. Conrad, A. M. Fremont, and S. Timmermans. Nashville, TN: Vanderbilt University Press.

Couzin-Frankel, J. 2009. Newborn Blood Collections. Science Gold Mine, Ethical Minefield. *Science* 324 (5924): 166–168.

Cowan, Ruth Schwartz. 2008. *Heredity and Hope: The Case for Genetic Screening.* Cambridge, MA: Harvard University Press.

Cox, Susan M., and William McKellin. 1999. "There's This Thing in Our Family": Predictive Testing and the Construction of Risk for Huntington's Disease. *Sociology of Health and Illness* 21 (5): 622–646.

Craig, Gillian, and Graham Scambler. 2006. Negotiating Mothering against the Odds: Gastrostomy Tube Feeding, Stigma, Governmentality and Disabled Children. *Social Science and Medicine* 62 (5): 1115–1125.

Crombez, Eric A., Stephen D. Cederbaum, Elaine Spector, Erica Chan, Denise Salazar, Julie Neidich, and Stephen Goodman. 2008. Maternal Glutaric Acidemia, Type I Identified by Newborn Screening. *Molecular Genetics and Metabolism* 94 (1): 132–134.

Daston, Lorraine, and Peter Galison. 2007. *Objectivity.* New York: Zone Books.

Davidson, Brad. 2001. Questions in Cross-Linguistic Medical Encounters: The Role of the Hospital Interpreter. *Anthropological Quarterly* 74 (4): 170–178.

Davis, Lennard. 1995. *Enforcing Normalcy: Disability, Deafness, and the Body.* New York: Verso.

Davis, Terry C., Sharon. G. Humiston, Connie L. Arnold, Joseph A. Bocchini Jr., Pat F. Bass III, Estela M. Kennem, Anna Bocchini, P. Kyler, and M. Lloyd-Puryear. 2006. Recommendations for Effective Newborn Screening Communication: Results of Focus Groups with Patients, Providers and Experts. *Pediatrics* 117 (5 Pt 2): S326–S340.

de Laet, Marianne, and Annemarie Mol. 2000. The Zimbabwe Bush Pump: Mechanics of a Fluid Technology. *Social Studies of Science* 30 (2): 225–263.

Detmar, Symone, Esther Hosli, Nynke Dijkstra, Niels Nijsingh, Marlies Rijnders, and Marcel Verweij. 2007. Information and Informed Consent for Neonatal Screening: Opinions and Preferences of Parents. *Birth* 34 (3): 238–44.

Dewey, John. 2005 [1910]. *How We Think.* New York: Barnes and Noble.

Dumit, Joe. 2006. Illnesses You Have to Fight to Get: Facts as Forces in Uncertain, Emergent Illnesses. *Social Science and Medicine* 62 (3): 577–590.

Duster, Troy. 1990. *Backdoor to Eugenics.* New York: Routledge.

Eastman, John W., Ruth Wong, Catherine L. Liao, and Daniel R. Morales. 1996. Automated HPLC Screening of Newborns for Sickle Cell Anemia and other Hemoglobinopathies. *Clinical Chemistry* 42 (5): 704–10.

Ehrich, Kathryn, and Clare Williams. 2010. A "Healthy Baby": The Double Imperative of Preimplantation Genetic Diagnosis. *Health* 14 (1): 41–56.

Elderkin-Thompson, Virginia, Roxanne Cohen Silver, and Howard Waitzkin. 2001.

When Nurses Double as Interpreters: A Study of Spanish-Speaking Patients in a US Primary Care Setting. *Social Science and Medicine* 52 (9): 1343–1358.

El-Hattab, Ayman W., Fang-Yuan Li, Joseph Shen, Berkley R. Powell, Erawati V. Bawle, Darius J. Adams, Erica Wahl, et al. 2010. Maternal Systemic Primary Carnitine Deficiency Uncovered by Newborn Screening: Clinical, Biochemical, and Molecular Aspects. *Genetics in Medicine* 12 (1): 19–24.

England, Paula. 2005. Emerging Theories of Care Work. *Annual Review of Sociology* 31: 381–399.

Epstein, Steven. 1995. The Construction of Lay Expertise: AIDS Activism and the Forging of Credibility in the Reform of Clinical Trials. *Science, Technology and Human Values* 20 (4): 408–437.

———. 1996. *Impure Science: AIDS, Activism, and the Politics of Knowledge.* Berkeley: University of California Press.

———. 1997. Activism, Drug Regulation, and the Politics of Therapeutic Evaluating in the AIDS Era: A Case Study of ddC and the "Surrogate Markers" Debate. *Social Studies of Science* 27 (3): 691–726.

———. 2007. *Inclusion: The Politics of Difference in Medical Research.* Chicago: University of Chicago Press.

Fadiman, Anne. 1997. *The Spirit Catches You and You Fall Down.* New York: Noonday Press.

Featherstone, Katie, Paul Atkinson, Aditya Bharadwaj, and Angus Clarke. 2006. *Risky Relations: Family, Kinship and the New Genetics.* Oxford, UK: Berg.

Featherstone, Katie, Joanna Latimer, Paul Atkinson, Daniella T. Pilz, and Angus Clarke. 2005. Dysmorphology and the Spectacle of the Clinic. *Sociology of Health and Illness* 27 (5): 551–574.

Ferzacca, Steve. 2000. "Actually I Don't Feel That Bad": Managing Diabetes and the Clinical Encounter. *Medical Anthropology Quarterly* 14 (1): 28–50.

Feuchtbaum, Lisa, Sunaina Dowray, and Fred Lorey. 2010. The Context and Approach for the California Newborn Screening Short- and Long-Term Follow-Up Data System: Preliminary Findings. *Genetics in Medicine* 12 (Suppl 12): S242–S250.

Feuchtbaum, Lisa, Fred Lorey, Lisa Faulkner, John Sherwin, Robert Ciurrier, Ajit Bhandal, and George Cunningham. 2006. California's Experience Implementing a Pilot Newborn Supplemental Screening Program Using Tandem Mass Spectrometry. *Pediatrics* 117 (5): S261–S269.

Finkler, Kaja. 2000. *Experiencing the New Genetics: Family and Kinship on the Medical Frontier.* Philadelphia: University of Pennsylvania Press.

———. 2005. Family, Kinship, Memory and Temporality in the Age of New Genetics. *Social Science and Medicine* 61 (5): 1059–1071.

Fitzgerald, Ruth. 2008. The Politics of Care: Rural Nurse Specialists, Clinical Practice and the Politics of Care. *Medical Anthropology Quarterly* 27 (3): 252–282.

Forss, Anette, Carol Tishelman, Catarina Widmark, and Lisbeth Sachs. 2004.

Women's Experiences of Cervical Cellular Changes: An Unintentional Transition from Health to Liminality? *Sociology of Health and Illness* 26 (3): 306–325.

Fost, Norma C. 1992. Ethical Implications of Screening Asymptomatic Individuals. *FASEB Journal* 6 (10): 2813–2817.

Foucault, Michel. 1976. *The Birth of the Clinic: An Archaeology of Medical Perception.* Translated by A. M. Sheridan. London: Tavistock.

Fox, Renee C. 1957. Training for Uncertainty. In *The Student Physician*, edited by R. K. Merton, G. Reader, and P. L. Kendall. Cambridge, MA: Harvard University Press.

———. 1980. The Evolution of Medical Uncertainty. *Milbank Memorial Fund Quarterly* 58 (1): 1–49.

———. 2000. Medical Uncertainty Revisited. In *The Handbook of Social Studies in Health and Medicine*, edited by G. L. Albrecht, R. Fitzpatrick and S. C. Scrimshaw. London: Sage.

Fox, Renee C., and Judith P. Swazey. 1974. *The Courage to Fail: A Social View of Organ Transplants and Dialysis.* Chicago: University of Chicago.

Frankenburg, William K., Burris R. Duncan, R. Wendell Coffelt, Richard Koch, James G. Coldwell, and Choon D. Son. 1968. Maternal Phenylketonuria: Implications for Growth and Development. *Journal of Pediatrics* 73 (4): 560–570.

Franklin, Sarah. 2003. Re-Thinking Nature-Culture: Anthropology and the New Genetics. *Anthropological Theory* 3 (1): 65–85.

Franklin, Sarah, and Jeanette Edwards. 1999. *Technologies of Procreation: Kinship in the Age of Assisted Conception.* London: Routledge.

Franklin, Sarah, Celia Lury, and Jackie Stacey. 2000. *Global Nature, Global Culture.* London: Sage.

Franklin, Sarah, and Celia Roberts. 2006. *Born and Made: An Ethnography of Preimplantation Genetic Diagnosis.* Princeton, NJ: Princeton University Press.

Freese, Jeremy, and Sara Shostak. 2009. Genetics and Social Inquiry. *Annual Review of Sociology* 35: 107–128.

Frisbie, Parker W., Seung-Eun Song, Daniel A. Powers, and Julie A. Street. 2004. The Increasing Racial Disparity in Infant Mortality: Respiratory Distress Syndrome and Other Causes. *Demography* 41 (4): 773–800.

Fromm-Reichmann, F. 1948. Notes on the Development of Treatment of Schizophrenics by Psychoanalytic Therapy. *Psychiatry: Journal for the Study of Interpersonal Processes* 11 (3): 263–273.

Fujimura, Joan, Troy Duster, and Ramya Rajagopalan. 2008. Race, Genetics and Disease: Questions of Evidence, Matters of Consequence. *Social Studies of Science* 38 (5): 643–656.

Fullwiley, Duana. 2007. Race and Genetics: Attempts to Define the Relationship. *BioSocieties* 2 (2): 221–237.

———. 2008. The Biological Construction of Race. *Social Studies of Science* 38 (5): 695–735.

Garg, Uttam, and Majed Dasouki. 2006. Expanded Newborn Screening of Inherited Metabolic Disorders by Tandem Mass Spectrometry: Clinical and Laboratory Aspects. *Clinical Biochemistry* 39 (4): 315–32.

Garro, Adrienne, S. Kenneth Thurman, MaryLouise E. Kerwin, and Joseph P. Ducette. 2005. Parent/Caregiver Stress during Pediatric Hospitalization for Chronic Feeding Problems. *Journal of Pediatric Nursing* 20 (4): 268–75.

Gill, Virginia T., and Douglas Maynard. 1995. On "Labeling" in Actual Interaction: Delivering and Receiving Diagnoses of Developmental Disabilities. *Social Problems* 42 (1): 11–37.

Gillespie, Chris. 2009. The Experience of Living with Measured Risk: The Cases of Elevated PSA and Cholesterol Levels as Proto-Illnesses, Unpublished PhD dissertation, Brandeis University.

Ginsburg, Faye, and Rayna Rapp. 1991. The Politics of Reproduction. *Annual Review of Anthropology* 20: 311–343.

Glaser, Barney G., and Anselm L. Strauss. 1965. *Awareness of Dying.* Chicago: Aldine.

Glazer, Nona Y. 1993. *Women's Paid and Unpaid Labor: The Work Transfer in Health Care and Retailing.* Philadelphia: Temple University Press.

Glendinning, Caroline. 1983. *Unshared Care: Parents and their Disabled Children.* London: Routledge.

Good, Byron. 1994. *Medicine, Rationality and Experience: An Anthropological Perspective.* Cambridge: Cambridge University Press.

Good, Byron, and Mary-Jo DelVecchio Good. 1994. In the Subjunctive Mode: Epilepsy Narratives in Turkey. *Social Science and Medicine* 38 (6): 835–842.

Good, Mary-Jo DelVecchio. 2007. The Biotechnical Embrace and the Medical Imaginary. In *Subjectivity: Ethnographic Investigations*, edited by J. Biehl, B. Good, and A. M. Kleinman. Berkeley: University of California Press.

Goodwin, Charles. 1994. Professional Vision. *American Anthropologist* 96 (3): 606–633.

Gordon, Elisa. 2000. Preventing Waste: A Ritual Analysis of Candidate Selection for Kidney Transplantation. *Anthropology and Medicine* 7 (3): 351–372.

Greene, Jeremy A. 2007. *Prescribing by Numbers.* Baltimore: Johns Hopkins University Press.

Gregersen, N., V. Winter, D. Curtis, T. Deufel, M. Mack, J. Hendrickx, P. J. Willems, et al. 1993. Medium-Chain Acyl-CoA Dehydrogenase (MCAD) Deficiency: The Prevalent Mutation G985 (K304E) Is Subject to a Strong Founder Effect from Northwestern Europe. *Human Heredity* 43 (6): 342–350.

Grineski, Sara E. 2009. Parental Accounts of Children's Asthma Care: The Role of Cultural and Social Capital in Health Disparities. *Sociological Focus* 42 (2): 107–132.

Grob, Rachel. 2011. *Testing Baby: The Transformation of Newborn Screening, Parenting, and Policymaking.* New Brunswick, NJ: Rutgers University Press.

Groce, Ellen Nora. 1985. *Everyone Here Spoke Sign Language*. Cambridge, MA: Harvard University Press.

Groopman, Jerome. 2004. *The Anatomy of Hope: How People Prevail in the Face of Illness*. New York: Random House.

―――. 2007. *How Doctors Think*. New York: Houghton Mifflin.

Grosse, Scott. 2009. Cost-Effectiveness as a Criterion for Newborn Screening Policy Decisions. In *Ethics and Newborn Genetic Screening*, edited by M. A. Baily and T. Murray. Baltimore: Johns Hopkins University Press.

Guillemin, Jeanne Harley, and Lynda Lytle Holstrom. 1986. *Mixed Blessings: Intensive Care for Newborns*. New York: Oxford University Press.

Gurian, Elizabeth A., Danile D. Kinnamon, Judith J. Henry, and Susan E. Waisbren. 2006. Expanded Newborn Screening for Biochemical Disorders: The Effect of a False-Positive Result. *Pediatrics* 117 (6): 1915–1921.

Guthrie, Robert. 1992. The Origin of Newborn Screening. *Screening* 1: 5–15.

Hacking, Ian. 1986. Making Up People. In *Reconstructing Individualism*, edited by T. Heller, S. Morton, and D. E. Wellberry. Stanford, CA: Stanford University Press.

―――. 1990. *The Taming of Chance*. Cambridge: Cambridge University Press.

―――. 1991. The Making and Molding of Child Abuse. *Critical Inquiry* 17: 253–288.

―――. 2004. Between Michel Foucault and Erving Goffman: Between Discourse in the Abstract and Face-to-Face Interaction. *Economy and Society* 33 (3): 277–302.

―――. 2007. Kinds of People: Moving Targets. *Proceedings of the British Academy* 151: 285–318.

Halpern, Sydney A. 2004. *Lesser Harms: The Morality of Risk in Medical Research*. Chicago: University of Chicago Press.

Han, Paul K., William M. Klein, and Neeraj K. Arora. 2011. Varieties of Uncertainty in Health Care: A Conceptual Taxonomy. *Medical Decision Making* 31 (6): 828–838.

Harrell, Heather. 2009. Currents in Contemporary Ethics: The Role of Parents in Expanded Newborn Screening. *Journal of Law and Medical Ethics* 37 (4): 846–51.

Harrington Meyer, Madonna, ed. 2000. *Care Work: Gender, Labor, and the Welfare State*. New York: Routledge.

Hasegawa, L. E., K. A. Fergus, N. Ojeda, and S. M. Au. 2010. Parental Attitudes toward Ethical and Social Issues Surrounding the Expansion of Newborn Screening Using New Technologies. *Public Health Genomics* 14 (4/5): 298–306.

Haug, Marie R., and B. Lavin. 1983. *Consumerism in Medicine*. Beverly Hills, CA: Sage.

Hedgecoe, Adam M. 2003. Expansion and Uncertainty: Cystic Fibrosis, Classification and Genetics. *Sociology of Health and Illness* 25 (1): 50–70.

————. 2004. *The Politics of Personalized Medicine*. Cambridge: Cambridge University Press.

Heimer, Carol A., and Lisa R. Staffen. 1998. *For the Sake of the Children: The Social Organization of Responsibility in the Hospital and the Home*. Chicago: University of Chicago Press.

Helmreich, Stefan. 2009. *Alien Ocean: Anthropological Voyages in Microbial Seas*. Berkeley: University of California Press.

Heritage, John, and Anna Lindstrom. 1998. Motherhood, Medicine, and Morality: Scenes from a Medical Encounter. *Research on Language and Social Interaction* 31 (3/4): 397–438.

HGSA-RACP. 2004. Newborn Blood-Spot Screening. Human Genetics Association of Australasia.

Hibbard, Judith H., and Edward C. Weeks. 1987. Consumerism in Health Care: Prevalence and Predictors. *Medical Care* 25 (11): 1019–1032.

Hinton, Cynthia F., Jelili A. Ojodu, Paul M. Fernhoff, Sonja A. Rasmussen, Kelley S. Scanlon, and W. Harry Hannon. 2010. Maternal and Neonatal Vitamin B12 Deficiency Detected through Expanded Newborn Screening—United States, 2003–2007. *Journal of Pediatrics* 157 (1): 162–163.

Hogle, Linda. 2005. Enhancement Technologies and the Body. *Annual Review of Anthropology* 34: 695–716.

————. 2009. Pragmatic Objectivity and the Standardization of Engineered Tissues. *Social Science and Medicine* 39 (5): 717–742.

Holtzman, Neil A. 2003. Expanding Newborn Screening: How Good Is the Evidence? *JAMA* 290 (19): 2606–2608.

Holtzman, Neil A., Allen G. Meek, and David E. Mellits. 1974. Neonatal Screening for Phenylketonuria. I. Effectiveness. *JAMA* 229 (6): 667–670.

Holtzman, Neil A., and Michael S. Watson. 1998. *Promoting Safe and Effective Genetic Testing in the United States: Final Report of the Task Force on Genetic Testing*. Baltimore: Johns Hopkins University Press.

Howell, R. Rodney. 2006a. Introduction: Newborn Screening. *Mental Retardation and Developmental Disabilities Research Reviews* 12 (4): 229.

————. 2006b. We Need Expanded Newborn Screening. *Pediatrics* 117 (5): 1800–1805.

Howse, Jennifer L., and M. Katz. 2000. The Importance of Newborn Screening. *Pediatrics* 106 (3): 595.

Howse, Jennifer L., Marina Weiss, and Nancy S. Green. 2006. Critical Role of the March of Dimes in the Expansion of Newborn Screening. *Mental Retardation and Developmental Disabilities Research Reviews* 12 (4): 280–287.

Howson, Alexandra. 1999. Cervical Screening, Compliance, and Moral Obligation. *Sociology of Health and Illness* 21 (4): 401–425.

————. 2001. Locating Uncertainties in Cervical Screening. *Health, Risk and Society* 3 (2): 177–187.

Hsieh, Elaine. 2007. Interpreters as Co-Diagnosticians: Overlapping Roles and Services Between Providers and Interpreters. *Social Science and Medicine* 64 (4): 924–937.

Hughes, Everett. 1971 [1945]. *The Sociological Eye: Selected Papers*. Chicago: Aldine-Atherton.

Hunt, Linda, and Nedal Arar. 2001. An Analytic Framework for Contrasting Patient and Provider Views of the Process of Chronic Disease Management. *Medical Anthropology Quarterly* 15 (3): 347–367.

Hutchinson, B. Lynne, Alistair Stewart, and Edwin Mitchell. 2009. Characteristics, Head Shape Measurements and Developmental Delay in 287 Consecutive Infants Attending a Plagiocephaly Clinic. *Acta Paediatrica* 98 (9): 1494–1499.

Iafolla, A. K., R. J. Thompson, and C. R. Roe. 1994. Medium-Chain Acyl-Coenzyme A Dehydrogenase Deficiency: Clinical Course in 120 Affected Children. *Journal of Pediatrics* 124 (3): 409–415.

James, Allison. 2004. The Standardized Child: Issues of Openness, Objectivity, and Agency in Promoting Childhood Health. *Anthropological Journal on European Cultures* 13: 93–110.

James, William. 1981 [1907]. *Pragmatism*. Cambridge, MA: Hackett.

Kaljee, Linda, and Robert Beardsley. 1992. Psychotropic Drugs and Concepts of Compliance in a Rural Mental Health Clinic. *Medical Anthropology Quarterly* 6 (3): 271–287.

Karpati, George, Stirling Carpenter, Andrew G. Engel, Gordon Watters, Jeffrey Allen, Stanley Rothman, Gerald Klassen, and Orval A. Mamer. 1975. The Syndrome of Systemic Carnitine Deficiency. Clinical, Morphologic, Biochemical, and Pathophysiologic Features. *Neurology* 25 (1): 16–24.

Kaufert, Patricia. 2000. Screening the Body: The Pap Smear and the Mammogram. In *Living and Working with the New Medical Technologies*, edited by M. Lock, A. Young, and A. Cambrosio. Cambridge: Cambridge University Press.

Kaufman, Sharon R. 2005. *. . . And a Time to Die: How American Hospitals Shape the End of Life*. New York: Scribner.

Keating, Peter, and Alberto Cambrosio. 2000. Real Compared to What? Diagnosing Leukemias and Lymphomas. In *Living and Working with the New Medical Technologies: Intersections of Inquiry*, edited by M. M. Lock, A. Young, and A. Cambrosio. Cambridge: Cambridge University Press.

———. 2003. *Biomedical Platforms: Realigning the Normal and Pathological in Late Twentieth Century Medicine*. Cambridge, MA: MIT Press.

Kelle, Helga. 2010. "Age-Appropriate Development" as Measure and Norm: An Ethnographic Study of the Practical Anthropology of Routine Pediatric Checkups. *Childhood* 17 (1): 9–25.

Kelly, Susan. 2002. "New" Genetics Meets the Old Underclass: Findings from a Study of Genetic Outreach Services in Rural Kentucky. *Critical Public Health* 12 (2): 169–186.

Kennedy, Shelley, Beth K. Potter, Kumanan Wilson, Lawrence Fisher, Michael Geraghty, Jennifer Milburn, and Pranesh Chakraborty. 2010. The First Three Years of Screening for Medium Chain Acyl-CoA Dehydrogenase Deficiency (MCADD) by Newborn Screening Ontario. *BMC Pediatrics* 10: 82.

Kent, Deborah. 2000. Somewhere a Mockingbird. In *Prenatal Testing and Disability Rights*, edited by E. Parens and A. Asch. Washington, DC: Georgetown University Press.

Kerr, Anne. 2003. Genetics and Citizenship. *Society* 40 (6): 44–50.

———. 2005. Understanding Genetic Disease in a Socio-Historical Context: A Case Study of Cystic Fibrosis. *Sociology of Health and Illness* 27 (7): 873–896.

Kerr, Anne, and Sarah Cunningham-Burley. 2000. On Ambivalence and Risk: Reflexive Modernity and the New Human Genetics. *Sociology* 34 (2): 283–304.

Kerruish, N. J., and S. P. Robertson. 2005. Newborn Screening: New Developments, New Dilemmas. *Journal of Medical Ethics* 31 (7): 393–398.

King, Nancy M. P. 2000. Defining and Describing Benefit Appropriately in Clinical Trials. *Journal of Law, Medicine, and Ethics* 28 (4): 332–343.

Kirk, Stuart A., and Herb Kutchins. 1992. *The Selling of the DSM: The Rhetoric of Science in Psychiatry*. Hawthorne, NY: Aldine De Gruyter.

Klawiter, Maren. 2009. *The Biopolitics of Breast Cancer*. Minneapolis: University of Minnesota Press.

Kleven, Daniel T., Christopher R. McCudden, and Monte S. Willis. 2008. Cystic Fibrosis: Newborn Screening in America. *MLO Medical Laboratory Observer* 40 (7): 16–27.

Koch, Jean J. 1997. *Robert Guthrie — the PKU Story: Crusade against Mental Retardation*. Pasadena, CA: Hope.

Koeberl, D. D., D. S. Millington, W. E. Smith, S. D. Weavil, J. Muenzer, S. E. McCandless, P. S. Kishnani, et al. 2003. Evaluation of 3-Methylcrotonyl-CoA Carboxylase Deficiency Detected by Tandem Mass Spectrometry Newborn Screening. *Journal of Inherited Metabolic Diseases* 26 (1): 25–35.

Koenig, Barbara, and Linda Hogle. 1995. Organ Transplantation (Re)examined? *Medical Anthropology Quarterly* 9 (3): 393–397.

Kolata, Gina. 2011. Considering When It Might Be Best Not to Know about Cancer. *New York Times*, October 30.

Kolker, Emily. 2004. Framing as a Cultural Resource in Health Social Movements: Funding Activism and the Breast Cancer Movement in the US 1990–1993. *Sociology of Health and Illness* 26 (6): 820–844.

Konrad, Monica. 2003. Predictive Genetic Testing and the Making of the Pre-Symptomatic Person: Prognostic Moralities amongst Huntington's-Affected Families. *Anthropology and Medicine* 10 (1): 23–49.

Kraszewski, Jennifer, Taylor Burke, and Sara Rosenbaum. 2006. Legal Issues in Newborn Screening: Implications for Public Health, Practice, and Policy. *Public Health Reports* 121 (1): 92–93.

Kuhn, Thomas. 1962. *The Structure of Scientific Revolutions*. 2nd ed. Chicago: University of Chicago Press.

Kuzawa, Christopher, and Elizabeth Sweet. 2009. Epigenetics and the Embodiment of Race: Developmental Origins of US Racial Disparities in Cardiovascular Health. *American Journal of Human Biology* 21 (1): 2–15.

Lakoff, Andrew. 2005. *Pharmaceutical Reason: Knowledge and Value in Global Psychiatry*. Cambridge: Cambridge University Press.

———. 2007. The Right Patients for the Drug: Managing the Placebo Effect in Antidepressant Trials. *BioSocieties* 2 (1): 57–71.

Lampl, Michelle, and Amanda Thompson. 2007. Growth Chart Curves Do Not Describe Individual Growth Biology. *American Journal of Human Biology* 19 (5): 643–653.

Landecker, Hannah. 2007. *Culturing Life: How Cells Became Technologies*. Cambridge, MA: Harvard University Press.

Landsman, Gail H. 1998. Reconstructing Motherhood in the Age of "Perfect" Babies: Mothers of Infants and Toddlers with Disabilities. *Signs* 24 (11): 69–99.

———. 2003. Emplotting Children's Lives: Developmental Delay vs. Disability. *Social Science and Medicine* 56 (9): 1947–1960.

———. 2009. *Reconstructing Motherhood and Disability in an Age of "Perfect" Babies*. London: Routledge.

Laraway, Kelly, Leann Birch, Michele Shaffer, and Ian Paul. 2010. Parent Perception of Healthy Infant and Toddler Growth. *Clinical Pediatrics* 49 (4): 343–349.

Latimer, Joanna. 2007. Diagnosis, Dysmorphology, and the Family: Knowledge, Motility, Choice. *Medical Anthropology* 26 (2): 97–138.

Latimer, Joanna, Katie Featherstone, Paul Atkinson, Angus Clarke, Daniela T. Pilz, and Alison Shaw. 2006. Rebirthing the Clinic: The Interaction of Clinical Judgment and Genetic Technology in the Production of Medical Science. *Science, Technology, and Human Values* 31 (5): 599–630.

Lauritzen, Sonja. 1997. Notions of Child Health: Mothers' Accounts of Health in their Young Babies. *Sociology of Health and Illness* 19 (4): 436–456.

Layne, Linda L. 1996. "How's the Baby Doing?" Struggling with Narratives of Progress in a Neonatal Intensive Care Unit. *Medical Anthropology Quarterly* 10 (4): 624–656.

Lee, Carol. 1993. Creating a Genetic Underclass: The Potential for Genetic Discrimination by the Health Insurance Industry. *Pace Law Review* 13 (1): 189–228.

Lee, Simon Craddock. 2010. Uncertain Futures: Individual Risk and Social Context in Decision-Making in Cancer Screening. *Health, Risk and Society* 12 (2): 101–117.

Leiter, Valerie. 2004. Dilemmas in Sharing Care: Maternal Provision of Professionally Driven Therapy for Children with Disabilities. *Social Science and Medicine* 58 (4): 837–849.

———. 2007. "Nobody's Just Normal, You Know": The Social Creation of Developmental Disability. *Social Science and Medicine* 65 (8): 1630–1641.

Lenke, Roger R., and Harvey L. Levy. 1980. Maternal Phenylketonuria and Hyperphenylalaninemia. An International Survey of the Outcome of Untreated and Treated Pregnancies. *New England Journal of Medicine* 303 (21): 1202–1208.

Levy, Harvey. 1982. Maternal PKU: Control of an Emerging Problem. *American Journal of Public Health* 72 (12): 1320–1321.

Lewis, Michelle H., Aaron Goldenberg, Rebecca Anderson, Erin Rothwell, and Jeffrey R. Botkin. 2011. State Laws Regarding the Retention and Use of Residual Newborn Screening Blood Samples. *Pediatrics* 127 (4): 703–712.

Lewis, Suzan, Carolyn Kagan, and Patricia Heaton. 2000. Dual-Earner Parents with Disabled Children: Family Patterns for Working and Caring. *Journal of Family Issues* 21 (8): 1031–1060.

Leydiker, K. B., J. A. Neidich, F. Lorey, E. M. Barr, R. L. Puckett, R. M. Lobo, and J. E. Abdenur. 2011. Maternal Medium-Chain acyl-CoA Dehydrogenase Deficiency Identified by Newborn Screening. *Molecular Genetics and Metabolism* 103 (1): 92–95.

Lin, Henry J., Julie A. Neidich, Denise Salazar, Evangela Thomas-Johnson, Barbara F. Ferreira, Alan M. Kwong, Amy M. Lin, et al. 2009. Asymptomatic Maternal Combined Homocystinuria and Methylmalonic Aciduria (cblC) Detected through Low Carnitine Levels on Newborn Screening. *Journal of Pediatrics* 155 (6): 924–927.

Lindee, Susan. 2005. *Moments of Truth in Genetic Medicine*. Baltimore: Johns Hopkins University.

Lippman, Abby. 1991. Prenatal Genetic Testing and Screening: Construcing Needs and Reinforcing Inequalities. *American Journal of Law and Medicine* 17 (1/2): 15–50.

Lipstein, Ellen A., Sienna Vorono, Marsha F. Browning, Nancy S. Green, Alex R. Kemper, A. Alixandra Knapp, Lisa A. Prosser, and James M. Perrin. 2010. Systematic Evidence Review of Newborn Screening and Treatment of Severe Combined Immunodeficiency. *Pediatrics* 125 (5): e1226–e1235.

Lloyd-Puryear, Michele A., and Amy Brower. 2010. Long-Term Follow-up in Newborn Screening: A Systems Approach for Improving Health Outcomes. *Genetics in Medicine* 12 (Suppl 12): S256–S260.

Lo, Y. M. Dennis, K. C. Allen Chan, Hao Sun, Eric Z. Chen, Peiyong Jiang, Fiona M. Lun, Yama W. Zheng, et al. 2010. Maternal Plasma DNA Sequencing Reveals the Genome-Wide Genetic and Mutational Profile of the Fetus. *Science Translational Medicine* 61 (2): 61ra91.

Lock, Margaret. 2000. Accounting for Disease and Distress: Morals of the Normal and the Abnormal. In *Handbook of Social Studies in Health and Medicine*, edited by G. Albrecht, R. Fitzpatrick, and S. Scrimshaw. London: Sage.

Lock, Margaret, and Vinh-Kim Nguyen. 2010. The Social Life of Organs. In *An Anthropology of Biomedicine*. West Sussex, UK: Wiley Blackwell.

Locke, Karen, Karen Golden-Biddle, and Martha S. Feldman. 2008. Making Doubt Generative: Rethinking the Role of Doubt in the Research Process. *Organization Science* 19 (6): 907–918.

Luker, Kristin. 1985. *Abortion and the Politics of Motherhood*. Berkeley: University of California Press.

Lupton, Deborah. 1995. *The Imperative of Health: Public Health and the Regulated Body*. London: Sage.

Lutfey, Karen, and Jeremy Freese. 2005. Toward Some Fundamentals of Fundamental Causality: Socioeconomic Status and Health in the Routine Clinic Visit for Diabetes. *American Journal of Sociology* 110 (5): 1326–1372.

MacDonald, Cameron. 2002. "It Shouldn't Have to Be a Trade:" Recognition and Redistribution in Care Work Advocacy. *Hypatia* 17 (2): 67–83.

MacDorman, Marian F., and T. J. Mathews. 2009. Behind International Rankings of Infant Mortality: How the United States Compares with Europe. *NCHS Data Brief* 23: 1–8.

Maier, Esther M., Bernhard Liebl, Wulf Roschinger, Uta Nennstiel-Ratzel, Ralph Fingerhut, Bernhard Olgemoller, Ulrich Busch, Nils Krone, Rüdiger v. Kries, and Adelbert A. Roscher. 2005. Population Spectrum of ACADM Genotypes Correlated to Biochemical Phenotypes in Newborn Screening for Medium-chain Acyl-CoA Dehydrogenase Deficiency. *Human Mutation* 25 (5): 443–452.

Malloy, Michael H., and Daniel H. Freeman. 2000. Respiratory Distress Syndrome Mortality in the United States, 1987 to 1995. *Journal of Perinatology* 20 (7): 414–420.

Mann, Michael. 1987. Ruling Class Strategies and Citizenship. *Sociology* 21 (3): 339–354.

Marcus, George E. 1998. *Ethnography through Thick and Thin*. Princeton, NJ: Princeton University Press.

Marsden, Deborah, Cecilia Larson, and Harvey L. Levy. 2006. Newborn Screening for Metabolic Disorders. *Journal of Pediatrics* 148 (5): 577–584.

Marshall, T. H. 1950. *Citizenship and Social Class and Other Essays*. Cambridge: Cambridge University Press.

Mattingly, Cheryl. 1998. In Search of the Good: Narrative Reasoning in Clinical Practice. *Medical Anthropology Quarterly* 12 (3): 273–297.

———. 2006. Pocahontas Goes to the Clinic: Popular Culture as Lingua Franca in a Cultural Borderland. *American Anthropologist* 108 (3): 494–501.

———. 2010. *The Paradox of Hope: Journeys through a Clinical Borderland*. Berkeley: University of California Press.

Mattingly, Cheryl, and Mary Lawlor. 2003. Disability Experience from a Family Perspective. In *Willard and Spackman's Occupational Therapy*, edited by E. Crepeau, E. Coh, and B. Schell. Philadelphia: Lippincott, Williams, and Wilkins.

McBride, Colleen. M., Deborah Bowen, Lawrence C. Brody, Celeste M. Condit, Robert T. Croyle, Marta Gwinn, Muin J. Khoury, et al. 2010. Future Health Applications of Genomics: Priorities for Communication, Behavioral, and Social Sciences Research. *American Journal Preventine Medicine* 38 (5): 556–565.

McCabe, Linda L., and Edward R. B. McCabe. 2002. Newborn Screening as a Model for Population Screening. *Molecular Genetics and Metabolism* 75: 299–307.

———. 2008. Expanded Newborn Screening: Implications for Genetic Medicine. *Annual Review of Medicine* 59: 163–175.

McCaman, M. W., and E. Robins. 1962. Fluorometric Method for the Determination of Phenylalaline in Serum. *Journal of Laboratory and Clinical Medicine* 59: 885.

McCoyd, Judith. 2010. Authoritative Knowledge, the Technological Imperative and Women's Responses to Prenatal Diagnostic Technologies. *Culture, Medicine and Psychiatry* 34 (4): 590–614.

McGhee, Sean A., E. Richard Stiehm, and Edward R. McCabe. 2005. Potential Costs and Benefits of Newborn Screening for Severe Combined Immunodeficiency. *Journal of Pediatrics* 147 (5): 603–608.

McGowan, Michelle L., Jennifer R. Fishman, and Marcie A. Lambrix. 2010. Personal Genomics and Individual Identities: Motivations and Moral Imperatives of Early Users. *New Genetics and Society* 29 (3): 261–290.

McHugh, David M., Cynthia A. Cameron, Jose E. Abdenur, Mahera Abdulrahman, Ona Adair, Shahira Ahmed Al Nuaimi, Henrik Ahlman, et al. 2011. Clinical Validation of Cutoff Target Ranges in Newborn Screening of Metabolic Disorders by Tandem Mass Spectrometry: A Worldwide Collaborative Project. *Genetics in Medicine* 13 (3): 230–254.

McKeever, Patricia, and Karen-Lee Miller. 2004. Mothering Children Who Have Disabilities: A Bourdieusian Interpretation of Maternal Practices. *Social Science and Medicine* 59 (6): 1177–1191.

McKie, John, and Jeff Richardson. 2003. The Rule of Rescue. *Social Science and Medicine* 56 (12): 2407–2419.

McKie, Linda, Sophia Bowlby, and Sue Gregory. 2004. Starting Well: Gender, Care and Health in the Family Context. *Sociology* 38 (3): 593–611.

McLaughlin, Janice. 2008. Seeking and Rejecting Certainty: Exposing the Sophisticated Lifeworlds of Parents of Disabled Babies. *Sociology* 42 (2): 317–335.

Meckel, Richard. 1998. *Save the Babies: American Public Health Reform and the Prevention of Infant Mortality 1850–1929*. Ann Arbor: University of Michigan Press.

Mesman, Jessica. 2005. The Origins of Prognostic Difference: A Topography of Experience and Expectation in a Neonatal Intensive Care Unit. *Qualitative Sociology* 28 (1): 49–66.

Miller, Fiona Alice, Catherine Ahern, Jacqueline Ogilvie, Mita Giacomini, and Lisa Schwartz. 2005. Ruling in and Ruling Out: Implications of Molecular Genetic

Diagnoses for Disease Classification. *Social Science and Medicine* 61 (12): 2536–2545.

Miller, Robert, and Sterling Clarren. 2000. Long-Term Developmental Outcomes in Patients with Deformational Plagiocephaly. *Pediatrics* 105 (2): E26.

Millington, D. S., N. Kodo, D. L. Norwood, and C. R. Roe. 1990. Tandem Mass Spectrometry: A New Method for Acylcarnitine Profiling with Potential for Neonatal Screening for Inborn Errors of Metabolism. *Journal of Inherited Metabolic Diseases* 13 (3): 321–324.

Mintz, Steven. 2006. *Huck's Raft: A History of American Childhood*. Cambridge, MA: Belknap Press.

Mol, Annemarie. 2002. *The Body Multiple: Ontology in Medical Practice*. Durham, NC: Duke University Press.

———. 2008. *The Logic of Care: Health and the Problem of Patient Choice*. London: Routledge.

Mollering, G. 2006. *Trust: Reason, Routine, Reflexivity*. Oxford, UK: Elsevier.

Montgomery, Kathryn. 2005. *How Doctors Think: Clinical Judgment and the Practice of Medicine*. Oxford: Oxford University Press.

Moreira, Tiago. 2005. Diversity in Clinical Guidelines: The Role of Repertoires of Evaluation. *Social Science and Medicine* 60 (9): 1975–1985.

Morgan, Lynn M. 2009. *Icons of Life: A Cultural History of Human Embryos*. Berkeley: University of California Press.

Morioka, D., M. Kasahara, R. Horikawa, S. Yokoyama, A. Fukuda, and A. Nakagawa. 2007. Efficacy of Living Donor Transplantation for Patients with Methylmalonic Acidemia. *American Journal of Transplantation* 7 (12): 2782–2787.

Morris, Jenny. 2001. Impairment and Disability: Constructing an Ethics of Care that Promotes Human Rights. *Hypatia* 16 (4): 1–16.

Morrison, D. R., and E. W. Clayton. 2011. False Positive Newborn Screening Results are not Always Benign. *Public Health Genomics* 14 (3): 173–177.

Moyer, Virginia A., Ned Calonge, Steven M. Teutsch, and Jeffrey R. Botkin. 2008. Expanding Newborn Screening: Process, Policy, and Priorities. *Hastings Center Report* 38 (3): 32–39.

Mykhalovskiy, Eric, and Lorna Weir. 2004. The Problem of Evidence-Based Medicine: Directions for Social Science. *Social Science and Medicine* 59 (5): 1059–1069.

Nader, Laura. 1972. Up the Anthropologist—Perspectives Gained from Studying Up. In *Reinventing Anthropology*, edited by D. H. Hymes. New York: Pantheon Books.

National Academy of Sciences. 1975. Genetic Screening: Programs, Principles, and Research. Washington, DC: National Academy of Sciences.

Natowicz, Marvin. 2005. Newborn Screening: Setting Evidence-Based Policy for Protection. *New England Journal of Medicine* 353 (9): 867–870.

Nelkin, Dorothy, and Lori Andrews. 1999. DNA Identification and Surveillance Creep. *Sociology of Health and Illness* 21 (5): 689–706.

Nelkin, Dorothy, and Laurence Tancredi. 1989. *Dangerous Diagnostics: The Social Power of Biological Information* New York: Basic Books.

Nelson, Alondra. 2008. Bio Science: Genetic Ancestry Testing and the Pursuit of African Ancestry. *Social Studies of Science* 38 (5): 759–783.

Nettleton, Sarah. 2006. "I Just Want Permission to Be Ill": Towards a Sociology of Medically Unexplained Symptoms. *Social Science and Medicine* 62 (5): 1167–1178.

Novas, Carlos, and Nikolas Rose. 2000. Genetic Risk and the Birth of the Somatic Individual. *Economy and Society* 29 (4): 485–513.

Olson, Steve, and Adam C. Berger. 2010. Challenges and Opportunities in Using Residual Newborn Screening Samples for Translational Research. Workshop Summary. Washington, DC: Institute of Medicine.

Ortner, Sherry B. 2010. Access: Reflections on Studying Up in Hollywood. *Ethnography* 11 (2): 211–233.

Oudshoorn, Nelly, and Trevor Pinch, eds. 2003. *How Users Matter*. Cambridge, MA: MIT Press.

Palladino, Paolo. 2002. Between Knowledge and Practice: On Medical Professionals, Patients, and the Making of the Genetics of Cancer. *Social Studies of Science* 32 (1): 137–165.

Pandor, A., J. Eastham, C. Beverley, J. Chilcott, and S. Paisley. 2004. Clinical Effectiveness and Cost-Effectiveness of Neonatal Screening for Inborn Errors of Metabolism Using Tandem Mass Spectrometry: A Systematic Review. *Health Technology Assessment* 8 (12): 1–121.

Parker, Steven, Barry Zuckerman, and Marilyn Augustyn. 2004. *Developmental and Behavioral Pediatrics: A Handbook for Primary Care*. Philadelphia: Lippincott, Williams, and Wilkins.

Parsons, Talcott. 1951. *The Social System*. Glencoe, IL: Free Press.

Parthasarathy, Shobita. 2005. Architectures of Genetic Medicine: Comparing Genetic Testing for Breast Cancer in the USA and the UK. *Social Studies of Science* 35 (1): 5–40.

Pass, Kenneth A., Peter A. Lane, Paul M. Fernhoff, Cynthia F. Hinton, Susan R. Panny, John S. Parks, Mary Z. Pelias, et al. 2000. US Newborn Screening System Guidelines II: Follow-Up of Children, Diagnosis, Management, and Evaluation. *Pediatrics* 137 (4): S1–S47.

Paul, Diane B. 1997. The History of Newborn Phenylketonuria Screening in the US. In *Promoting Safe and Effective Genetic Testing in the United States: Final Report of the Taskforce on Genetic Testing*, edited by N. A. Holtzman and M. S. Watson. Bethesda, MD: National Institutes of Health.

Paul, Diane B., and Jeffrey P. Brosco. Forthcoming. *PKU: The Biography*. Baltimore: Johns Hopkins University Press.

Petryna, Adriana. 2002. *Life Exposed: Biological Citizens after Chernobyl*. Princeton, NJ: Princeton University Press.

————. 2009. *When Experiments Travel: Clinical Trials and the Global Search for Human Subjects*. Princeton, NJ: Princeton University Press.

Phenylketonuria: Screening and Management. NIH Consensus Statement. 2000. October 16–18; 17 (3): 1–27.

Pollitt, R. J. 2006. International Perspectives on Newborn Screening. *Journal of Inherited Metabolic Disease* 29 (2–3): 390–396.

Porter, Theodore. 1995. *Trust in Numbers: Objectivity in Science and Public Life*. Princeton, NJ: Princeton University Press.

Powell, Kimberly, Kim Van Naarden Braun, Rani Singh, Stuart K. Shapira, Richard S. Olney, and Marshalyn Yeargin-Allsopp. 2010. Prevalence of Developmental Disabilities and Receipt of Special Education Services among Children with an Inborn Error of Metabolism. *Journal of Pediatrics* 156 (3): 420–426.

Powers, Elizabeth. 1999. Child Disability and Maternal Labor Force Participation. Working Paper of the Institute of Government and Public Affairs of the University of Illinois at Urbana-Champaign. http://igpa.uillinois.edu/system/files/WP79-childDisability.pdf.

President's Council on Bioethics. 2008. The Changing Moral Focus of Newborn Screening: An Ethical Analysis by the President's Council on Bioethics. Washington, DC.

Press, Nancy, Carole Browner, Diem Tran, Christine Morton, and Barbara LeMaster. 1998. Provisional Normalcy and "Perfect Babies": Pregnant Women's Attitudes Toward Disability in the Context of Prenatal Testing. In *Reproducing Reproduction: Kinship, Power, and Technological Innovation*, edited by S. Franklin and H. Ragone. Philadelphia: University of Pennsylvania Press.

Prosser, Helen, and Tom Walley. 2006. New Drug Prescibing by Hospital Doctors: The Nature and Meaning of Knowledge. *Social Science and Medicine* 62 (7): 1565–1578.

Rabeharisoa, Vololona. 2006. Towards a New Form of Medical Work in Psychiatry Genetics: The Case of Autism. *Sciences Sociales et Sante* 24 (1): 83–116.

Rabeharisoa, Vololona, and Pascale Bourret. 2009. Staging and Weighting Evidence in Biomedicine: Comparing Clinical Practices in Cancer Genetics and Psychiatric Genetics. *Social Studies of Science* 39 (5): 691–715.

Rabinow, Paul. 1996. Artificiality and Enlightenment: From Sociobiology to Biosociality. In *Essays on the Anthropology of Reason*, edited by P. Rabinow. Princeton, NJ: Princeton University Press.

Rapp, Rayna. 2000a. Extra Chromosomes and Blue Tulips: Medico-Familial Interpretations. In *Living and Working with the New Medical Technologies*, edited by M. Lock, A. Young, and A. Cambrosio. Cambridge: Cambridge University Press.

————. 2000b. *Testing Women, Testing the Fetus: The Social Impact of Amniocentesis in America*. New York: Routledge.

Raspberry, Kelly, and Debra Skinner. 2007. Experiencing the Genetic Body:

Parents' Encounters with Pediatric Genetics. *Medical Anthropology* 26 (4): 355–391.

———. 2011. Enacting Genetic Responsibility: Experiences of Mothers Who Carry the Fragile X Gene. *Sociology of Health and Illness* 33 (3): 420–433.

Raz, Aviad. 2009. Eugenic Utopias/Dystopias, Reprogenetics, and Community Genetics. *Sociology of Health and Illness* 31 (4): 602–616.

Raz, Aviad, and Yafa Vizner. 2008. Carrier Matching and Collective Socialization in Community Genetics: Dor Yeshorim and the Reinforcement of Stigma. *Social Science and Medicine* 67 (9): 1361–1369.

Reardon, Jennifer. 2005. *Race to the Finish: Identity and Governance in the Age of Genomics*. Princeton, NJ: Princeton University Press.

Reichertz, J. 2007. Abduction: The Logic of Discovery in Grounded Theory. In *Handbook of Grounded Theory*, edited by A. Bryant and K. Charmaz. London: Sage.

Remenick, Larissa. 2006. The Quest for a Perfect Baby: Why Do Israeli Women Seek Prenatal Genetic Testing? *Sociology of Health and Illness* 28 (1): 21–53.

Robins, Cynthia. 2001. Generating Revenues: Fiscal Changes in Public Mental Health Care and the Emergence of Moral Conflicts among Care-Givers. *Culture, Medicine, and Psychiatry* 25 (4): 457–466.

Rose, Nikolas. 1999. *Governing the Soul: The Shaping of the Private Self*. London: Free Association Books.

———. 2007. *The Politics of Life Itself: Biomedicine, Power, and Subjectivity in the Twenty-First Century*. Princeton, NJ: Princeton University Press.

———. 2009. Normality and Pathology in a Biomedical Age. *Sociological Review* 52 (Suppl 2): 66–83.

———. 2010. "Screen and Intervene": Governing Risky Brains. *History of the Human Sciences* 23 (1): 79–105.

Rosenberg, Charles E. 1979. Towards an Ecology of Knowledge: On Discipline, Contexts and History. In *The Organization of Knowledge in Modern America*, edited by A. Oleson and J. Voss. Baltimore: Johns Hopkins University Press.

———. 2007. *Our Present Complaint: American Medicine, Then and Now*. Baltimore, MD: Johns Hopkins University Press.

Ross, Friedman Lainie. 2011. Mandatory versus Voluntary Consent for Newborn Screening? *Kennedy Institute of Ethics Journal* 20 (4): 299–328.

Rothman, Barbara Katz. 1993. *The Tentative Pregnancy: How Amniocentesis Changes the Experience of Motherhood*. New York W. W. Norton.

Rothshild, Joan. 2005. *The Dream of the Perfect Child*. Bloomington: Indiana University Press.

Rothwell, Erin, Rebecca Anderson, and Jeffrey R. Botkin. 2010. Policy Issues and Stakeholder Concerns Regarding the Storage and Use of Residual Newborn Dried Blood Samples for Research. *Policy, Politics, and Nursing Practice* 11 (1): 5–12.

Rothwell, Erin W., Rebecca A. Anderson, Matthew J. Burbank, Aaron J. Golden-
    berg, Michelle H. Lewis, Louisa A. Stark, Bob Wong, and Jeffrey R. Botkin.
    2011. Concerns of Newborn Blood Screening Advisory Committee Members
    Regarding Storage and Use of Residual Newborn Screening Blood Spots.
    *American Journal of Public Health* 101 (11): 2111–2116.

Rouse, B. M. 1966. Phenylalanine Deficiency Syndrome. *Journal of Pediatrics* 69
    (2): 246–249.

Rouse, Carolyn. 2010. Patient and Practitioner Noncompliance: Rationing, Thera-
    peutic Uncertainty, and the Missing Conversation. *Anthropology and Medicine*
    17 (2): 187–200.

Sachs, Lisbeth. 1995. Is There a Pathology of Prevention? The Implications of Visu-
    alizing the Invisible in Screening Programs. *Culture, Medicine and Psychiatry* 19
    (4): 503–525.

Sarangi, Srikant, Kristina Bennert, Lucy Howell, and Angus Clarke. 2003. "Rela-
    tively Speaking": Relativisation of Genetic Risk in Counselling for Predictive
    Testing. *Health, Risk, and Society* 5 (2): 155–170.

Sarangi, Srikant, and Angus Clarke. 2002. Zones of Expertise and the Manage-
    ment of Uncertainty in Genetics Risk Communication. *Research on Language
    and Social Interaction* 35 (2): 139–171.

Saukko, Paula M., Suzanne H. Richards, Maggie H. Shepherd, and John L. Camp-
    bell. 2006. Are Genetic Tests Exceptional? Lessons from a Qualitative Study on
    Thrombophilia. *Social Science and Medicine* 63 (7): 1947–1959.

Saunders, Barry. 2008. *CT Suite: The Work of Diagnosis in the Age of Noninvasive
    Cutting*. Durham, NC: Duke University Press.

Schaffer, Rebecca, Kristine Kuczynski, and Debra Skinner. 2008. Producing
    Genetic Knowledge and Citizenship through the Internet: Mothers, Pediatric
    Genetics, and Cybermedicine. *Sociology of Health and Illness* 30 (2): 145–159.

Scheper-Hughes, Nancy. 2003. Rotten Trade: Millenial Capitalism, Human Values,
    and Global Justice Organ Trafficking. *Journal of Human Rights* 2 (2): 197–226.

———. 2004. Parts Unknown: Undercover Ethnography of the Organs-Trafficking
    Underworld. *Ethnography* 5 (1): 29–73.

Schimmenti, Lisa A., Eric A. Crombez, Bernd C. Schwahn, Bryce A. Heese,
    Timothy C. Wood, Richard J. Schroer, Kristi Bentler, et al. 2007. Expanded
    Newborn Screening Identifies Maternal Primary Carnitine Deficiency. *Molecu-
    lar Genetics and Metabolism* 90 (4): 441–445.

Schweitzer-Krantz, Susanne. 2003. Early Diagnosis of Inherited Metabolic Dis-
    order Towards Improving Outcome: The Controversial Issue of Galactosaemia.
    *European Journal of Pediatrics* 162 (Suppl 1): S50–S53.

Scott, S., Lindsay Prior, F. Wood, and J. Gray. 2005. Repositioning the Patient: The
    Implications of Being "At Risk." *Social Science and Medicine* 60 (8): 1869–1879.

Scriver, Charles R. 2007. The PAH Gene, Phenylketonuria, and a Paradigm Shift.
    *Human Mutation* 28 (9): 831–845.

Sewell, William H. Jr. 1992. A Theory of Structure: Duality, Agency, and Transformation. *American Journal of Sociology* 98 (1): 1–29.

Shakespeare, Tom. 2005. Disability, Genetics, and Global Justice. *Social Policy and Society* 4 (1): 87–95.

Shim, Janet K. 2002. Understanding the Routinized Inclusion of Race, Socioeconomic Status and Sex in Epidemiology: The Utility of Concepts from Technoscience Studies. *Sociology of Health and Illness* 24 (2): 129–150.

———. 2010. Cultural Health Capital. *Journal of Health and Social Behavior* 51 (1): 1–15.

Shoji, Yutaka, Akio Koizumi, Tsuyoshi Kayo, Tomoaki Ohata, Tsutomo Takahashi, Kenji Harada, and Goro Takada. 1998. Evidence for Linkage of Human Primary Systemic Carnitine Deficiency with D5S436: A Novel Gene Locus on Chromosome 5q. *American Journal of Human Genetics* 63 (1): 101–108.

Shostak, Sara, Peter Conrad, and Allan Horwitz. 2008. Sequencing and Its Consequences: Path Dependence and the Relationships between Genetics and Medicalization. *American Journal of Sociology* 114 (S1): S287–S316.

Sia, Calvin, Thomas F. Tonniges, Elizabeth Osterhus, and Sharon Taba. 2004. History of the Medical Home Concept. *Pediatrics* 113 (Suppl 5): 1473–1478.

Silverman, Chloe. 2012. *Understanding Autism: Parents, Doctors, and the History of a Disorder*. Princeton, NJ: Princeton University Press.

Simon, Christian, Stephen Zyzanski, Ellen Duran, Xavier Jimenez, and Eric Kodish. 2006. Interpreter Accuracy and Informed Consent among Spanish-Speaking Families with Cancer. *Journal of Health Communication* 11 (5): 509–522.

Skinner, Debra, Summer Choudhury, John Sideris, Sonia Guarda, Allen Buansi, Myra Roche, Cynthia Powell, and Donald B. Bailey Jr. 2011. Parents' Decisions to Screen Newborns for FMR1 Gene Expansions in a Pilot Research Project. *Pediatrics* 127 (6): e1455–e1463.

Skinner, Debra, William Lachicotte, and Linda Burton. 2007. Childhood Disability and Poverty: How Families Navigate Health Care and Coverage. In *Child Poverty in America Today*, edited by B. A. Arrighi and D. J. Maume. Westport, CT: Praeger.

Skinner, Debra, and Thomas Weisner. 2007. Sociocultural Studies of Families of Children with Intellectual Disabilities. *Mental Retardation and Developmental Disabilities Research Reviews* 13 (4): 302–312.

Smith, Emily H., Cheryl Thomas, David McHugh, Dimitar Gavrilov, Kimiyo Raymond, Piero Rinaldo, Silvia Tortorelli, Dietrich Matern, W. Edward Highsmith, and Devin Oglesbee. 2010. Allelic Diversity in MCAD Deficiency: The Biochemical Clasification of 54 Variants Identified during 5 Years of ACADM Sequencing. *Molecular Genetics and Metabolism* 100 (3): 241–250.

Stanley, Charles A. 2004. Carnitine Deficiency Disorders in Children. *Annals of the New York Academy of Sciences* 1033: 42–51.

Star, Susan Leigh. 1991a. Power, Technologies, and the Phenomenology of Conventions: On Being Allergic to Onions. In *A Sociology of Monsters: Essays on Power, Technology and Domination*, edited by J. Law. London: Routledge.

———. 1991b. The Sociology of the Invisible: The Primacy of Work in the Writings of Anselm Strauss. In *Social Organization and Social Process*, edited by D. R. Maines. New York: Aldine de Gruyter.

———. 1994. Misplaced Concretism and Concrete Situations: Feminism Method and Information Technology. Gender-Nature-Culture Working Paper No. 11. Odense University, Department of Feminist Studies.

———, ed. 1995. *Ecologies of Knowledge*. Albany: State University of New York Press.

Star, Susan Leigh, and Elihu M. Gerson. 1986. The Management and Dynamics of Anomalies in Scientific Work. *Sociological Quarterly* 28 (2): 147–169.

Starr, Paul. 1982. *The Social Transformation of American Medicine: The Rise of a Sovereign Profession and the Making of a Vast Industry*. New York: Basic Books.

Steinbok, Paul, David Lam, Swati Singh, Patricia Mortenson, and Ashutosh Singhai. 2007. Long Term Outcomes of Infants with Positional Occipital Plagiocephaly. *Child's Nervous System* 23 (11): 1275–1283.

Stewart, Moira, Judith B. Brown, W. Wayne Weston, Ian McWhinney, Carol McWilliam, and Thomas Freeman. 1995. *Patient-Centred Medicine: Transforming the Clinical Method*. London: Sage.

Stinchcombe, Arthur L. 2001. *When Formality Works: Authority and Abstraction in Law and Organizations*. Chicago: University of Chicago Press.

Stockl, Andrea. 2007. Complex Syndromes, Ambivalent Diagnosis, and Existential Uncertainty: The Case of Systemic Lupus Erythematosis. *Social Science and Medicine* 65 (7): 1549–1559.

Stone, Deborah. 1986. The Resistible Rise of Preventive Medicine. *Journal of Health Politics, Policy, and Law* 11 (4): 671–696.

Strathern, Marilyn. 1992. *After Nature: English Kinship in the Late Twentieth Century*. Lanham, MD: Rowman and Littlefield.

Strathmann, Cynthia, and Cameron Hay. 2009. Working the Waiting Room: Managing Fear, Hope and Rage at the Clinic Gate. *Medical Anthropology* 28 (3): 212–234.

Strauss, Anselm L., S. Fagerhaugh, B. Suczek, and C. Wiener. 1985. *The Social Organization of Medical Work*. Chicago: University of Chicago Press.

Suchman, Lucy. 2007. *Human-Machine Reconfigurations: Plans and Situated Actions*. 2nd ed. Cambridge: Cambridge University Press.

Sulik, Gayle A. 2009. Managing Biomedical Uncertainty: The Technoscientific Illness Identity. *Sociology of Health and Illness* 30 (7): 1059–1076.

Tamai, Ikumi, Rikiya Ohashi, Jun-Ichi Nezu, Hikaru Yabuuchi, Asuka Oku, Miyuki Shimane, Yoshimichi Sai, and Akira Tsuji. 1998. Molecular and Functional Identification of Sodium Ion-dependent, High Affinity Human Carnitine Transporter OCTN2. *Journal of Biological Chemistry* 273 (32): 20378–20382.

Tardy, Rebecca W. 2000. "But I Am a Good Mom:" The Social Construction of Motherhood through Health-Care Conversations. *Journal of Contemporary Ethnography* 29 (4): 433–473.

Tarini, Beth A. 2007. The Current Revolution in Newborn Screening. *Archive of Pediatrics and Adolescent Medicine* 161 (8): 767–772.

Taussig, Karen Sue. 2009. *Ordinary Genomes: Science, Citizenship, and Genetic Identitites*. Durham, NC: Duke University Press.

Taussig, Karen-Sue, Rayna Rapp, and Deborah Heath. 2003. Flexible Eugenics: Technologies of the Self in the Age of Genetics. In *Genetic Nature/Culture: Anthropology and Science Beyond the Two-Culture Divide*, edited by A. Goodman, D. Heath, and M. S. Lindee. Berkeley: University of California Press.

Taylor, Janelle. 2008. *The Public Life of the Fetal Sonogram: Technology, Consumption, and the Politics of Reproduction*. New Brunswick, NJ: Rutgers University Press.

Teach, Stephen J., Kathleen A. Lillis, and Mauro Grossi. 1998. Compliance with Pennicillin Prophylaxis in Patients with Sickle Cell Disease. *Archive of Pediatrics and Adolescent Medicine* 152 (3): 274–278.

Therrell, Bradford L. Jr. 2001. U.S. Newborn Screening Policy Dilemmas for the Twenty-First Century. *Molecular Genetics and Metabolism* 74 (1/2): 64–74.

Timmermans, Stefan. 1999a. Mutual Tuning of Multiple Trajectories. *Symbolic Interaction* 21 (4): 225–240.

———. 1999b. *Sudden Death and the Myth of CPR*. Philadelphia: Temple University Press.

———. 2002. Cause of Death vs. Gift of Life: Maintaining Jurisdiction in Death Investigation. *Sociology of Health and Illness* 24 (5): 550–574.

———. 2011. The Joy of Science: Finding Success in a "Failed" Randomized Clinical Trial. *Science, Technology and Human Values* 36 (4): 549–573.

Timmermans, Stefan, and Alison Angell. 2001. Evidence-Based Medicine, Clinical Uncertainty, and Learning to Doctor. *Journal of Health and Social Behavior* 42 (4): 342–359.

Timmermans, Stefan, and Marc Berg. 1997. Standardization in Action: Achieving Local Universality through Medical Protocols. *Social Studies of Science* 26 (4): 769–799.

———. 2003a. *The Gold Standard: The Challenge of Evidence-Based Medicine and Standardization in Health Care*. Philadelphia: Temple University Press.

———. 2003b. The Practice of Medical Technology. *Sociology of Health and Illness* 25 (3): 97–114.

Timmermans, Stefan, and Mara Buchbinder. 2010. Patients-in-Waiting: Living between Sickness and Health in the Genomics Era. *Journal of Health and Social Behavior* 51 (4): 408–423.

———. 2011. Improving Newborn Screening: A Reply to Watson, Howell, and Rinaldo. *Journal of Health and Social Behavior* 52 (2): 279–281.

————. 2012. Expanded Newborn Screening: Articulating the Ontology of Diseases with Bridging Work in the Clinic. *Sociology of Health and Illness* 34 (2): 208–220.

Timmermans, Stefan, and Betina Freidin. 2007. Caretaking as Articulation Work: The Effects of Taking up Responsibility for a Child with Asthma on Labor Force Participation. *Social Science and Medicine* 65 (7): 1351–1364.

Timmermans, Stefan, and Iddo Tavory. 2007. Advancing Ethnographic Research through Grounded Theory Practice. In *Handbook of Grounded Theory*, edited by A. Bryant and K. Charmaz. London: Sage.

Toiv, Helene F., Janina Austin, Emily G. Gardiner, Ann Tynan, Ariel Hill, Kevin Milne, Cindy Moon, and Susan Lawes. 2003. Newborn Screening: Characteristics of State Programs. Washington, DC: US General Accounting Office.

Traustadottir, Rannveig. 1991. Mothers Who Care: Gender, Disability, and Family Life. *Journal of Family Issues* 12 (2): 211–228.

Trostle, James. 1988. Medical Compliance as an Ideology. *Social Science and Medicine* 27 (12): 1299–1308.

Tutton, Richard. 2010. *Biobanking: Social, Political and Ethical Aspects*. London: John Wiley.

United States General Accounting Office. 2003. Newborn Screening: Characteristics of State Programs. Washington, DC: GAO.

Vailly, Joelle. 2008. The Expansion of Abnormality and the Biomedical Norm: Neonatal Screening, Prenatal Diagnosis and Cystic Fibrosis in France. *Social Science and Medicine* 66 (12): 2532–2543.

Vaughan, Diane. 1996. *The Challenger Launch Decision: Risky Technology, Culture and Deviance at NASA*. Chicago: University of Chicago Press.

————. 2004. Theorizing Disaster: Analogy, Historical Ethnography, and the Challenger Accident. *Ethnography* 5 (3): 315–347.

Vijay, S., A. Patterson, S. Olpin, M. J. Henderson, S. Clark, C. Day, G. Savill, and J. H. Walter. 2006. Carnitine Transporter Defect: Diagnosis in Asymptomatic Adult Women Following Analysis of Acylcarnitines in their Newborn Infants. *Journal of Inherited Metabolic Disease* 29 (5): 627–630.

Waddell, Leigh, Veronica Wiley, Kevin Capenter, Bruce Bennetts, Lyn Angel, Brage S. Andresen, and Bridget Wilcken. 2006. Medium-Chain Acyl-COA Dehydrogenase Deficiency: Genotype-biochemical Phenotype Correlations. *Molecular Genetics and Metabolism* 87 (1): 32–39.

Wailoo, Keith, Julie Livingston, Steven Epstein, and Robert A. Aronowitz, eds. 2010. *Three Shots at Prevention: The HPV Vacine and the Politics of Medicine's Simple Solutions*. Baltimore: Johns Hopkins University Press.

Wailoo, Keith, and Keith Pemberton. 2006. *The Troubled Dream of Genetic Medicine*. Baltimore: Johns Hopkins University Press.

Waisbren, Susan E., Simone Albers, Steve Amato, Mary Ampola, Thomas G. Brewster, Laurie Demmer, Roger B. Eaton, et al. 2003. Effect of Expanded Newborn

Screening for Biochemical Genetic Disorders on Child Outcomes and Parental Stress. *JAMA* 290 (19): 2564–2572.

Waldby, Catherine. 2000. *Tissue Economies: Blood, Organs, and Cell Lines in Late Capitalism.* Durham, NC: Duke University Press.

Watson, Michael S. 2006. Current Status of Newborn Screening: Decision-Making about the Conditions to Include in Screening Programs. *Mental Retardation and Developmental Disabilities Research Reviews* 12 (1): 230–235.

Watson, Michael S., R. Rodney Howell, and Piero Rinaldo. 2011. A Disservice to Advances in Newborn Genetic Screening: Comment on Timmermans and Buchbinder. *Journal of Health and Social Behavior* 52 (2): 277–278.

Watson, Michael S., Michele A. Lloyd-Puryear, Marie Y. Mann, Piero Ronaldo, and R. Rodney Howell. 2006. Newborn Screening: Toward a Uniform Screening Panel and System. *Genetics in Medicine* 8 (Suppl 5): 12S–252S.

Weaver, Meredith A., Alissa Johnson, Rani H. Singh, William R. Wilcox, M. Lloyd-Puryear, and Michael Watson. 2010. Medical Foods: Inborn Errors of Metabolism and the Reimbursement Dilemma. *Genetics in Medicine* 12 (6): 364–369.

Weimer, David L. 2007. Public and Private Regulation of Organ Transplantation: Liver Allocation and the Final Rule. *Journal of Health Politics, Policy, and Law* 32 (1): 9–49.

Weiss, Meira. 1994. *Conditional Love: Parents' Attitudes toward Handicapped Children.* Westport, CT: Greenwood.

White, Susan. 2002. Accomplishing "the Case" in Paediatrics and Child Health: Medicine and Morality in Interprofessional Talk. *Sociology of Health and Illness* 24 (2): 409–435.

Whitmarsh, Ian. 2009. Medical Schismogenics: Compliance and "Culture" in Caribbean Biomedicine. *Anthropological Quarterly* 82 (2): 447–475.

Whitmarsh, Ian, Arlene M. Davis, Debra Skinner, and Donald B. Bailey Jr. 2007. A Place for Genetic Uncertainty: Parents Valuing an Unknown in the Meaning of Disease. *Social Science and Medicine* 65 (6): 1082–1093.

Widhalm, Kurt, and Kiran Virmani. 1994. Long-Term Follow-Up of 58 Patients with Histidinemia Treated with a Histidine-Restricted Diet: No Effect of Therapy. *Pediatrics* 94 (6 Pt 1): 861–866.

Wilcken, Bridget. 2008. The Consequences of Extended Newborn Screening Programmes: Do We Know Who Needs Treatment? *Journal of Inherited Metabolic Disease* 31 (2): 173–177.

———. 2010. Fatty Acid Oxydation Disorders: Outcome and Long-Term Prognosis. *Journal of Inherited Metabolic Disease* 33 (5): 501–506.

Wilson, J. M. G., and G. Jungner. 1968. *Principles and Practice of Screening for Disease.* Geneva: World Health Organization.

Wong, James. 1994. On the Very Idea of the Normal Child, Unpublished PhD Dissertation, University of Toronto.

Wood, Fiona, Lindsay Prior, and Jonathon Gray. 2003. Translations of Risk: Decision Making in a Cancer Genetics Service. *Health, Risk and Society* 5 (2): 185–198.

Woolf, Louis, and D. B. Vulliamy. 1951. Phenylketonuria with a Study of the Effect upon It of Glutamic Acid. *Archives of Disease in Childhood* 26 (130): 487–494.

Woolgar, Steve. 1991. Configuring the User: The Case of Usability Trials. In *A Sociology of Monsters: Essays on Power, Technology, and Domination*, edited by J. Law. London: Routledge.

Wu, Xiang, Puttur D. Prasad, Frederick H. Leibach, and Vadivel Ganapathy. 1998. cDNA Sequence, Transport Function, and Genomic Organization of Human OCTN2, A New Member of the Organic Cation Transporter Family. *Biochemical and Biophysical Research Communications* 246 (3): 589–95.

Yang, Zi, Patrick E. Lantz, and Jamal A. Ibdah. 2007. Post-Mortem Analysis for Two Prevalent Beta Oxidation Mutations in Sudden Infant Death. *Pediatrics International* 49 (6): 883–887.

Yusopov, Roman, David N. Finegold, E. W. Naylor, Inderneel Sahai, Susan E. Waisbren, and Harvey L. Levy. 2010. Sudden Death in Medium Chain Acyl-Coenzyme A Dehydrogenase Deficiency (MCADD) despite Newborn Screening. *Molecular Genetics and Metabolism* 101 (1): 33–39.

Zelizer, Viviana. 1994. *Pricing the Priceless Child: The Changing Social Value of Children*: Princeton, NJ: Princeton University Press.

# Index

3-MCC (3-methylcrotonyl-coenzyme): clinical relevance, 80; as condition not disease, 79; expansion of screening, 60; maternal diagnosis, 113; questionable value of newborn screening for, 183; recalcitrant traction, 91

abductive analysis, 30, 151, 227–229
abortion, 226, 233
access to health care: citizenship, 195–197; health insurance, 197–202
ACMG (American College of Medical Genetics), 263–264n62
Advanced Liquid Logic, 239
advocacy: affective economy, 47, 225–226; clinical realities, 236–238; genetics clinics in, 235; lay organizations, 44–45; legislative success of, 48; power of the public, 41, 239; by providers of screening technology, 48; science, 35, 41, 45, 57; statistics, 47; testimonials, 45–48, 59–60, 218, 225–226
Affordable Care Act, 231
Ahmed, Sara, 47
Aleccia, JoNel, 214, 218, 236
Alzheimer's disease, 26
AMA (American Medical Association), 38
American Academy of Pediatrics, 38, 44–45, 49–50, 59
American College of Medical Genetics (ACMG), 263–264n62. See also American College of Medical Genetics (ACMG) report
American College of Medical Genetics (ACMG) report: beneficiaries of screening, 51–53; criticism of, 56–58, 60; on

false positives, 214; implementation of recommendations of, 59–61; leadership of, 239, 261n10; multiplex testing and recommendations of, 53, 54–55; number of screening targets, 62; on potential for successful treatment, 188–189; report on newborn screening by, 8, 48–58; scoring system of, 52, 54–55, 56, 248n87; uniform screening panel, 34, 50, 52, 54, 56, 109; unscientific basis for recommendations of, 50–51; weak evidentiary base for recommendations, 55–58, 248n87. See also American College of Medical Genetics (ACMG)
American Medical Association (AMA), 38
amniocentesis, 241n13, 253n28
Anspach, Renee, 181, 231
Arc of the United States, 35, 44–45
arginase deficiency, 189
Armstrong, David, 229–230
Arnold family, 136
Aronowitz, Robert, 20, 218–219
Association of Women's Health, Obstetric and Neonatal Nurses, 59
autism, 193

Bailey Baio Angel Foundation, 1, 5, 6
Baily, Mary Ann, 262n28
Baio family: cutoff values, 19; false positive, 1–6, 219; marital challenges, 9, 83; mutation analysis, 185; uncertainty, 12, 16
Baker, Maxine, 38
Beaudet, Arthur, 232–233
Beck, Ulrich, 241n18
Becker, Howard, 84, 90

Ben-Joseph, Elana, 253n35
Berns-Bonniau family, 103–104
bioethics: Human Genome Project, 44; informed consent, 216, 237–238, 248n106
biotin deficiency, 71
biotinidase deficiency, 49, 86, 189
blindness, 252n3
bonding, parent-infant, 3, 61, 241n13
Bonilla/Lancerio family, 74–76, 82, 109–112, 140–141
Bosk, Charles, 32, 249n12
Botkin, Jeffrey, 217
Bourret, Pascale, 254n41
breast cancer, 218–219, 226, 229. *See also* mammograms
breastfeeding, 69, 82–83
bridging work, 63–64, 117, 236, 238
British National Health Service, 57–58
Broderick/Thompson family. *See* Thompson/ Broderick family
Brosco, Jeffrey, 216
Bruner, Jerome, 146
bubble boy disease. *See* SCID (Severe Combined Immunodeficiency Disorder)
Buchanan family, 108, 139–140, 162, 189–195, 259n17

California Children's Services (CCS), 171, 199–201, 202
California Department of Public Health, 197–198
Cambrosio, Albert, 99
Campos family, 129
Canada, 245n1
cancer screening, 218–219
Canguilhem, Georges, 124
caregiving: articulation work, 194; chronic illness management, 255–256n18; day care, 163–164; developmental therapies, 176–177; family reorganization for, 180; gender of caregivers, 158, 165; grandmothers, 164–165; growth charts, 140; in-home nursing, 163; during hospitalizations, 165–166; logistical hurdles, 204; mothers' disproportionate role in, 163; paid employment, 163–164; parental diligence required for, 189–195; relentlessness of, 187; respite care, 157; stratified reproduction, 255n16; uncooperative fathers, 164

carnitine deficiency and carnitine transporter deficiency: antibiotics, 251n41; family history, 83–84; glutaric acidemia type 1 (GA1), 259n32; health insurance, 198, 200, 201; maternal diagnosis, 112–117, 198, 201; muscle weakness, 71; normality and normalization, 139; paternal diagnosis, 116–117; questionable value of newborn screening for, 183; treatment for, 114–116, 189
CCS (California Children's Services), 171, 199–201, 202
Centerwall, Willard, 36
charity: transportation challenges, 206
Chen family, 114–115
Chernobyl disaster, 196
Child Protective Services (CPS), 173, 224
Children's Hospital, Boston, 185
Chin, Lucy: health insurance, 198, 211; medical foods, 202; noncompliance with dietary regimen, 174; role of at clinic, 31; transplantation, 178
chorionic villus sampling (CVS), 86
Christakis, Nicholas, 222–225, 262n31
chromatography, 53, 247n76
chronic illness management: acceptance of knowledge gaps, 256n20; care versus patient choice in, 255–256n18; long-term doctor-patient relationships, 166–167; precarious beginnings, 159–163; stabilization and routinization of care, 163–168; timing of notification, 161–163. *See also* clinic-patient relationship; dietary management for metabolic disorders; follow-up visits
churches: transportation challenges, 206
citizenship, biological, 196–197
citrullinemia, 130, 162
class. *See* socioeconomic status
clinic-patient relationship: abductive reasoning in, 227–229; accommodation of patient preferences, 168, 256n21; ambivalence about screening, 221–222; biomedical uncertainty, 15–16, 223–224; Child Protective Services, 173, 224; clinical team meetings, 257n40; collaboration in, 167–168, 195; dietary negotiation, 171–175; dietary regimens, 169–170; dyadic versus team-based, 242n34; emotional expression in, 226–227; long-term,

166–167; noncompliance, 168–169; physicians' emotions, 262n38; public health policy, 235–236; rhetoric of suspicion, 175

cobalamin C deficiency, 113, 183

Collins, Francis, 23

communication: diversity of study participants, 153; withholding of information, 12. *See also* notification of parents

congenital adrenal hyperplasia, 49, 234

congenital hypothyroidism. *See* hypothyroidism

consanguinity, 106, 207–208, 251n33, 254n2

Council of Regional Networks for Genetic Services, 39

Cowan, Ruth Schwartz, 255n9

CPS (Child Protective Services), 173, 224

Crick, Francis, 23

culture: cultural health capital, 172, 191; noncompliance with medical advice, 174

cutoff values: Baio family, 19; changing of, 111; false negatives and positives, 41, 236–237; for inclusion in screening panel, 56; misplaced concretism, 77; natural history of disease, 56; state-to-state variation in, 237; target ranges, 264n64

CVS (chorionic villus sampling), 86

Cyprus, genetic screening in, 232, 255n9

cystic fibrosis, 49, 241n11, 249n8

Darlington family, 90–91

Daston, Lorraine, 253n29

Dati, Jean-Pierre: on asymptomatic children, 186; carnitine deficiency case, 112; doubts about value of newborn screening, 182–183, 220, 221; follow-up visits, 131, 141; hyperprolinemia case, 74–75, 110–112; inconclusive test results, 182; maternal diagnosis, 115–116; MCADD cases, 79–80, 88; paternal diagnosis, 116–117; role of at clinic, 31, 32

developmental disability: developmental therapies, 175–177; maple syrup urine disease (MSUD), 157; origins of newborn screening, 35–36; PKU, 40–41; positional plagiocephaly, 254n43; social implications of, 253n32; social support, 37–38

De Vries, Ella, 32, 78–79, 94, 105, 174

Dewey, John, 66–67

diagnosis: biochemical versus phenotypical, 101–102; blissful ignorance in absence of, 184, 258n3; clinical relevance, 79–81; condition versus disease, 79; geneticists' modus operandi, 76; maternal, 112–117, 185, 198, 201, 212, 221, 228, 251n51; before notification of screening results, 154–155, 159; odyssey of, 65–66, 184; overcall, 89; paternal, 116–117, 251n51; swiftness of, 162; time required for, 93; uncertainty after screening, 66, 71, 92, 93–95

dietary management for metabolic disorders: Child Protective Services, 173; cornstarch treatment, 101, 108, 190–192; death and, 257n33; dietary supplements, 114–115; diet diaries, 256n31; doctor-patient relationship, 169–170, 171–175; education, 171; expired prescriptions, 171; g-tubes, 205; health insurance, 202–203; medical foods, 202; negative outcomes because of screening, 186; noncompliance, 172–174, 175; parental vigilance, 191–194; special dietary use of food, 256n24; versus transplantation, 177–178; unclear relationship of to health status, 174–175

dietitian: attitudes toward families' class, 172; education of families, 171; patient relations, 169

disability, social model of, 206

discrimination, health insurance, 15, 231

disease: bureaucratic disease entities, 81; versus condition, 79; between health and, 92–95; hidden, 230; tinkering with categories of, 117, 119–120. *See also* ontology of disease

DNA sequencing, 75–76, 104–105

doctor-patient relationship. *See* clinic-patient relationship

doctor shopping, 15

Down syndrome, 142

Dowshen, Steven, 253n35

Duarte galactosemia, 80, 82–83

Duster, Troy, 26

Early Start, 204

emergency letters, 81–82, 107, 161

emotion: affective economy, 47, 225–226; expression of in clinic, 226–227, 262n38

endocrine disorders, 241n11

ethnicity: amniocentesis and, 253n28; consanguinity and, 106, 251n33, 254n2; growth charts and, 140, 253n37; hospitals as border zones and, 153–154; MCADD and, 101, 105–106; SCID and, 260n2; of study participants, 153; Tay-Sachs disease and, 232

ethnography, "us" and "them" in, 32

eugenics, 26, 196, 259n20

evidence-based medicine, 13

expansion of newborn screening, 34–64; addition of new tests, 39; anomalous findings, 109; arguments for, 8–9; beneficiaries of, 51–53; changing assumptions, 119; conditions selected for screening, 50; consensus on advisability of, 42–44; consequences of for families, 61; controversy surrounding, 37–38; creation of disease, 120; degree of, 61; diagnostic uncertainty, 93–94; do-it-yourself evidence, 55–58; genomics, 229–230; health care infrastructure, 41, 43–44, 55, 56, 58, 63; implementation of ACMG recommendations, 59–61; implementation problems, 35; inevitability of, 60–61; logic of prevention, 181; MCADD, 100; natural history of disease, 55–56; new technology, 34; number of screening targets, 62; PKU (phenylketonuria), 35–37, 39–48; popular advocacy, 44–45, 225–226; properties of screened conditions, 62–63, 66; relative significance of, 214, 237, 263–264n62; response to authors' research, 263–264n62; tandem mass spectrometry, 53–55; timing of implementation, 41. *See also* newborn screening

Fadiman, Anne, 174

false negatives, 20, 41, 236–237, 257n2

false positives: anxiety due to, 218; breast cancer screening, 218–219; bridging work, 238; cutoff values, 41, 236–237; failure to thrive, 186; health insurance, 198; limbo between pathology and normality, 75; versus maternal-infant link, 113–114; misunderstandings about

importance of testing, 253n28; mutation analysis, 78; parents' support for screening, 219; passage of time, 92–93; patients-in-waiting, 67, 72; public responses to, 213–214, 261n10; rate of, 260nn1–2; sensitivity of screening, 20; statistics on, 212; success of newborn screening, 217, 236; two-tiered screening, 39

family: access to health insurance, 231–232; blood ties and medical scrutiny, 26; changing models of, 244n98; clinical versus familial worldviews, 180; developmental therapies, 177; hospitalizations, 165–166; parental conflict over care, 191; routines, 165; visible differences, 255n17

fetal remains, 27–28, 244n105

fetal surgery, 233

Flores, Gabriel: assurances from, 122; difficult cases, 182; doubts about value of newborn screening, 220–221; follow-up visits, 138; glutaric acidemia type 1 (GA1) cases, 77–78, 201, 210; Goldilocks syndrome, 169; hyperprolinemia case, 75; on international disease incidence variations, 105–106; "knocking on wood," 222; maple syrup urine disease (MSUD) case, 155, 157; maternal diagnosis, 115–116; MCADD cases, 103; messages to families from, 82; noncompliance with dietary regimen, 173–174; on rare diseases, 69; role of at clinic, 31, 32; Spanish language and, 161, 206; on success of early intervention, 179; uncertainty about best clinical action, 167–168

follow-up visits: changing triggers for, 19; funding for, 197–198; growth charts, 131; health insurance, 200–202, 211; older children, 121; parental reports, 129–132; physical examination, 135–138; prognoses, 142; statistics on, 212; structure of, 121, 126–128; travel for, 127; waiting room, 126, 253n27

Foucault, Michel, 131, 135, 151

founder effect, 101

Fox, Renee, 13, 228

fragile X gene, 14

Franklin, Sarah, 221

future of newborn screening: abductive reasoning, 227–229; biomedical uncertainty,

222–225; clinical realities, 234–239; collateral damage, 218–222; emotion, 225–227; five omens of, 212–215; public health genomics, 229–234; success as a contested category, 216–218

GA1. *See* glutaric acidemia type 1
GA2. *See* glutaric acidemia type 2
galactosemia, 49, 62, 189, 202
Galison, Peter, 253n29
Gamboa family, 105–106
gay marriage, 196
Genetic Alliance, 246n43
genetic counseling, 15
geneticists: advocacy for screening, 226; anomalous findings, 118–119; clinical domain of practice, 249n12; collective learning process among, 95, 118, 258n5; diagnostic uncertainty, 93–95; disciplinary eye of, 136; doubts about value of screening among, 182–183, 186, 220–221; families' trust in, 95; "knocking on wood," 222–223, 262n31; long-term patient relationships, 166–167; resistance to parental wishes, 181; training of, 136; as transplantation gatekeepers, 179; uncertainty about best clinical action, 167–168
genetics: ambiguous test results, 76; carriers, 12; clinical relevance, 102–104; context of information receipt, 24–25; counseling value of testing, 102; definition of, 23; diagnosis and, 76; genetic stratification, 23–28, 232; genotype, 24; laboratory-clinic relationship, 99; multiple bases of disease, 25; mutation analysis, 77–78, 102–104; new group formation, 25–26; of race, 26, 196; social differentiation, 26–27. *See also* genomics
*Genetics in Medicine* (journal), 212
genomics: genomic services, 14; guidelines for screening, 41; normality and normalization, 125; personalized medicine, 233; promise of, 23, 24, 234; public health and, 229–234; routinization of, 24, 25
genotype-phenotype link, variability of, 62
Giddens, Anthony, 241n18
Gill, Virginia, 253n32
glutaric acidemia type 1 (GA1): Baio family, 1–6; carnitine deficiency and, 259n32;

clinical signs of, 137–138; death from, 207–210; Honan family, 76–79; inconclusive test results, 182; maternal diagnosis, 113, 201; medical supervision, 84, 88–89; mutation analysis, 77–78, 185; positive outcome regardless of screening, 185; potential for successful treatment, 189; sibling death and, 160, 207; symptomatic versus nonsymptomatic, 186
glutaric acidemia type 2 (GA2), 62, 71
Goldilocks syndrome, 169
Gonzales/Ramos family: developmental delays, 176; follow-up visits, 138; fragile beginnings, 153–158; paid employment, 156, 163; as success story of intervention, 179, 220; timing of screening notification, 162; uncertainty about best clinical action, 167–168
Good, Byron, 146
Good, Mary-Jo DelVecchio, 146
Goodwin, Charles, 254n40
Grob, Rachel, 249n8
Groopman, Jerome, 256n21
growth charts: ethnicity and, 140, 254n37; medical gaze and, 256n31; metabolic disorders, 148–149; as misleading, 252–253n20; normalization, 124–125, 127, 131, 132–135, 139–141; parental understanding of, 253n35
Guthrie, Robert, 35–39

H1N1 virus, 190, 193–194, 259n17
Hacking, Ian: on feedback in categorization, 27, 28; on interactive diagnostic classification, 119; on normality, 125; on personhood, 24; on statistical thinking, 252n3
Hay, Cameron, 253n27
health care system: articulation work in, 194; citizenship rights, 197; costliness of, 211; cultural health capital in, 172; expansion of screening, 41, 43–44, 55, 56, 58; immigrants' access to, 177–179; inequities in, 183, 187, 195, 211; medical home in, 44; Obama reform, 259n26; prescription authorizations, 171; rationing concerns, 58; sociopolitical screening infrastructure, 63; study participants' trouble with, 163–164. *See also* access to health care; health insurance

health insurance: access to, 197–202; consequences of screening, 10; discrimination in, 15, 231; effect of false positive on, 198; family structure and, 231–232; HMOs, 199, 200–201; job loss, 164; medical foods, 202–203; PPOs, 199; precariousness of, 201–202; preexisting conditions, 231, 255n15; public, 199–200, 255n14; rationing of care, 198–199, 211; special diets, 170; stifling restrictions in, 16; study participants' trouble with, 255n15; treatment of adults, 117
Health Resources and Services Administration (HRSA), 49–50, 237
health/sickness binary, 22
Healthy Families program (California), 199
hematological disorders, 241n11
hereditary conditions, sibling-to-sibling spillover, 86–87
Heritage, John, 244n109
Hidalgo family: child care, 164; death in, 184–185, 257n33; developmental delays, 176; genetics team and, 160; hospitalizations, 162; language barrier, 161, 204; noncompliance, 173–174; transplantation, 177; unpredictability of illness, 165
high blood pressure, 97
histidinemia, 186
history, shifting health policy, 20–21
HIV/AIDS, 97, 226, 230
Hogle, Linda, 257n42
Holt family, 130, 175
homocystinuria, 49, 113
homosexuality, shifting ontology of disease, 97
Honan family, 76–79, 94, 185
hope: uncertainty and, 15, 151; 254–255n4
hospitalization, roller coaster experience of, 254–255n4
Howell, Rodney, 263–264n62
Howse, Jennifer, 45
HRSA (Health Resources and Services Administration), 49–50, 237
Hughes, Everett, 29, 66
Human Genome Project, 23, 24, 44
human papillomavirus vaccine, 19
Huntington's disease, 15, 199
hyperplasia, 39
hyperprolinemia: access to services, 82; clinical relevance, 75, 80, 117; DNA sequencing, 76; ontology, 109; schizophrenia and, 71; screening panels, 249n11; types of, 74–75
hypoglycemia, 101
hypothyroidism, 39, 49, 189, 234

iatrogenic harm, 186
identity formation, genetic basis for, 25–26, 27
immigration. See ethnicity
immunophenotyping, 99
infant mortality, US rate of, 233
informed consent: advisory bodies on, 43; American College of Medical Genetics (ACMG), 52; bioethics, 216, 237–238, 248n106; bypassing of, 39, 216; exceptions to, 43; lack of, 61; retention and use of screening samples, 214–215, 237–238; untreatable conditions, 53
innovation, creation of needs, 242n40
Institute of Medicine (IOM), 41–43, 215
Internet, 3, 12, 71, 242n34
intuition, versus science, 12–13
IOM (Institute of Medicine), 41–43, 215
isovaleric acidemia, 45
Izenberg, Neil, 253n35

Jacek-Love family, 219–220
James, William, 11
Johnston/Walker family. See Walker/Johnston family
Jungner, Gunnar, 42, 43, 51, 55

Kaufert, Patricia, 262n45
Keating, Peter, 99
Kelly, Susan, 231
Kennedy, John F., 37
Kent, Deborah, 252n3
kinship, shared genetic traits, 26–27
"knocking on wood," 222–225, 262n31
knowledge: curtailed future, 15; ecologies of, 117–120, 151; frustration with gaps in, 256n20; information overload, 15; versus intuition, 12–13; from laboratory to clinic, 28; in-the-making, 101; parents' self-education, 74; perceptual practices, 254n40; preventive action, 11–12; relief in, 24–25; uncertainty, 12, 13–14, 224–225; will to know, 14–15
Koenig, Barbara, 257n42

Kuhn, Thomas, 119
Kuvan (medication), 249n10

Lampl, Michelle, 252–253n20
Lancerio/Bonilla family. *See* Bonilla/
    Lancerio family
language and interpretation: access to ser-
    vices and, 206; ambiguous test results, 74;
    dietary regimens and, 170; limitations of,
    160–161; seriousness of disorders and,
    92; therapeutic services and, 204
laryngomalacia, 155
Latimer, Joanna, 99, 131, 254n41
Layne, Linda L., 254–255n4
Lee, Lia, 174
Lee family, 162, 177–179, 257n36, 257n41
Levinson family, 68–72, 86, 135
Levy-Fisch, Jill, 258n5
lifesaving potential of newborn screening:
    access to health care, 195; authors' posi-
    tion on, 183–184; chain of survival, 210;
    versus death in spite of, 207–210; epidemi-
    ological outcomes, 233; expiration of ser-
    vices, 204; factors affecting, 184, 191, 207,
    211, 232; four possible outcomes, 184–187;
    geneticists' doubts, 182–183, 220–221;
    genome sequencing, 234; health insurance,
    197–202, 211; inequities in health care sys-
    tem, 183, 187; language challenges, 204,
    206; limited data on outcomes, 183–184;
    medical foods and special formulas, 202–
    204; met and unmet opportunities, 210;
    negative outcomes because of screening,
    186, 189; negative outcomes regardless of
    screening, 184–185, 257n2, 258n5; parental
    diligence, 189–195; PKU experience, 187–
    188; positive outcomes because of screen-
    ing, 187; positive outcome regardless of
    screening, 185–186; success as contested
    category, 216–218, 220–221; therapeutic
    services, 203–204; transportation chal-
    lenges and, 205–206; window of oppor-
    tunity, 187–189, 225, 232
Lloyd-Puryear, Michele, 264n67
Lopez family, 139
Lorey, Fred, 213, 217
Luminex, 239

Mabini family, 140
Malvern, Sarah, 122; difficult cases, 221; on

DNA sequencing, 104; hyperprolinemia
    case, 112; normalization, 139; role of at
    clinic, 31, 32; SCADD case, 80; trans-
    plantation, 178
mammograms, 20, 21, 262n45. *See also*
    breast cancer
maple syrup urine disease (MSUD): devel-
    opmental delay, 157; fragile beginnings,
    155; potential for successful treatment,
    189; state-to-state variations in screening
    for, 49; treatment for, 157
March of Dimes Foundation: ACMG report,
    59; advocacy, 44–45; lobbying days of, 59,
    60; screening recommendations of, 2; tes-
    timonials, 225–226; uniform screening, 50
Martin family, 102, 107, 200–201
Massachusetts Newborn Screening Advi-
    sory Committee, 50
Mattingly, Cheryl, 153, 172, 253n27, 256n26
Maynard, Douglas, 253n32
Mayo Clinic, 104–105, 263–264n62
MCADD (medium-chain acyl-coenzyme
    A dehydrogenase deficiency): breast-
    feeding and, 83; changing management
    of, 224; clinical relevance, 79–80; com-
    mon disease identity, 117; cornstarch
    treatment, 191–192; cost-effectiveness
    of screening for, 58; deaths of children
    with, 185, 258n5; diagnosis, 101–104,
    150n24, 150n28; dietary management,
    107, 191–193; emergency room visits,
    118; ethnicity and, 101; fading vigilance,
    88; follow-up visits, 127; genetic marker
    for, 62; geographical health disparities,
    34; health insurance and, 198, 200–201;
    inevitability of negative results, 258n5;
    international variations in, 105–106;
    lifesaving treatment, 162; marital chal-
    lenges, 83, 191; maternal diagnosis, 113;
    medical effects of, 100; mutation anal-
    ysis, 103–104, 200–201; ontology of, 100–
    109; outcomes, 108–109; parental dili-
    gence required with, 189–195; potential
    for successful treatment, 189; prescreen-
    ing morbidity and mortality from, 118;
    rarity of, 62; recalcitrant traction, 90–91;
    severity and incidence of, 104–106, 107,
    150n27; sudden death and, 71, 100; treat-
    ment for, 101, 106–108, 112; value of
    newborn screening for, 183

McAllister family, 86–87
MCKAT (medium-chain ketoacyl-coenzyme A thiolase deficiency), 62
Medicaid, 199, 259n32, 260n39
Medi-Cal, 199, 201, 202, 261–262n23
medical foods: health insurance and, 260n39
medical gaze: compulsory schooling, 124; diet diaries, 256n31; disciplinary objectivity, 136; mobilization versus reassurance, 138
medical home, 44
Medicare, 197
medium-chain acyl-coenzyme A dehydrogenase deficiency. See MCADD
medium-chain ketoacyl-coenzyme A thiolase deficiency (MCKAT), 62
mental retardation. See developmental disability
metabolic disorders: children's cooperation with treatment, 170; clinical relevance, 79–81; clinical versus familial worldviews, 180; creation of, 120; developmental therapies for, 175–177; everyday clinical management of, 180; genetics and, 23; growth and, 122; honeymoon period, 143, 145; knowledge explosion and, 119; late diagnosis, 65; limits of prevention, 152, 179–181; Listserv for specialists in, 80; metabolic tightrope, 169; noncompliance with treatment, 168–169, 170, 172–174, 175; pediatricians' lack of knowledge about, 118; regression after crisis, 176–177; state-to-state variations in screening for, 49; therapeutic odyssey, 180; transplantation, 177–179. See also dietary management for metabolic disorders
methylmalonic acidemia. See MMA
Miner family, 112, 115–116, 117, 221
MMA (methylmalonic acidemia): death from, 257n33; developmental delays, 176; future expectations, 166; limits of prevention, 181; maternal diagnosis, 113; normal development and, 257n36; normalization and difference, 146–147; potential for successful treatment, 189; questionable value of screening for, 182–183; sibling death and, 160; timing of screening for, 162; transplantation and, 177–179

Mol, Annemarie, 255–256n18
Molloy v. Meier et al., 59
Monaco, Jana, 45–47
morality: clinical team deliberations, 257n40; normalization, 139–141
Morgan, Lynn, 27–28
Moskowitz, Denise, 31, 157, 167, 204–206, 211
MSUD. See maple syrup urine disease
Muñoz family, 160, 162, 204
mutation analysis: glutaric acidemia type 1 (GA1), 77–78; health insurance and, 200–201; positive outcome regardless of screening, 185; VLCADD and, 86–87
mutations, splice site, 258n12

National Academy of Sciences, 38, 41, 45
National Association for Retarded Children (NARC), 35, 38. See also Arc of the United States
National Coalition for PKU and Allied Disorders, 45
National Human Genome Research Institute, 42, 229
National Institute of Child Health and Human Development, 229
National Institutes of Health (NIH), 110, 229, 239. See also National Human Genome Research Institute
Nazif, Anippe, 32, 134, 251n33
newborn screening: ambiguity of success of, 179–181; authors' position on, 6, 183–184; as benefit to others, 42–43; biological citizenship and, 196; as biomedical platform, 234, 263n60; with blood versus urine, 36–37; blunting sharp edges of, 238; commercially available, 54; cost of, 21, 50, 57–58, 213, 217–219, 261–262n23; delayed processing of, 258n5; democratic nature of, 187, 197; federal legislation for, 48; funding for, 197, 261–262n23; illnesses detected by, 241n11; inconclusive retesting, 75–79; increased medical consumption, 198; mandatory, 7, 38, 43, 61; medicalization, 221; metaphors for positive results of, 227; opportunity cost, 262n28; opposition to, 38–39; origins of, 35–39; overt resistance to, 92; parental consent, 7; parents' preferences, 6; PKU success story, 44–48; ver-

sus prenatal screening, 255n9; process of, 53–54; public knowledge about, 61; rates of various results of, 212, 260n2; reproductive decisions and, 43; retention and use of screening samples, 214–215, 218, 261n12; as science project, 119; secondary prevention and, 152; state-to-state variations in, 34, 37–39, 48–49, 59, 213; statistics on, 212, 237, 264n63; success story of, 179; system components of, 39; timing of screening, 41; treatability and, 51–52; two-tiered, 39; in United Kingdom, 57–58; universal, 28, 45, 216; voluntary, 38. *See also* expansion of newborn screening; future of newborn screening; lifesaving potential of newborn screening; notification of parents; prenatal screening

NIH. *See* National Institutes of Health

normality and normalization: creativity in, 150–151; critics of, 125; cultural schemas of, 130–131; definition of, 123, 252n4; developmental therapies, 175–176; of deviance, 58; disciplinary objectivity, 135–138, 144; doubled discourse, 142, 149–150; as foreshadowing work, 141–149; Foucauldian legacy, 151; geneticists' reassurances, 122, 128; growth charts and, 124–125, 127, 132–135, 139–141, 148–149; in historical perspective, 123–126; mechanical objectivity, 132–135, 137–138, 141; morality, 125, 139–141, 144, 147; mutual pretense, 252n3; narrative objectivity, 129–132; normalizing judgment, 131; objective developmental standards, 123; ongoing follow-up visits, 121–122; precarious, 142–149; production of difference, 141–142, 150; prognosis, 123; relativity, 141, 144; renorming, 150; social order, 125; stage model of human development, 124; standardized norms, 128–138; subjunctivity, 145–147, 150, 223; unstable meaning of, 150

notification of parents: contradictory messages, 70; cystic fibrosis and, 249n8; disease onset preceding, 154–155, 159, 161–162, 180, 255n9; family context, 71–72; reactions to, 70; timing of, 69–70, 219

Novas, Carlos, 24

Obama, Barack, 259n26

objectivity: clinical judgment, 254n41; developmental standards, 123; disciplinary, 135–138, 144; mechanical, 132–135, 137–138, 141, 254n41; types of, 253n29

ontology of disease: actions facilitated by, 97–98; anomalies, 98–100; carnitine deficiency and, 112–117; examples of shifts in, 97; hyperprolinemia and, 109–112; knowledge ecologies, 117–120, 151; laboratory-clinic relationship, 99–100; MCADD and, 100–109; technology and, 97–98

Organic Acidemia Association, 45

Pap smears, 20, 262n45

parental consent, 7, 241n8

patients-in-waiting: clinical relevance, 79–81; clinic visits, 72–75; contradictory messages, 67; diagnostic odyssey, 65–66, 180; fading vigilance, 87–89; family relationships, 81–85; between health and disease, 92–96; implied imperfection and, 66; interactive diagnostic classification, 119; logic of increased pathology, 77; marital challenges, 83; medicalization and, 221; normality and normalization, 150; ongoing medical supervision, 85–87, 88; onset of status of, 68–72; parents and infants as, 67–68; proto-disease states, 95–96; recalcitrant traction, 89–92; repeat testing, 75–79; resistance to change in, 84; side bets, 84, 90; success of newborn screening and, 236; trajectories of, 72–74, 92–93

Peirce, Charles S., 10

PerkinElmer Genetics, 54, 239

personhood: mutation and, 24

Petryna, Adriana, 196

PGD (preimplantation genetic diagnosis), 221

pharmaceutical industry, 20, 239, 264n70

phenylketonuria. *See* PKU

PKU (phenylketonuria): access to medical foods and, 203; age at treatment initiation, 188; breastfeeding and, 69; cautionary tale of screening for, 39–44, 47; clear diagnostic picture, 94; as commonly screened for, 3; cost-effectiveness of screening for, 57–58; diagnosis of, 68–69,

PKU (phenylketonuria) (*continued*)
71; dietary restrictions, 170; genetics
and, 23, 62, 246n19; high standard for
treatment, 62; versus hyperphenylalanine, 41; lifesaving promise of newborn
screening, 187–188; maternal, 40, 113;
mental retardation and, 41, 233, 246n19;
negative outcomes because of screening, 186; origins of newborn screening,
35–36; as screening success story, 44–48,
234; shame and, 173; siblings with, 186;
testing methods for, 36–37, 245n6; timing of screening for, 41; treatment for,
36, 37, 40–41, 249n10; universal screening for, 49
policy. *See* public health policy
Porter, Ted, 137
positional plagiocephaly, 254n43
pragmatist theory, 9–11
preimplantation genetic diagnosis (PGD),
221
prenatal screening: future of, 232–233, 239;
versus newborn screening, 255n9; preimplantation genetic diagnosis, 221; reproductive decisions and, 59. *See also* newborn screening
President's Commission for the Study of
Ethical Problems in Medicine and Biomedical and Behavioral Research, 43
prevention, secondary, 2, 9, 152–153
problem-solving: abductive insights, 11
prognosis, normality, 123
propionic acidemia, 143–145, 181, 183, 189
prostate cancer, 21
PSA screening, 21
public health policy: bridging work, 63–64,
236; clinical realities, 225–229, 232, 234–
239, 263–264n62; eugenics and, 259n20;
genomics and, 229–234; historical shifts
in, 20–21; international variations in,
34, 245n1, 245n7; medical consumption markets, 239, 264n70; in nineteenth
century, 124; public health genetics, 230,
262–263n46; surveillance medicine, 230;
uncertainty about results of screening, 29

Rabeharisoa, Vololona, 254n41
Rabinow, Paul, 25, 244n88
race and racism: clinicians' speech about
differences, 256n26; genetics of race, 26,

196; health disparities and, 254n2; race
as biological construct, 106, 196; race of
study participants, 153; sickle cell screening, 21–22, 42; stigmatizing taxonomy
of, 172; variations in disease incidence
and, 106
Ramos/Gonzales family. *See* Gonzales/
Ramos family
Rapp, Rayna, 142, 149, 255n17
Raspberry, Kelly, 150
Regional Genetics and Newborn Screening
Collaboratives, 237
regulation: bioethics and, 44; consequences
of screening, 10; marriage and, 196;
model regulations, 49; of newborn
screening in California, 31; technology
adoption, 18; of transplantation, 257n41
reproductive decisions, 51, 66
reproductive technologies, 244n98
research methods, 8–11, 29–33, 244–
245nn109–110
Reyes family, 134, 139
Rinaldo, Piero, 263–264n62
risk management, 20, 89
Roberts, Celia, 221
Rockford, Maryland, workshop on newborn
screening, 229, 232, 239
Roddick family, 170
Rodriguez family, 162, 164–166, 176, 204
roller coaster experiences: hospitalizations, 254–255n4; notification of screening results, 69–70; patients-in-waiting,
72–73, 86
Rosales, Rocio, 30, 206, 244n109
Rose, Nikolas, 24, 124, 125
Rosenberg, Charles, 95
Rothman, Barbara Katz, 241n13

Sanchez family: beginning of treatment, 162;
children's deaths, 160, 207–210, 257n37,
258n5; day care, 163–164; developmental
delays, 176; family life, 165; health insurance, 163–164, 255n14; language barrier, 204; paid employment, 164; Spanish
interpretation, 160–161
Save Babies Through Screening Foundation,
Inc., 2, 48, 258n5, 261n20
SCADD (short-chain acyl-coenzyme A
dehydrogenase), 62, 80, 139, 219–220
Schaffer family, 115, 131

Scheper-Hughes, Nancy, 257n41
schizophrenia, 71, 193
Schubert, Nathan, 59–60
Schubert family, 91
SCID (Severe Combined Immunodeficiency
    Disorder), 212–213, 217, 206n2, 260–
    261n7, 261n20
science: advocacy, 35, 41, 45; versus intuition,
    12–13; standards of evidence, 57
screening: adult onset diseases, 229; argu-
    ments against, 21; beneficiaries of, 51–53;
    benefit to others, 42–43; for carriers,
    232–233; companies and universities
    offering, 48; compulsory, 19, 22; conse-
    quences of, 9–11; meanings of, 19–20, 22;
    motivations for participation in, 21–22;
    normalization and, 252n3; payment for,
    19; points of consensus about, 42–44;
    proactive versus reactive, 53; process of,
    6–8, 36–37; rates of, 7; sensitivity ver-
    sus specificity of, 20; state-to-state dis-
    crepancies in, 1–2; timing of, 232–233.
    See also newborn screening; prenatal
    screening
Sebelius, Kathleen, 212–213
Secretary's Advisory Committee on Heri-
    table Disorders in Newborns and Chil-
    dren, 45, 59, 217, 260–261nn6–7, 263–
    264n62
Severe Combined Immunodeficiency Dis-
    order. See SCID
Shim, Janet, 131
short-chain acyl-coenzyme A dehydroge-
    nase (SCADD), 62, 80, 139, 219–220
siblings: carnitine deficiency and, 116; death
    of, 160, 207; hyperprolinemia and, 111;
    VLCADD and, 86–87
sickle cell disease: access to treatment,
    63; carriers of, 42; controversy over
    screening for, 21–22, 40; racism and, 42;
    selective screening, 197; state-to-state
    variations in screening for, 49; testing
    methods for, 247n76
SIDS (sudden infant death syndrome), 100,
    254n43
Silverman, Mark: 3-MCC case, 79; advo-
    cacy and, 235; on ambiguity of success
    of treatment, 181; collaboration with
    families, 168; collegial consultations,
    137; developmental therapies, 175–176;

dismissiveness of, 191–192; on DNA
    sequencing, 104–105; doubts about
    value of screening, 185–186, 220, 221; on
    Duarte galactosemia, 80; follow-up visits,
    129–130, 135–136, 139–140, 143–148,
    190; giving bad news to parents, 160; glu-
    taric acidemia type 1 (GA1) death and,
    207–210; health insurance and, 200–201,
    203; inconclusive test results and, 76; on
    Internet message boards, 71; "knock-
    ing on wood," 222; on logic of PKU
    prevention, 188; long-term patient rela-
    tionships, 166, 167; markers of class in
    speech of, 210, 256n29; maternal diag-
    nosis and, 113–115, 116, 228; MCADD
    testing and, 102–103, 107; medicaliza-
    tion concerns of, 253n32; messages to
    parents from, 82; on need for further
    research, 118; normalizing subjunctiv-
    ity and, 145, 146–148; ongoing medical
    supervision, 85–89, 249n19; on paren-
    tal diligence, 194; parent's avoidance of,
    259n17; paternal diagnosis and, 116–117;
    personality of, 31; recalcitrant traction
    and, 90–91; relationship with research-
    ers, 32–33; role of at clinic, 31; Spanish
    language and, 206; speech delays, 175,
    253n32; transplantation and, 177–178,
    179; transportation to appointments,
    205; uncooperative fathers and, 164; on
    upsetting the applecart with screening,
    223; on value of newborn screening, 183;
    weight gain and, 174–175
Skinner, Debra, 150
Social Security, 156
socioeconomic status: clinicians' speech
    about, 210, 256n29; cultural health
    capital and, 172; genetic stratification
    and, 23–28, 231–232; health disparities
    and, 153, 254n2; literacy and, 171, 172;
    logistical challenges and, 205; noncom-
    pliance, 172; of study participants, 153;
    tolerance of uncertainty and, 256n20;
    transplantation and, 257n42
speech therapy, 253n32
Spirit Catches You and You Fall Down, The
    (Fadiman), 174
Spock, Benjamin, 124
Star, Leigh, 44
Stardust family, 85–86, 137–138, 254n42

Starr, Paul, 233
stigma: of predictive testing, 15
Stone, Deborah, 218
Strathmann, Cynthia, 253n27
subjunctivity, normalizing, 145–147, 150, 223
success as contested category, 216–218
sudden infant death syndrome (SIDS), 100, 254n43
surveillance medicine, 20–21, 230
Susi, Ada, 36
swine flu. *See* H1N1 virus
symptomatic patients. *See* chronic illness management

Taboada, Arianna, 30
Tadwell family, 83–84
tandem mass spectrometry: cost-effectiveness, 58; diagnostic uncertainty, 66; display of results from, 22; early uses of, 242n40; expansion of screening and, 16, 53–55; genetic technology and, 23
Task Force on Genetic Testing, 42, 43
Tay-Sachs disease, 232
technology: bridging from designers to users, 63–64, 117; chemistry of, 54; clinical implementation, 99–100; cultural logic, 231; expansion of screening, 34, 43; flexibility versus rule-following with, 17–18; interlinked parties involved in, 18–19; multiple biomarkers in blood samples, 16–17; multiplex testing, 43, 53; shifting ontology of disease, 97–98; stimulation of new markets and, 53
terminal illnesses: relief in knowing, 24–25
thalassemia, 232, 255n9
Thompson, Amanda, 252–253n20
Thompson/Broderick family: developmental delays and, 176; doctor-patient relationship, 166, 167; family life, 165; follow-up visits, 130–131; health insurance, 255n15; hospitalizations, 165–166; notification of screening results, 161; paid employment, 164; physical therapy, 175; precarious normality and, 142–145; subjunctive normality and, 146; weight gain, 175
throughput, 54, 247n82
T lymphocyte disorders, 261n20
Torres family, 160–161, 163, 166, 176–177, 205

toxoplasmosis, 39
transplantation: black market, 248n97; clinical deliberations, 257n40; international variation in, 257n41; live donor, 257n41; normalization of deviance in, 58; socioeconomic status and, 257n42; stem cells, 213; transplant tourism, 257n41
trust: complexity in medicine and, 242n34; successful screening program and, 215
tyrosinemia, 49, 189

uncertainty: about best clinical action, 167–168; about policy consequences of screening, 29; acting under, 11–16; alleviation of diagnostic, 180; ambiguous test results, 72–74; asymptomatic versus symptomatic patients, 256n20; clinical relevance, 79–81; continuum of certainty and, 93; dietary management and health status and, 174–175; expansion of newborn screening, 93–94; forms of, 14; genetic counseling and, 15, 35; hope and, 15, 151; as inventive force, 16; "knocking on wood," 222–225; knowledge and, 224–225; limbo between pathology and normality, 75; maladaptive parental reactions to, 53; management of, 15; medical profession and, 13, 228, 242n34; modern life and, 241n18; mutations and, 104; normalization and, 126; normalizing subjunctivity and, 151; parent-infant bonding and, 61; patient-clinician interaction and, 15–16; patients-in-waiting and, 66–67; prognosis and, 123, 153, 159; recursive nature of, 13, 223, 225; relief in knowing versus, 24–25; time since diagnosis and, 91; triggers of, 16–17; vigilance, 109; will to know, 14–15
United Kingdom, cost-effectiveness and screening in, 57–58
US Armed Forces Pathology Laboratory, 215
US Children's Bureau, 36–37
US Food and Drug Administration, 256n24
US Health Resources and Services Administration, 45
US Preventive Services Task Force, 57

Velazquez, Rosario. *See* Rodriguez family
Vennick family, 115

Venter, Craig, 24
very long-chain acyl-coenzyme A dehydro-
    genase. *See* VLCADD
Vetter, David, 213
VLCADD (very long-chain acyl-coenzyme
    A dehydrogenase), 62, 86–87, 189

Walker/Johnston family: child care, 164;
    developmental delays and, 176; doctor-
    patient relationship, 168; early medical
    crisis, 159, 160; neglect claim, 173; nor-
    malization and difference and, 146–148;
    receipt of screening results, 161; timing
    of notification, 162, 163; transplantation
    and, 177
Watson, James D., 23
Watson, Michael, 261n10, 263–264n62
Weiss, Meira, 255n17
*What to Expect When You're Expecting*
    (Murkoff and Mazel), 124

White, Susan, 257n40
WHO (World Health Organization), 42
WIC (Women, Infants, and Children), 156
Wilson, JMG (Max), 42, 43, 51, 55
Women, Infants, and Children (WIC), 156
Wong, James, 123
Wong family, 185–186, 203
World Health Organization (WHO), 42
Wu, Monica: on ambiguity of success of
    treatment, 181; collegial consultations,
    137; health insurance and, 76, 198, 201,
    203, 211; on iatrogenic harm, 186; logis-
    tical assistance from, 209; MCADD
    cases and, 103, 109; medical foods and,
    202–203; on noncompliance with dietary
    regimen, 174; role of at clinic, 30–31, 167;
    on supply of special food, 171; on timing
    of screening, 162

Zimbabwe Bush Pump, 17–18